Current Controversies in Cancer Care for the Surgeon

Katherine A. Morgan

Editors

Current Controversies in Cancer Care for the Surgeon

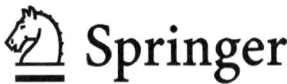 Springer

Editor
Katherine A. Morgan
Division of Gastrointestinal and Laparoscopic Surgery
Medical University of South Carolina
Charleston, SC, USA

ISBN 978-3-319-16204-1   ISBN 978-3-319-16205-8   (eBook)
DOI 10.1007/978-3-319-16205-8

Library of Congress Control Number: 2015953841

Springer Cham Heidelberg New York Dordrecht London
© Springer International Publishing Switzerland 2016

Printed on acid-free paper

Springer International Publishing AG Switzerland is part of Springer Science+Business Media (www.springer.com)

Preface

Miley Cyrus once said, "I like controversy because that's what sells." And while her affinity for dissention drew her at times in a wayward direction, her comment was spot-on. Controversies are the fuel of progress, particularly in medicine. The modern surgeon understands that challenging the standard, seeking evidence for traditional practices, is essential to best practice surgery. This book is intended to summarize the existing standards and evidence in the surgical management of oncologic disease, while also highlighting the areas of current debate and innovation.

Charleston, SC   Katherine A. Morgan

Contents

Contributors

Shuja Ahmed Department of Surgery, Louisiana State University Health Sciences Center, New Orleans, LA, USA

Kanza Aziz Department of Surgery, Johns Hopkins University School of Medicine, Baltimore, MD, USA

Megan K. Baker Department of Surgery, Roper St. Francis Health Care System, Charleston, SC, USA

Kevin E. Behrns Department of Surgery, University of Florida, Gainesville, FL, USA

Michelle L. Bryan Department of Surgery, Wake Forest School of Medicine, Winston-Salem, NC, USA

E. Ramsay Camp Department of Surgery, Medical University of South Carolina, Charleston, SC, USA

Ralph H. Johnson VA Medical CenterMedical University of South Carolina, Charleston, SC, USA

John D. Christein Division of Gastrointestinal Surgery, Department of Surgery, University of Atlanta at Birmingham, Birmingham, AL, USA

Michael I. D'Angelica Department of Surgery, Memorial Sloan Kettering Cancer Center, Weill School of Medicine, Cornell University, New York, NY, USA

Daniel Delitto Department of Surgery, University of Florida, Gainesville, FL, USA

Keith A. Delman Division of Surgical Oncology, Emory University Hospital, Atlanta, GA, USA

Jeremiah L. Deneve Division of Surgical Oncology, University of Tennessee Health Science Center, Memphis, TN, USA

Ammar Asrar Javed The Center for Surgical Trials and Outcomes Research, Johns Hopkins University School of Medicine, Baltimore, MD, USA

Department of Surgery, Johns Hopkins University School of Medicine, Baltimore, MD, USA

Julie N. Leal Division of Hepatopancreatobiliary Surgery, Department of Surgery, Memorial Sloan Kettering Cancer Center, Weill School of Medicine, Cornell University, New York, NY, USA

Edward A. Levine Department of Surgery, Wake Forest School of Medicine, Winston-Salem, NC, USA

Robert C.G. Martin II Division of Surgical Oncology, Department of Surgery, University of Louisville, Louisville, KY, USA

Pinckney J. Maxwell IV Department of Surgery, Medical University of South Carolina, Charleston, SC, USA

The Ralph H. Johnson VA Medical Center, Charleston, SC, USA

John C. McAuliffe Department of Surgery, Memorial Sloan Kettering Cancer Center, New York, NY, USA

Nancy D. Perrier Department of Surgical Oncology, The University of Texas MD Anderson Cancer Center, Houston, TX, USA

Neda Rezaee Department of Surgery, Johns Hopkins University, Baltimore, MD, USA

Georgios Rossidis Department of Surgery, University of Florida, Gainesville, FL, USA

Maria C. Russell Division of Surgical Oncology, Department of Surgery, Emory University Hospital, Atlanta, GA, USA

Perry Shen Department of Surgery, Wake Forest School of Medicine, Winston-Salem, NC, USA

Travis Spaulding Division of Surgical Oncology, Department of Surgery, University of Louisville, Louisville, KY, USA

John H. Stewart IV Department of Surgery, Duke University School of Medicine, Durham, LC, USA

Chee-Chee H. Stucky Department of Surgical Oncology, University of Texas MD Anderson Cancer Center, Houston, TX, USA

Konstantinos I. Votanopoulos Department of Surgery, Wake Forest School of Medicine, Winston-Salem, NC, USA

Christopher L. Wolfgang Department of Surgery, Johns Hopkins University School of Medicine, Baltimore, MD, USA

Department of Pathology, Johns Hopkins University School of Medicine, Baltimore, MD, USA

The Sidney Kimmel Comprehensive Cancer Center, Johns Hopkins University School of Medicine, Baltimore, MD, USA

The Skip Viragh Center for Pancreatic Cancer, Johns Hopkins University School of Medicine, Baltimore, MD, USA

The Sol Goldman Pancreatic Cancer Center, Johns Hopkins University School of Medicine, Baltimore, MD, USA

Gastric Cancer

Georgios Rossidis

Epidemiology

Despite a steady decrease in incidence and mortality, gastric cancer remains a major health burden worldwide. Almost one million new cases of stomach cancer were estimated to have occurred in 2012 (952,000 cases, 6.8 % of the total), making it the fifth most common malignancy in the world, after cancers of the lung, breast, colorectum and prostate (Fig. 1) [1]. In contrast, in 1975, gastric cancer was the most common neoplasm. The highest incidence rates are reported in East Asia, especially China, with annual incidence rates between 40 and 60 per 100 000 inhabitants. Other areas of high incidence are in the Andes Mountains and in Central and Eastern Europe (Fig. 2).

Stomach cancer is the third leading cause of cancer death in both sexes worldwide (723,000 deaths, 8.8 % of the total) third to lung and liver malignancies. The highest estimated mortality rates are in Eastern Asia (24 per 100,000 in men, 9.8 per 100,000 in women), and the lowest are in Northern America (2.8 and 1.5, respectively) [2]. High mortality rates are also present in both sexes in Central and Eastern Europe, and in Central and South America.

Gender-specific incidence and mortality are double in men compared to women.

GLOBOCAN 2012 shows the trend in both incidence and mortality since 1975 and the tendency is towards a marked decline in nearly all populations, irrespective of whether the population is at high risk (Japanese males) or low risk (US white females). This can be attributed to changes in food handling, refrigeration, abundance of fresh fruit and vegetables, the decrease in the use of tobacco and salt, but above all the decreased exposure to a ubiquitous risk factor, *H. pylori*.

G. Rossidis, M.D. (✉)
Department of Surgery, University of Florida, P.O. Box 100286, Gainesville, FL 32610, USA

3036 SW 93rd Street, Gainesville, FL 32608, USA
e-mail: georgios.rossidis@surgery.ufl.edu

© Springer International Publishing Switzerland 2016
K.A. Morgan (ed.), *Current Controversies in Cancer Care for the Surgeon*, DOI 10.1007/978-3-319-16205-8_1

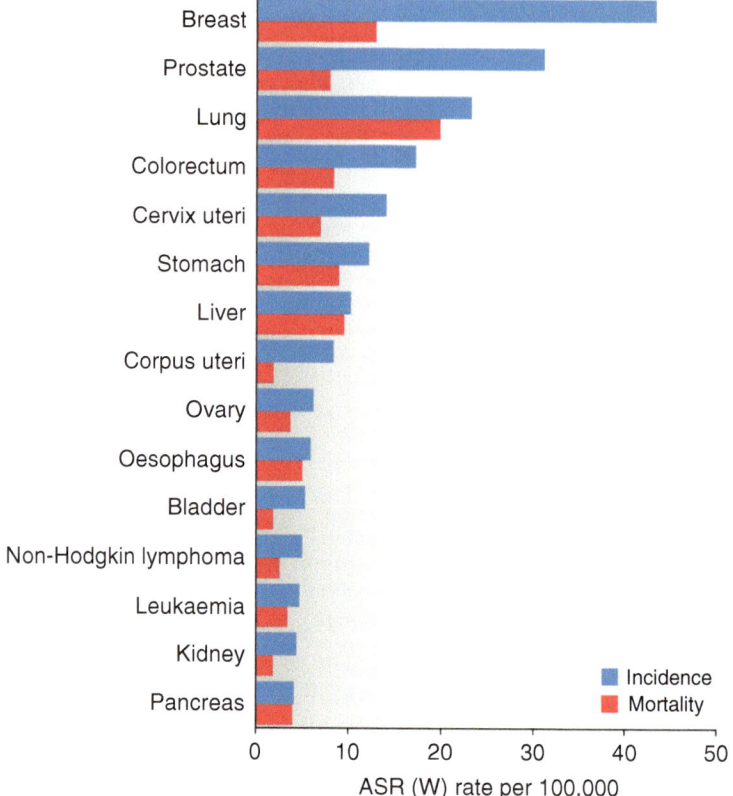

Fig. 1 Incidence and mortality of different malignancies GLOBOCAN 2012 Ferlay J IARC Internet based

Risk Factors/Pathogenesis

Helicobacter pylori

H. pylori is gram-negative bacterium that colonizes the stomach, and even though the majority of infections are asymptomatic, *H. pylori* is associated with peptic ulcer disease, chronic gastritis, gastric mucosa-associated lymphoid tissue (MALT) lymphoma, and gastric adenocarcinoma. It is thought that *H. pylori* was once ubiquitous to mankind but its prevalence is declining in successive generations, and is now very rare in Western Europe, North America, Australia and Japan [3]. The decreased incidence and prevalence in these developed countries can be explained by the fact that infection risk is associated with overcrowding, poor sanitation and low socioeconomic status [4, 5]. The decreased prevalence of *H. pylori* is matched to the decline in incidence and mortality of gastric cancer.

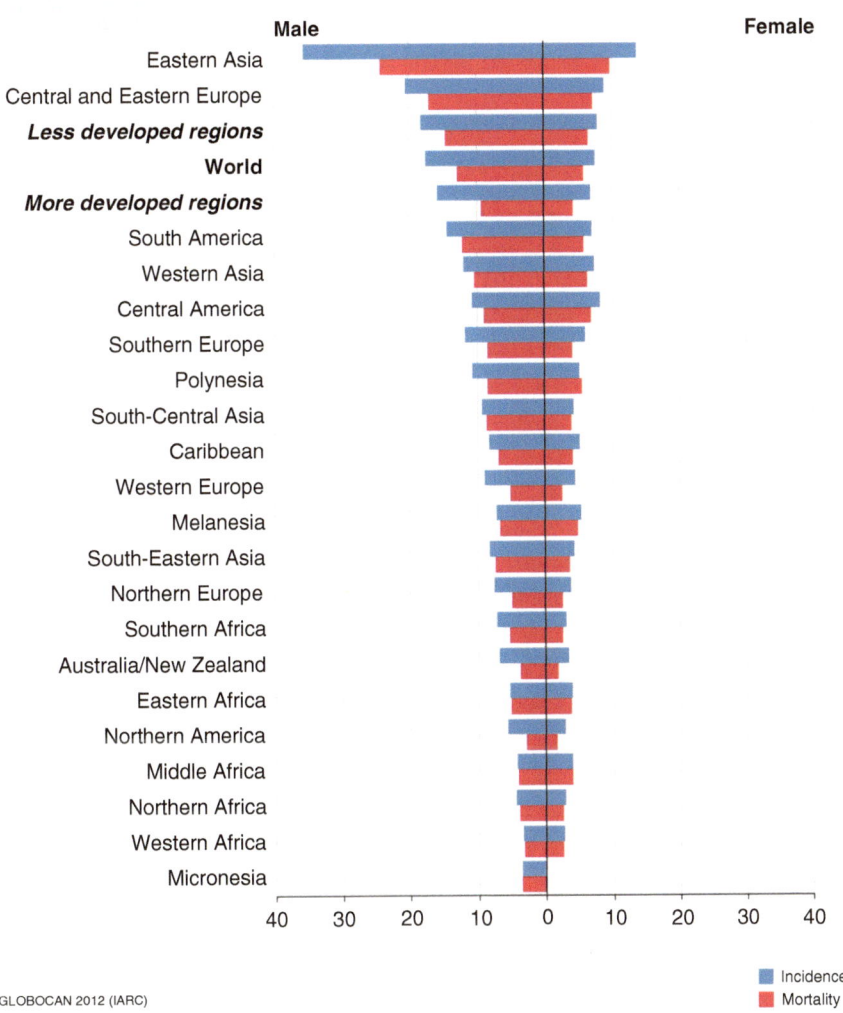

Fig. 2 Incidence and mortality of gastric cancer per region. GLOBOCAN 2012 Ferlay J IARC Internet based

The International Agency for Research on Cancer (IARC) classified infection with *H. pylori* as carcinogenic in 1994 based on its association to gastric cancer and MALT [6]. This conclusion was confirmed by IARC in 2009 stating that *H. pylori* causes non-cardiac gastric cancer due to the confinement of *H. pylori* to the distal part of the stomach [7]. The best estimate of relative risk for *H. pylori* and gastric cancer comes from the Helicobacter and Cancer Collaborative Group which performed a pooled analysis of 12 prospective studies, including 762 cases of non-cardiac cancer and 2250 controls. The odds ratio for *H. pylori* was 2.97 [8].

The same study included 274 cases of cardia gastric cancer and 827 controls with an odds ratio of 0.99 for *H. pylori* infection.

H. pylori is genomically highly diverse and this diversity may contribute to the clinical outcome of the infection. Several genetic factors associated with *H. pylori* colonization and virulence (cagA, acA) have been identified. The genetic marker that has attracted the most attention in epidemiologic studies is the presence of the cag pathogenicity island, a DNA sequence of 40 kbp that is present in 70 % of *H. pylori* strains in Europe and North America, but is ubiquitous in Asia and most of Africa. CagA-positive strains are associated with higher risk of gastric cancer than CagA negative strains. A meta-analysis of 16 cohort and case–control studies including 778 cases of non-cardia gastric cancer and 1409 matched controls found an elevated risk of CagA-positive *H. pylori* infections, with an OR of 2.01 for CagA-positivity among all *H. pylori*-infected individuals [8].

Socioeconomic Status

Less developed countries exhibit higher incidence and mortality of gastric cancer, presumably secondary to untreated prevalent *H. pylori* infection. But even within a given country or population, non-cardia cancer is seen much more commonly in individuals with surrogates associated with a lower socioeconomic status (lower education, number of siblings, crowding) [9, 10].

Tobacco and Alcohol Abuse

A meta-analysis performed by Ladeiras-Lopes et al. showed that the summary risk estimate of gastric cancer was 1.62 in male smokers and 1.2 in female smokers compared to nonsmokers [11]. The risk for cancer is known to increase significantly with increasing numbers of cigarettes per day, pack-years, or duration of smoking [12]. Although alcohol is considered a risk factor for gastric cancer, prospective studies have failed to show an increased relative risk compared to the control group [13].

Body Mass Index and Physical Activity

A meta-analysis by Yang et al. has shown increased risk for cardia gastric cancer in patients with a BMI above 30 with a relative risk estimate of 2.6 [14]. With non-cardia gastric cancers, however, cohort studies have failed to show an increased risk in obese patients [15]. Regular physical activity is known to be associated with decreased risk of gastric cancer, and two prospective studies, one from Norway and one from the USA studying physical activity and gastric and esophageal cancer have shown a protective effect [16, 17].

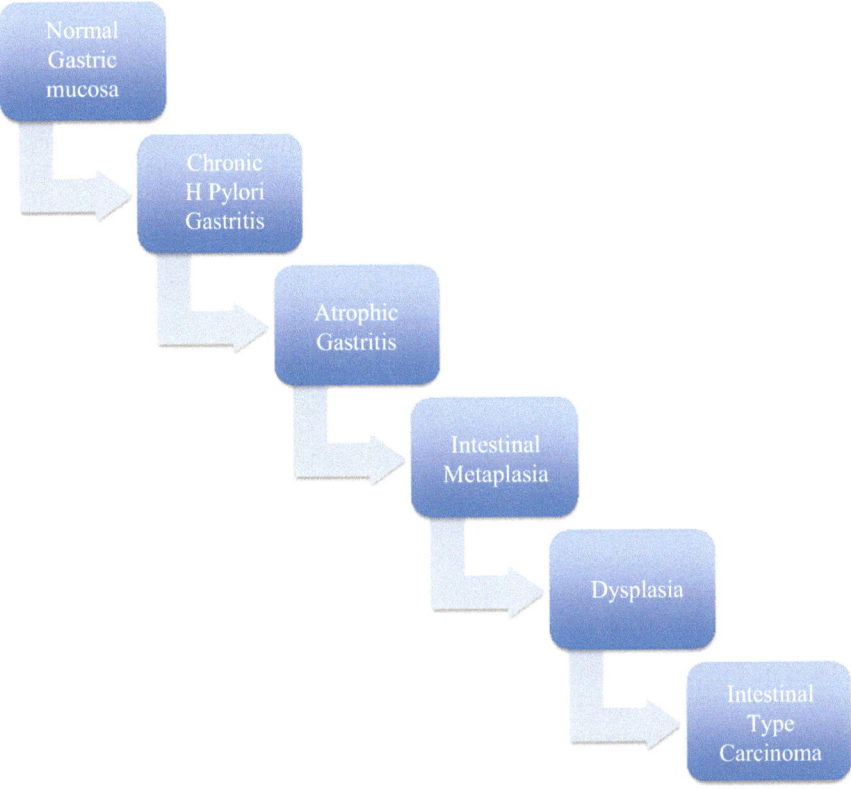

Fig. 3 Correra model of intestinal type gastric cancer carcinogenesis

Pathogenesis

There are two models of carcinogenesis in gastric cancer, the Correa pathway for the intestinal type [18, 19] and the Carneiro pathway for the diffuse type of adenocarcinoma [20]. Figure 3 summarizes the Correa pathway, a multistep process with multiple genetic and epigenetic alterations that may take years to decades to develop. Chronic *H. pylori* gastritis leads to genomic instability (dysfunction of the DNA mismatch repair system) and through DNA methylation leads to atrophic gastritis, defined as the loss of normal glandular epithelium, and the lost glandular epithelium is replaced by intestinal epithelium, leading to metaplasia. There are two main types of metaplastic cells. The first are spasmolytic polypeptide-expressing metaplasia (SPEM) cells, found in 68 % of patients with *H. pylori* infection and associated with 90 % of gastric cancers. Therefore SPEM may be a step in neoplastic progression. The second type of metaplasia is intestinal metaplasia, which may arise in the background of SPEM or in the native gastric epithelium. Intestinal metaplasia is also associated with increased risk of gastric cancer as well as gastric ulcers and chronic gastritis. Mutations in tumor suppressor genes (APC, TP53) lead to dysplasia, which then is followed by loss of heterozygosity at the DCC (deleted in colon cancer) locus and APC (adenomatous polyposis coli) gene mutation, leading to intestinal type carcinoma.

The Carneiro pathway is based on germline mutations in the E-cadherin gene CDH1. Mutations of CDH1 gene are responsible for 30–40 % of hereditary diffuse gastric cancer syndrome. The second hit occurs in most cases by epigenetic silencing of CDH1 promoter by methylation, leading to signet ring carcinoma in situ and ultimately to invasive signet ring carcinoma [20].

Classification

There are different classification schemes for gastric cancer, based on anatomic location within the stomach, histological subtype, as well as degree of invasion.

Anatomic Classification

Based on the location of the carcinoma, gastric cancer can be divided into **cardia** (proximal stomach) and **distal** (non-cardia). The incidence of distal tumors has decreased in recent decades; in contrast, the occurrence of proximal tumors has increased, especially in industrialized countries, apparently related to gastroesophageal reflux disease. Adenocarcinomas of the cardia display a far more aggressive behavior, invading the gastric and esophageal walls and metastasizing to local lymph nodes; the 5-year survival rate is less than 15 % in the USA.

Of clinical interest is the distinction between distal esophageal and proximal gastric cancers and the management of those lesions. The Siewert classification divides the lesions into three types:

Type I: adenocarcinoma of the distal part esophagus (tumor center located between 1 and 5 cm above the anatomic gastroesophageal junction (GEJ)).
Type II: adenocarcinoma of the true gastric cardia (within 1 cm above and 2 cm below the GEJ).
Type III: adenocarcinoma of the subcardial stomach (2–5 cm below the GEJ) [21].

Siewert proposed esophagectomy as the procedure of choice for Type I lesions and total gastrectomy with extension into the esophagus for Type II and III lesions [22]. The American Joint Commission on Cancer Classification (AJCC) considers tumors of the gastroesophageal junction including the esophagus and the proximal 5 cm of the stomach as esophageal carcinomas and recommends the clinical management of these tumors follow the guidelines for esophageal cancer [23]. A lesion with its center within 5 cm of the GEJ but without extension into the esophagus, and a lesion with its center greater than 5 cm away from the GEJ are staged using gastric carcinoma criteria [24].

Degree of Invasion

Based on the degree of invasion gastric cancer can be classified as **early** or **advanced**. Early cancers are those limited to the mucosa and submucosa irrespective of lymph node involvement. The 5-year survival rate is 85–100 % for early gastric cancers. Advanced gastric cancers are those invading beyond the submucosa and are divided according to the Borrmann classification to (1) polypoid, (2) ulcerated, (3) ulcerated infiltrating, and (4) diffusely infiltrating (also known as linitis plastica). The 5-year survival for advanced cancers is 5–20 %.

Histologic Classification

The Lauren classification is the most commonly used histologic classification system, and it divides the tumors into two types: **intestinal** and **diffuse**.

Intestinal type is so named due to the glandular forming neoplastic epithelium, with cellular cohesion. Intestinal is the most common histologic type, found in high-incidence populations.

Diffuse-type gastric cancer histologically is notable for a lack of cellular cohesion, with independent cellular islands of tissue invasion. Signet ring cells are classified as diffuse type [25].

Presentation

The most common symptoms at initial diagnosis of gastric cancer are weight loss (62 %) and persistent abdominal pain (52 %). Weight loss is often secondary to insufficient caloric intake that may be attributable to anorexia, nausea, early satiety, and dysphagia. Dysphagia is present in 26 % of patients and is a common symptom in cancers arising in the proximal stomach. Abdominal pain tends to be epigastric, vague and mild in early disease but more severe and constant as disease progresses. Nausea (34 %) is present in patients with linitis plastica with poor gastric distensibility or patients with gastric outlet obstruction due to an advanced distal tumor. Occult gastrointestinal bleeding is not uncommon and can be accompanied by iron deficiency anemia [26].

Diagnosis

Tissue diagnosis and anatomic localization of the primary tumor are best obtained by upper gastrointestinal endoscopy. Although more invasive and more costly, upper endoscopy is also more sensitive and specific for diagnosing a variety of gastric, esophageal, and duodenal lesions than alternative diagnostic strategies (such as barium studies). The early use of upper endoscopy in patients presenting with gastrointestinal complaints may be associated with a higher rate of detection of early gastric cancers.

The ability to perform biopsy during endoscopy adds to the clinical utility of this modality. As up to 5 % of malignant ulcers appear benign grossly, it is imperative that all such lesions be evaluated by biopsy and histologic assessment [27]. A barium exam may be more useful is in patients with linitis plastica. The decreased distensibility of the stiff, "leather-flask"-appearing stomach is more apparent on a radiographic study, while the endoscopic appearance may be relatively normal.

Staging

The most widely used staging system in gastric cancer was developed jointly by the American Joint Committee on Cancer (AJCC) and the International Union Against Cancer (UICC). This classification system is most often used in the Western hemisphere and now commonly in Asian countries as well. The seventh edition was introduced in 2010 and the major differences compared to the sixth edition involved the depth of tumor invasion. Table 1 summarizes the TNM staging system for gastric cancer. Table 2 shows the 5-year survival rate according to stage.

Table 1 TNM classification of gastric cancer based on 7th Edition of the AJCC Cancer Staging Manual

T stage	N stage	M stage	Stage
T0: No evidence of tumor	N0: No regional lymph node metastasis	M0: No distant metastasis	
Tis: Carcinoma in situ	N1: 1–2 lymph nodes	M1: Distant metastasis	0: TisN0
		Positive cytology is M1 disease	
T1a: Lamina propria	N2: 3–6 lymph nodes		IA: T1N0
T1b: Submucosa			IB: T2N0
T2: Muscularis propria	N3a: 7–15 lymph nodes		IIA: T3N0, T2N1, T1N2
	N3b: >15 lymph nodes		IIB: T4aN0, T3N1, T2N2, T1N3
T3: Subserosa			IIIA: T4aN1, T3N2, T2N3
			IIIB: T4bN0, T4bN1, T4aN2, T3N3
			IIIC: T4bN2, T4bN3, T4aN3
T4a: Perforates serosa			IV: Any T, any N, M1
T4b: Invades adjacent organ			

Table 2 Five-year survival according to stage

Stage	5-year survival rate (%)
IA	70.8
IB	57.4
IIA	45.5
IIB	32.8
IIIA	19.8
IIIB	14
IIIC	9.2
IV	4

Clinical staging is of high importance as it dictates the management of gastric carcinoma: Stage I–III tumors are potentially curable while stage IV disease is referred for palliative therapy based on the symptoms and functional status of the patient. All stages are best managed by a multidisciplinary team.

CT scan of the chest abdomen and pelvis is performed early in the preoperative evaluation after diagnosis of gastric cancer is made. It is best suited to stage the cancer, assessing for degree of local involvement as well as for metastatic disease (hepatic or adnexal metastases, ascites). Peritoneal metastases smaller than 5 mm are frequently missed by CT scan, even when using modern CT technology [28]. Burke et al. compared staging laparoscopy to CT in 103 patients with gastric adenocarcinoma and no evidence of metastatic disease on CT scan. In 31 % of the patients, laparoscopy identified biopsy-proven metastatic disease. The sensitivity and specificity of staging laparoscopy was 94 % and 100 %, respectively [29]. Karanicolas and colleagues reviewed the SEER database to analyze frequency of staging laparoscopy in the general population in the period between 1998 and 2005. Of 6388 patients, only 506 (8 %) underwent staging laparoscopy. Use of staging laparoscopy increased over time (5.5 % in 1998 to 11.1 % in 2005, $P<0.01$), and patients tended to be young and white, living in the Northeast, and with proximal cancers, and they had fewer comorbidities than those who did not undergo staging laparoscopy. Although increasing in use, staging laparoscopy seems to remain underutilized in its potential benefit of avoiding unnecessary laparotomy [30].

Endoscopic ultrasonography (EUS) is considered the most reliable nonsurgical method available for evaluating the depth of invasion of gastric cancers [31]. The accuracy of EUS for differentiation of individual tumor stages (T1–T4) ranges from 77 to 93 %, with the experience of the operator markedly influencing these rates [32]. EUS is a more accurate predictor of the T stage compared to CT [33], although the accuracy for nodal staging is only slightly greater [34]. The advantage of EUS in the assessment of the nodal status is the ability to perform fine needle aspiration of suspicious nodes and areas, which adds to the accuracy of nodal staging.

The role of positron emission tomography (PET) is still in evolution. PET is more sensitive than CT scan in the detection of distant metastases [36]. An important caveat is that the sensitivity of PET scanning for peritoneal carcinomatosis is only 50 % [37]. Therefore PET cannot adequately replace staging laparoscopy for detection of peritoneal metastases. NCCN guidelines for preoperative evaluation of gastric cancer suggest integrated PET/CT. However, gastric cancer is not a reimbursable diagnosis for PET scanning in the US Medicare program.

Extent of Gastric Resection

Distal Disease

One of the biggest controversies in surgical treatment of gastric cancer is the extent of the resection for distal lesions, i.e., whether a subtotal gastrectomy (SG) would provide similar oncologic outcomes when compared to total gastrectomy (TG). Gouzi et al. were the first to address this issue. In their prospective randomized study 169 patients underwent either SG or TG. The perioperative morbidity (34 % vs. 33 %) and mortality (3.2 % vs. 1.6 %) were similar. The overall 5-year survival was 48 %, and the extent of resection was NOT associated with different survival. Factors that determined survival were serosal invasion and lymph node involvement [38]. Even underpowered, the study showed that SG was a viable treatment option for distal lesions. A larger study by Bozzetti and colleagues included 624 patients compared patients undergoing SG (320 patients) to TG (304 patients). In this study perioperative mortality was the same between SG and TG (1.3 % vs. 2.3 %), although morbidity was greater in the TG group (15.5 % vs. 10.3 % P=0.05). Mean length of stay was improved in the SG group (13.8 days vs. 15.4 days P=0.001) [39] and the 5-year survival as published subsequently was comparable between the two groups (65.3 % vs. 62.4 %) [40]. One of the primary arguments in favor of SG over TG is long term quality of life. Davies and colleagues evaluated 47 consecutive patients who underwent potential R0 resection for gastric cancer. TG was performed for lesions of the proximal and middle thirds of the stomach and SG was performed for those of the distal third. D2 dissection was performed, and the spleen and pancreas were preserved when possible. No patient received adjuvant chemotherapy. Quality of life was assessed preoperatively and at 1, 3, 6, and 12 months postoperatively using five validated questionnaires. The Rotterdam symptom checklist and the Troidl index achieved a statistically significant difference between the SG and TG groups through 12 months postoperatively, with improved quality of life in the SG group as compared to the TG group [41]. Based on approximately equivalent long-term survival rates, potentially higher operative morbidity of TG, and improved quality of life for patients undergoing SG, SG is favored for distal gastric cancer, provided that adequate proximal margins of 5–6 cm are obtained.

Proximal Disease

Another controversy in gastric cancer is the oncologic and functional adequacy of proximal gastrectomy (PG) vs. total gastrectomy (TG) for malignancies of the proximal third of the stomach. Kim and colleagues retrospectively reviewed patients who underwent either PG or TG for proximal gastric cancer. PG was performed only when the cancer was limited to the proximal one-third. Between 1992 and 2000, 43 patients underwent PG and 104 underwent TG. The groups were fairly well matched for tumor characteristics, including size and differentiation, although all T4 lesions were resected via TG. The majority of the PG group underwent D1 dissection, whereas the majority of the TG group underwent at least D2 dissection. The PG group experienced higher perioperative morbidity (48.8 % vs. 14.4 %), most commonly anastomotic strictures, and higher rate of recurrence (39.5 % vs. 4.8 %). Overall 5-year survival was similar (48.6 % in TG vs. 46.0 % in PG). This survival equivalence held for stage I or stage II disease; however for stage III disease, 5-year survival after TG was significantly improved (38.4 % vs. 17.1 %). Therefore, the authors concluded that PG is best applied in early gastric cancer with achievable margins and limited nodal involvement [42].

An et al. investigated the outcomes of PG compared to TG in patients with proximal early gastric cancer. From 2000 to 2005, 423 patients underwent PG (89 patients) or TG (334 patients) for stage I or stage II proximal gastric adenocarcinoma. The TG group had larger tumors (4.0 cm vs. 2.5 cm) and more mean lymph nodes harvested (39.1 vs. 22.4). PG was associated with higher morbidity (61.8 % vs. 12.6 %), most often anastomotic stenosis and esophageal reflux, and these were successfully treated with balloon dilatation. 5-year survival was similar between the two groups (99.2 % in PG vs. 98.5 % in TG), as were long-term body weight and nutritional markers. Due to the higher perioperative morbidity the authors did not recommend proximal gastrectomy even for early gastric malignancies.

Laparoscopic Gastric Resection

After the initial introduction of laparoscopic gastrectomy for gastric cancer by Kitano et al. in 1993, the procedure has evolved significantly and is now considered one of the standard minimally invasive procedures for the treatment of early gastric cancer. There is a growing volume of literature comparing laparoscopic to open gastrectomy for early gastric cancer in the distal stomach. The first randomized studies published by Kitano, Huscher, Hayashi, and Lee were underpowered, with the number of patients recruited less than 50 [44–47], but with the same results and the same theme. The laparoscopic distal gastrectomy (LADG) group had less operative blood loss, shorter length of stay, quicker return to diet compared to the open distal gastrectomy group (ODG), and the perioperative morbidity and mortality as well as long-term survival was comparable in both laparoscopic and open gastrectomies. The largest and most notable randomized controlled study of laparoscopic vs. open distal gastrectomy for early gastric cancer is the Korean multicenter trial named KLASS (Korean Laparoendoscopic Gastrointestinal Surgery Study). Included were patients with clinical stage I gastric adenocarcinoma. The primary endpoint was overall survival, and the secondary endpoints were disease-free survival, morbidity, mortality, quality of life, inflammatory and immune responses, and cost-effectiveness. A distal gastrectomy with D1 + β or D2 LN dissection was performed in both groups. Reconstruction was performed by Billroth I or Billroth II or Roux-en-Y fashion, depending on surgeon preference. To assure high surgical quality, surgery was performed by 15 surgeons, who had performed at least 50 cases each of LADG and ODG, at 12 high-volume institutions, which had performed more than 80 cases of distal gastrectomy per year. From February 2006 to August 2010, 1415 patients (704 LADG and 711 ODG) were enrolled, and the final results are expected to be reported in September 2015 [48]. The interim analysis of this KLASS-01 trial was published in 2010. A total of 342 patients were randomized (179 LADG and 161 ODG). There were no significant differences between the two groups concerning patient demographics. The postoperative complication rates of LADG and ODG groups were 10.5 % (17/179) and 14.7 % (24/163, $p=0.137$). The postoperative mortality was 1.1 % (2/179) and 0 % (0/163) in the LADG and ODG groups ($p=0.497$). The authors concluded that there was no significant difference in the morbidity and mortality between the two groups [49]. Another important Korean single-center RCT, conducted by Kim et al. [16], was published in 2008. This study aimed to evaluate the quality of life after LADG compared to ODG ($n=82$ in each group) in patients with EGC. The LADG group showed better functional and symptom scales of EORCT QLQ-C30 and QLQ-STO22 at 3 months after surgery. Also, intraoperative blood loss, total amount of postoperative analgesics, and postoperative hospital stay were significantly less in the LADG group. The authors concluded that LADG resulted in improved quality of life outcomes after surgery in EGC patients compared to ODG. To evaluate the long term results of LADG Strong et al. from Memorial Sloan-Kettering Cancer Center reported a retrospective case–control study comparing 30 LADG with 30 ODG. Controls were matched for stage, age, and gender from 2005 to 2008. The mean number of resected LNs was 18 (range: 7–36) in the LADG group and 21 (range: 7–44) in the ODG group ($p=0.03$). There were four recurrences (13.3 %) in the LADG group during 11 months of follow-up and five recurrences (16.6 %) in the ODG group during 13.8 months of follow-up ($p=0.71$).

Laparoscopic Gastrectomy for Advanced Gastric Cancer

As the sophistication of available technology has improved and laparoscopic experience has evolved, laparoscopic resections with extensive lymphadenectomy for advanced gastric cancer (AGC) have emerged. A recent meta-analysis, including seven case–control studies with 1271 AGC patients (626 LADG and 645ODG), showed that LADG patients had longer operative time but less estimated blood loss, less analgesic requirement, and a shorter hospital stay compared with patients undergoing ODG. There were no significant differences between the two groups in number of LN harvested, postoperative mortality, overall complications, and 3-year overall survival rate. Therefore, the authors concluded that the oncologic outcomes of LADG for AGC patients were comparable with an open approach [50]. Based on this data the KLASS two trial was launched in October 2011 to compare LADG to ODG for advanced gastric cancer. The estimated sample size is 1050 and the primary endpoint is 3-year disease-free survival rate. As the surgical quality may emerge as an important issue in this clinical trial, surgeons are required to undergo a quality assessment before joining the trial. On February 2013, 18 surgeons at 11 institutes had been approved, and 316 patients out of 1050 (30.1 %) were enrolled for the last year. The results of this trial are eagerly anticipated.

Extent of Lymph Node Dissection

One of the most controversial areas in the surgical management of gastric cancer is the optimal extent of lymph node dissection. Japanese surgeons routinely perform extended lymphadenectomy, a practice that some suggest at least partially accounts for the better survival rates in Asian as compared to Western series. The term "extended lymphadenectomy" variably refers to either a D2 or a D3 lymph node dissection. Table 3 shows the different gastric lymph node stations, divided according to the Japanese classification [51]. Stations 1–6 are perigastric, and the remaining ten are located adjacent to major vessels, behind the pancreas, and along the aorta.

- D1 lymphadenectomy refers to a limited dissection of only the perigastric lymph nodes.
- D2 lymphadenectomy is an extended lymph node dissection, entailing removal of nodes along the hepatic, left gastric, celiac, and splenic arteries as well as those in the splenic hilum (stations 1–11).
- D3 dissection is an extensive lymphadenectomy. The term has been used by some to describe a D2 lymphadenectomy plus the removal of nodes within the porta hepatis and periaortic regions (stations 1–16), while others use the term to denote a D2 lymphadenectomy plus periaortic nodal dissection (PAND) alone. Most Western surgeons (and the AJCC/UICC TNM staging classification) classify disease in these regions as distant metastases and do not routinely remove nodes in these areas during a potentially curative gastrectomy.

The arguments in favor of extended lymphadenectomy (i.e., D2 or D3 vs. D1) are that removing a larger number of nodes more accurately stages disease extent and that failure to remove these nodes leaves behind disease (failure of therapy) in as many as one-third of patients [52]. A consequence of more accurate staging is to minimize stage migration [53, 54]. The resulting improvement in stage-specific survival may explain, in part, the better results in Asian patients.

The influence of total lymph node count on stage-specific survival was studied in a series of 3814 patients undergoing gastrectomy for T1-3N0-1 (classified according to the 1997 AJCC gastric cancer staging system and reported to the Surveillance, Epidemiology and End Results (SEER) database between 1973 and 2000) [55]. For every stage subgroup (T1/2N0, T1/2N1, T3N0, T3N1), survival was significantly better as more nodes were examined. Although cut point analysis revealed the greatest survival difference when ten lymph nodes were examined, there were significant survival differences for cut points up to 40 nodes examined, always in favor of a greater number of nodes in the specimen.

Table 3 Gastric lymph node stations, according to Japanese classification of gastric carcinoma: 3rd English edition. Gastric Cancer. 2011 Jun;14(2):101–12

Lymph node station	Definition
1	Right paracardial LNs, including those along the first branch of the ascending limb of the left gastric artery
2	Left paracardial LNs including those along the esophagocardiac branch of the left subphrenic artery
3a	Lesser curvature LNs along the branches of the left gastric artery
3b	Lesser curvature LNs along the second branch and distal part of the right gastric artery
4sa	Left greater curvature LNs along the short gastric arteries (perigastric area)
4sb	Left greater curvature LNs along the left gastroepiploic artery (perigastric area)
4d	Rt. greater curvature LNs along the second branch and distal part of the right gastroepiploic artery
5	Suprapyloric LNs along the first branch and proximal part of the right gastric artery
6	Infrapyloric LNs along the first branch and proximal part of the right gastroepiploic artery down to the confluence of the right gastroepiploic vein and the anterior superior pancreatoduodenal vein
7	LNs along the trunk of left gastric artery between its root and the origin of its ascending branch
8a	Anterosuperior LNs along the common hepatic artery
8p	Posterior LNs along the common hepatic artery
9	Celiac artery LNs
10	Splenic hilar LNs including those adjacent to the splenic artery distal to the pancreatic tail, and those on the roots of the short gastric arteries and those along the left gastroepiploic artery proximal to its first gastric branch
11p	Proximal splenic artery LNs from its origin to halfway between its origin and the pancreatic tail end
11d	Distal splenic artery LNs from halfway between its origin and the pancreatic tail end to the end of the pancreatic tail
12a	Hepatoduodenal ligament LNs along the proper hepatic artery, in the caudal half between the confluence of the right and left hepatic ducts and the upper border of the pancreas
12b	Hepatoduodenal ligament LNs along the bile duct, in the caudal half between the confluence of the right and left hepatic ducts and the upper border of the pancreas
12p	Hepatoduodenal ligament LNs along the portal vein in the caudal half between the confluence of the right and left hepatic ducts and the upper border of the pancreas
13	LNs on the posterior surface of the pancreatic head cranial to the duodenal papilla
14v	LNs along the superior mesenteric vein
15	LNs along the middle colic vessels
16a1	Para-aortic LNs in the diaphragmatic aortic hiatus
16a2	Para-aortic LNs between the upper margin of the origin of the celiac artery and the lower border of the left renal vein
16b1	Para-aortic LNs between the lower border of the left renal vein and the upper border of the origin of the inferior mesenteric artery

There are two main arguments against the routine use of an extended lymphadenectomy: the higher associated morbidity (particularly if splenectomy is performed in order to achieve extended lymphadenectomy) and the lack of a survival benefit for extended lymphadenectomy in most large randomized trials.

Although retrospective reports suggest that extended lymphadenectomy improves survival [56–58], this survival benefit failed to materialize in multiple prospective randomized trials both in Asian and Western populations, and a meta-analysis failed to show an overall survival benefit with D2 vs. D1 lymphadenectomy [59–63] or with D3 compared to D2 lymphadenectomy [64]. The range of findings can be illustrated by the three largest trials.

The Medical Research Council (MRC) randomly assigned 400 patients undergoing potentially curative resection to a D1 or a D2 lymphadenectomy [61]. Postoperative morbidity was significantly greater in the D2 group (46 % vs. 28 %), as was operative mortality (13 % vs. 6 %). The excess morbidity and mortality were clearly associated with the use of splenectomy and distal pancreatectomy to achieve complete node dissection. In a later follow-up, 5-year survival rates were no better for patients undergoing D2 compared to D1 dissection (33 % vs. 35 %) [65].

The largest randomized trial came from the Dutch Gastric Cancer Group and compared D1 with D2 lymphadenectomy in 711 patients who were treated with curative intent [62, 66]. This trial relied heavily upon input from a Japanese surgeon, who trained 11 Dutch surgeons in the technique of radical lymph node dissection and monitored the operative procedures. Despite these efforts to maintain quality control of the surgical procedures, both under removal and over removal of required nodal stations occurred, somewhat blurring the distinction between the groups.

As was shown in the MRC trial, both postoperative morbidity (43 % vs. 25 %) and mortality (10 % vs. 4 %) were higher in the D2 group. Moreover, a statistically significant survival advantage in the radical dissection group was not observed, both in the initial report and with longer follow-up [67], despite a significantly lower risk of recurrence. This was attributed to the detrimental impact of increased operative mortality in this group.

The conclusion of the Dutch trial (and its accompanying editorial [68]) was that D2 lymph node dissection could not be routinely recommended.

Many clinicians consider that both the Dutch and the MRC trials are flawed. The design of the Dutch trial was based upon the assumption that radical lymph node dissection would increase the survival rate from 20 to 32 %, likely an overestimation of benefit. Furthermore, 40 % of enrolled patients had early gastric cancer, an unexpectedly high proportion that was not anticipated when the trial was designed.

Moreover, both the MRC and the Dutch studies were relatively underpowered for the group of patients most likely to benefit from the extended dissection. If the proportion of patients with N2 disease is approximately 30 %, and only approximately one-fourth of these patients survive 5 years after a potentially curative D2 lymphadenectomy, less than 8 % of patients benefit long term. These results indicate that one additional life might be saved for every 13 patients undergoing a D2 dissection and that much larger sample sizes are needed. Thus, the benefit of D2 versus D1 dissection (particularly using safer spleen-preserving D2 dissection techniques) remains controversial.

The Dutch trial has been updated with 15-year follow-up [67]. The survival curves have continued to separate, although the difference in overall survival is still not statistically significant (22 % vs. 28 % in the D1 and D2 arms, respectively, $p = 0.34$). However, the gastric cancer-related death rate is significantly higher in the D1 arm (48 % versus 37 %) while death rates due to other causes were not different. This supports the concept that if the D2 dissection can be done with low operative mortality, similar to that of a D1 dissection (as occurs in high volume centers), there will be a positive survival impact. This mirrors the conclusion of the latest Dutch trial paper that D2 dissection is recommended in patients with potentially curable gastric cancer. In summary, given the apparent impact of D2 lymphadenectomy on disease specific survival, most major cancer centers are performing a D2 as compared to a D1 dissection. Treatment guidelines published by the National Comprehensive Cancer Network recommend that D2 lymph node dissection is preferred over a D1 dissection. However, in view of the higher reported rates of operative morbidity when this procedure has been performed in randomized trials, this recommendation is valid in high-volume centers.

If there is a survival benefit to be gained by extended lymphadenectomy, it requires that there be no added operative morbidity. A pancreas and spleen-preserving D2 lymphadenectomy provides superior staging information and may provide a survival benefit while avoiding its excess morbidity. Splenectomy during gastric resection for tumors not adjacent to or invading the spleen or the tail of the pancreas increases morbidity without improving survival. Thus it is not recommended unless there is direct tumor extension.

The debate between D3 and D2 lymph node dissection was addressed by the Japan Clinical Oncology Group (JCOG) study 9501. The study randomly assigned 523 patients to D2 versus D3 (D2 with para-aortic lymph nodes) dissection. The overall perioperative complication rate in the D3 group was significantly higher (28.1 % vs. 20.9 %), although there were no differences in major complications (anastomotic leak, pancreatic fistula, abdominal abscess, pneumonia) and perioperative mortality was very low (0.8 %) in both groups [64]. Five-year recurrence-free (approximately 63 % in both groups) and overall survival (70 % vs. 69 %) were no better after extended lymphadenectomy [69].

A meta-analysis of the JCOG trial and two other smaller randomized trials of D2 versus D3 (with PAND) dissection [70, 71] concluded that resection of the para-aortic nodes was inferior to a D2 dissection in terms of safety and without any survival benefit [72]. Thus, para-aortic lymphadenectomy should not be considered a routine practice for surgical treatment of gastric cancer.

Adjuvant Therapy

Adjuvant Chemotherapy

More than 30 randomized trials have compared adjuvant systemic chemotherapy to surgery alone in resectable gastric cancer, with variable, mostly negative results when overall survival is considered as the primary endpoint. While some of the trials were clearly underpowered to detect a significant survival difference, others utilized inferior surgical techniques, or much of the planned chemotherapy was not given because of prolonged recovery from surgery. The GASTRIC Group (Global Advanced/Adjuvant Stomach Tumor Research International Collaboration) identified 31 eligible trials from 1970 to 2009 and was able to obtain Individual Patient Data (IPD) from 17 of them [73]. An examination of the eligible studies does not indicate any bias with respect to studies for which the authors were and were not able to obtain the IPD. These authors used a fixed effects model and determined that there was a modest advantage of postoperative chemotherapy for OS (hazard ratio [HR] 0.82, 95 % CI 0.76–0.90; $p\backslash 0.001$) based on 17 trials, and for disease-free survival (HR 0.82, 95 % CI 0.75–0.90; $p\backslash 0.001$) based on 14 trials.

Adjuvant Chemoradiotherapy

The largest and most recent trial, US Intergroup INT0116, provides the most compelling data in support of adjuvant chemoradiotherapy following complete surgical resection, particularly since it used contemporary radiation therapy (RT) techniques and concurrently administered fluoropyrimidine radiosensitization [74]. Following potentially curative resection of gastric or EGJ cancer (T1-4, N0-1), 556 patients were randomly assigned to observation alone or adjuvant combined chemoradiotherapy. Treatment consisted of one cycle of FU and leucovorin calcium daily for 5 days, followed 1 month later by RT (45 Gy in daily 1.8 Gy fractions) given with concurrent FU and leucovorin calcium on days 1 through 4, and on the last 3 days of RT. Radiation treatment volumes were subject to centralized pretreatment review. Two more 5-day cycles of chemotherapy were given at monthly intervals beginning 1 month after completion of chemoradiotherapy.

The majority of tumors were T3/T4 (68 % and 69 % of the treated and control groups, respectively), and 85 % had nodal metastases. Three-year disease-free (48 % vs. 31 %) and overall survival rates (50 % vs. 41 %) were significantly better with combined modality therapy, and median survival was significantly longer (36 months vs. 27 months). Benefits were maintained with longer follow-up (5-year overall survival 43 % vs. 28 %, hazard ratio [HR] for survival 1.32 (95 % CI 1.10–1.60)) [75].

This study has shaped the treatment of gastric cancer in the United States and adjuvant chemoradiotherapy is now the standard of care. A criticism of this trial was the limited extent of the surgical procedure in most cases. Although D2 lymph node dissection was recommended, it was only performed in 10 % of cases, and 54 % did not even have clearance of the D1 nodal regions. This noncompliance likely contributed to inferior survival and a 64 % relapse rate in the surgery alone arm.

Chemotherapy vs. Chemoradiotherapy

In the largest trial, the ARTIST trial, 458 patients with complete resected gastric cancer and a D2 lymph node dissection were randomly assigned to six courses of postoperative capecitabine plus cisplatin (XP) or two courses of postoperative XP followed by chemoradiotherapy (45 Gy RT with concurrent daily capecitabine [825 mg/m^2 twice daily]) and two additional courses of XP [76]. Compared to chemotherapy alone, the addition of RT to XP chemotherapy did not significantly reduce recurrence rates, although in unplanned subgroup analysis, *patients with nodal metastases* had superior disease-free survival with combined therapy as compared to XP alone. Overall survival, a secondary endpoint, was not analyzed.

In the latest update, presented at the 2014 annual ASCO meeting, at a median follow-up of 84 months, 3-year disease-free survival (the primary endpoint) was not significantly better in patients who received combined modality therapy (hazard ratio [HR] 0.74, 95 % CI 0.52–1.05), although unplanned subset analysis did indicate a significantly better outcome with chemoradiotherapy in those with node-positive disease (3-year DFS 76 % versus 72 %, $p=0.004$) [77]. Overall survival, a secondary endpoint, was also not significantly different (HR 1.13, 95 % CI 0.775–1.647).

The hypothesis that adjuvant chemoradiotherapy may represent a better approach than adjuvant chemotherapy for patients with node-positive disease will be tested in a successor trial, the ARTIST-II trial.

Neoadjuvant Therapy

In contrast to the situation in the USA, the standard of care for treatment of gastric cancer in many parts of Europe is neoadjuvant or perioperative (preoperative plus postoperative) chemotherapy. In Japan and Southern Europe, patients routinely receive postoperative chemotherapy alone, although this practice seems to be changing, given the better tolerability of preoperative chemotherapy.

Neoadjuvant chemotherapy may be administered as a means of "downstaging" a locally advanced tumor prior to an attempt at curative resection. This approach has been applied to patients thought to have resectable disease as well as those with apparently unresectable but nonmetastatic disease. Another benefit of neoadjuvant chemotherapy is that patients who are at high risk of developing distant metastases (e.g., those with bulky T3/T4 tumors, visible perigastric nodes by preoperative imaging studies including endoscopic ultrasound, a linitis plastica appearance, or positive peritoneal cytology in the absence of visible peritoneal disease) may be spared the morbidity of unnecessary gastrectomy if evidence of distant metastases emerges after chemotherapy.

The MAGIC (Medical Research Council Adjuvant Gastric Infusional Chemotherapy) trial reported by Cunninghamet et al. [78] in 2006 is the largest trial incorporating preoperative therapy to date and the only randomized trial with a perioperative approach. A total of 503 patients were randomized to preoperative and postoperative epirubicin, cisplatin, fluorouracil (ECF), or surgery alone. Patients with adenocarcinoma of the stomach or lower third of the esophagus who had stage II or higher (M0) disease or locally advanced inoperable disease were included. It should be noted that only 68 % of patients underwent curative surgery, while the remaining patients had palliative surgery, no surgery, or surgery of unknown intent. Of the patients assigned to perioperative ECF, 41.6 % completed all six cycles of chemotherapy, and 49.5 % of the patients who completed preoperative ECF also completed postoperative therapy. Despite the fact that only 42 % of the patients were able to complete the protocol treatment, overall survival was significantly better in the chemotherapy group (hazard ratio [HR] for death 0.75, 95 % CI 0.60–0.93) as was progression-free survival (PFS, HR for progression 0.66). The 25 % reduction in the risk of death favoring chemotherapy translated into an improvement in 5-year survival from 23 to 36 %. Local failure occurred in 14 % of the chemotherapy-treated patients compared to 21 % of those undergoing surgery alone. Distant metastases developed in 24 % and 37 % of patients, respectively.

A similar benefit for perioperative chemotherapy was noted in a French multi-center trial (FNLCC/FFCD trial) in which 224 patients with potentially resectable stage II or greater adenocarcinoma of the stomach ($n=55$), EGJ ($n=144$) or distal esophagus ($n=25$) were randomly assigned to two to three cycles of preoperative chemotherapy (infusional FU plus cisplatin on day 1 or 2, every 4 weeks) or surgery alone. Patients in the chemotherapy arm were to receive three to four cycles of postoperative chemotherapy as well. Patients undergoing neoadjuvant chemotherapy were significantly more likely to undergo R0 (microscopically complete) resection (84 % vs. 73 %), and there was a statistically insignificant trend toward fewer node-positive tumors (67 % vs. 80 %, $p=0.054$) that favored this group as well. Among the patients who received at least one cycle of preoperative chemotherapy, only one-half received any postoperative chemotherapy. With a median 5.7-year follow-up, perioperative chemotherapy was associated with a significant 35 % reduction in the risk of disease recurrence (5-year disease-free survival 34 % vs. 19 %) and a significant, 31 % lower risk of death (5-year survival 38 % vs. 24 %) [79].

Studies comparing postoperative chemoradiotherapy to perioperative chemotherapy are not available, and thus the recommendations for adjuvant therapy are outlined in a systematic review and practice guideline by Knight et al. [80]:

- Postoperative 5-fluorouracil (5-FU)-based chemoradiotherapy (CRT) based on the Macdonald approach [74] or perioperative epirubicin/cisplatin/5-FU (ECF) chemotherapy based on the Cunningham/Medical Research Council Adjuvant

Gastric Infusional Chemotherapy (MAGIC) approach [78] are both acceptable standards of care in North America. Choice of treatment should be made on a case-by-case basis.

- Adjuvant chemotherapy is a reasonable option for those patients for whom the Macdonald and MAGIC protocols are contraindicated.
- Patients with resectable gastric cancer should undergo a pretreatment multidisciplinary assessment to determine the best plan of care. In addition to surgery, all patients should be considered for neoadjuvant and/or adjuvant therapy.

Follow-Up and Surveillance

Based on NCCN guidelines, follow-up should include a complete history and physical examination every 3–6 months for the first 2 years, every 6–12 months for 3–5 years, and then annually thereafter. Routine surveillance for asymptomatic recurrence is not currently supported by data. Thus, imaging and endoscopy are reserved for symptomatic patients. Patients who have undergone surgical resection should be monitored and treated as indicated for vitamin B12 and iron deficiency.

References

1. Rodrigues G, Prabhu R, Ravi B. Small bowel carcinoid: a rare cause of bowel obstruction. BMJ Case Rep. 2013;2013.
2. Siegel R, Ma J, Zou Z, Jemal A. Cancer statistics, 2014. CA Cancer J Clin. 2014;64(1):9–29.
3. Herrera V, Parsonnet J. Helicobacter pylori and gastric adenocarcinoma. Clin Microbiol Infect. 2009;15:971–6.
4. Palli D, Galli M, Caporaso NE, et al. Family history and risk of stomach cancer in Italy. Cancer Epidemiol Biomarkers Prev. 1994;3:15–8.
5. Rothenbacher D, Bode G, Berg G, et al. Helicobacter pylori among preschool children and their parents: evidence of parent-child transmission. J Infect Dis. 1999;179:398–402.
6. IARC Working Group on the Evaluation of Carcinogenic Risks to Humans. Schistosomes, liver flukes and Helicobacter pylori. IARC Monogr Eval Carcinog Risks Hum. 1994;61:1–241.
7. IARC Working Group on the Evaluation of Carcinogenic Risks to Humans. Biological agents. A review of human carcinogens. IARC Monogr Eval Carcinog Risks Hum. 2012;100(Pt B):1–441.
8. Helicobacter and Cancer Collaborative Group. Gastric cancer and Helicobacter pylori: a combined analysis of 12 case control studies nested within prospective cohorts. Gut. 2001; 49:347–53.
9. Hemminki K, Zhang H, Czene K. Socioeconomic factors in cancer in Sweden. Int J Cancer. 2003;105:692–700.
10. Power C, Hypponen E, Smith GD. Socioeconomic position in childhood and early adult life and risk of mortality: a prospective study of the mothers of the 1958 British birth cohort. Am J Public Health. 2005;95:1396–402.

11. Ladeiras-Lopes R, Pereira AK, Nogueira A, et al. Smoking and gastric cancer: systematic review and meta-analysis of cohort studies. Cancer Causes Control. 2008;19:689–701.
12. IARC Working Group on the Evaluation of Carcinogenic Risks to Humans. Personal habits and indoor combustions. Volume 100 E. A review of human carcinogens. IARC Monogr Eval Carcinog Risks Hum. 2012;100:1–538.
13. IARC Working Group on the Evaluation of Carcinogenic Risks to Humans. Alcohol consumption and ethyl carbamate. IARC Monogr Eval Carcinog Risks Hum. 2010;96:3–1383.
14. Yang P, Zhou Y, Chen B, et al. Overweight, obesity and gastric cancer risk: results from a meta-analysis of cohort studies. Eur J Cancer. 2009;45:2867–73.
15. Lukanova A, Bjor O, Kaaks R, et al. Body mass index and cancer: results from the Northern Sweden Health and Disease Cohort. Int J Cancer. 2006;118:458–66.
16. Sjodahl K, Jia C, Vatten L, et al. Body mass and physical activity and risk of gastric cancer in a population-based cohort study in Norway. Cancer Epidemiol Biomarkers Prev. 2008;17:135–40.
17. Leitzmann MF, Koebnick C, Freedman ND, et al. Physical activity and esophageal and gastric carcinoma in a large prospective study. Am J Prev Med. 2009;36:112–9.
18. Correa P. A human model of gastric carcinogenesis. Cancer Res. 1988;48:3554–60.
19. Correa P. Human gastric carcinogenesis: a multistep and multifactorial process – First American Cancer Society Award lecture on cancer epidemiology and prevention. Cancer Res. 1992;52:6735–40.
20. Carneiro F, Huntsman DG, Smyrk TC, et al. Model of the early development of diffuse gastric cancer in E-cadherin mutation carriers and its implications for patient screening. J Pathol. 2004;203:681–7.
21. Siewert JR, Stein HJ. Classification of adenocarcinoma of the oesophagogastric junction. Br J Surg. 1998;85:1457–9.
22. Von Rahden BH, Stein HJ, Siewert JR. Surgical management of esophagogastric junction tumors. World J Gastroenterol. 2006;12(41):6608–13.
23. Rice TW, Blackstone EH, Rusch VW. 7th edition of the AJCC Cancer Staging Manual: esophagus and esophagogastric junction. Ann Surg Oncol. 2010;17(7):1721–4.
24. Washington K. 7th edition of the AJCC Cancer Staging Manual: stomach. Ann Surg Oncol. 2010;17(12):3077–9.
25. Lauren P. The two histological main types of gastric carcinoma: diffuse and so called intestinal-type carcinoma. An attempt at a histo-clinical classification. Acta Pathol Microbiol Scand. 1965;64:31–49.
26. Wanebo HJ, Kennedy BJ, Chmiel J, et al. Cancer of the stomach. A patient care study by the American College of Surgeons. Ann Surg. 1993;218:583.
27. Graham DY, Schwartz JT, Cain GD, et al. Prospective evaluation of biopsy number in the diagnosis of esophageal and gastric carcinoma. Gastroenterology. 1982;82:228.
28. Kim SJ, Kim HH, Kim YH, et al. Peritoneal metastasis: detection with 16- or 64-detector row CT in patients undergoing surgery for gastric cancer. Radiology. 2009;253:407.
29. Burke EC, Karpeh MS, Conlon KC, et al. Laparoscopy in the management of gastric adenocarcinoma. Ann Surg. 1997;225(3):262–7.
30. Karanicolas PJ, Elkin EB, Jacks LM, et al. Staging laparoscopy in the management of gastric cancer: a population-based analysis. J Am Coll Surg. 2011;213(5):644–51.
31. Yoshida S, Tanaka S, Kunihiro K, et al. Diagnostic ability of high-frequency ultrasound probe sonography in staging early gastric cancer, especially for submucosal invasion. Abdom Imaging. 2005;30:518.
32. Byrne MF, Jowell PS. Gastrointestinal imaging: endoscopic ultrasound. Gastroenterology. 2002;122:1631.
33. Botet JF, Lightdale CJ, Zauber AG, et al. Preoperative staging of gastric cancer: comparison of endoscopic US and dynamic CT. Radiology. 1991;181:426.
34. Willis S, Truong S, Gribnitz S, et al. Endoscopic ultrasonography in the preoperative staging of gastric cancer: accuracy and impact on surgical therapy. Surg Endosc. 2000;14:951.

35. Chang KJ, Katz KD, Durbin TE, et al. Endoscopic ultrasound-guided fine-needle aspiration. Gastrointest Endosc. 1994;40:694.

36. Chen J, Cheong JH, Yun MJ, et al. Improvement in preoperative staging of gastric adenocarcinoma with positron emission tomography. Cancer. 2005;103:2383.

37. Yoshioka T, Yamaguchi K, Kubota K, et al. Evaluation of 18F-FDG PET in patients with advanced, metastatic, or recurrent gastric cancer. J Nucl Med. 2003;44:690.

38. Gouzi JL, Huguier M, Fagniez PL, et al. Total versus subtotal gastrectomy for adenocarcinoma of the gastric antrum. A French prospective controlled study. Ann Surg. 1989;209(2):162–6.

39. Bozzetti F, Marubini E, Bonfanti G, et al. Total versus subtotal gastrectomy: surgical morbidity and mortality rates in a multicenter Italian randomized trial. The Italian Gastrointestinal Tumor Study Group. Ann Surg. 1997;226(5):613–20.

40. Bozzetti F, Marubini E, Bonfanti G, et al. Subtotal versus total gastrectomy for gastric cancer: five-year survival rates in a multicenter randomized Italian trial. Italian Gastrointestinal Tumor Study Group. Ann Surg. 1999;230(2):170–8.

41. Davies J, Johnston D, Sue-Ling H, et al. Total or subtotal gastrectomy for gastric carcinoma? A study of quality of life. World J Surg. 1998;22(10):1048–55.

42. Kim JH, Park SS, Kim J, et al. Surgical outcomes for gastric cancer in the upper third of the stomach. World J Surg. 2006;30(10):1870–6.

43. An JY, Youn HG, Choi MG, et al. The difficult choice between total and proximal gastrectomy in proximal early gastric cancer. Am J Surg. 2008;196(4):587–91.

44. Kitano S, Shiraishi N, Fujii K, et al. A randomized controlled trial comparing open vs laparoscopy-assisted distal gastrectomy for the treatment of early gastric cancer: an interim report. Surgery. 2002;131:S306–11.

45. Hayashi H, Ochiai T, Shimada H, et al. Prospective randomized study of open versus laparoscopy-assisted distal gastrectomy with extraperigastric lymph node dissection for early gastric cancer. Surg Endosc. 2005;19:1172–6.

46. Huscher CG, Mingoli A, Sgarzini G, et al. Laparoscopic versus open subtotal gastrectomy for distal gastric cancer: five-year results of a randomized prospective trial. Ann Surg. 2005;l 241:232–7.

47. Lee JH, Han HS, Lee JH. A prospective randomized study comparing open vs laparoscopy-assisted distal gastrectomy in early gastric cancer: early results. Surg Endosc. 2005;19: 168–73.

48. Kim HH, Han SU, Kim MC, et al. Korean Laparoscopic Gastrointestinal Surgery Study (KLASS) Group: prospective randomized controlled trial (phase III) to comparing laparoscopic distal gastrectomy with open distal gastrectomy for gastric adenocarcinoma (KLASS 01). J Korean Surg Soc. 2013;84:123–30.

49. Kim HH, Hyung WJ, Cho GS, et al. Morbidity and mortality of laparoscopic gastrectomy versus open gastrectomy for gastric cancer: an interim report – a phase III multicenter, prospective, randomized trial (KLASS Trial). Ann Surg. 2010;251:417–20.

50. Qiu J, Pankaj P, Jiang H, Zeng Y, Wu H. Laparoscopy versus open distal gastrectomy for advanced gastric cancer: a systematic review and meta-analysis. Surg Laparosc Endosc Percutan Tech. 2013;23:1–7.

51. Japanese Gastric Cancer Association. Japanese classification of gastric carcinoma: 3rd English edition. Gastric Cancer. 2011;14:101.

52. Roukos DH, Kappas AM. Targeting the optimal extent of lymph node dissection for gastric cancer. J Surg Oncol. 2002;81:59.

53. Bunt AM, Hermans J, Smit VT, et al. Surgical/pathologic-stage migration confounds comparisons of gastric cancer survival rates between Japan and Western countries. J Clin Oncol. 1995;13:19.

54. De Manzoni G, Verlato G, Roviello F, et al. The new TNM classification of lymph node metastasis minimises stage migration problems in gastric cancer patients. Br J Cancer. 2002;87:171.

55. Smith DD, Schwarz RR, Schwarz RE. Impact of total lymph node count on staging and survival after gastrectomy for gastric cancer: data from a large US-population database. J Clin Oncol. 2005;23:7114.

56. Noguchi Y, Imada T, Matsumoto A, et al. Radical surgery for gastric cancer. A review of the Japanese experience. Cancer. 1989;64:2053.
57. Maruyama K, Okabayashi K, Kinoshita T. Progress in gastric cancer surgery in Japan and its limits of radicality. World J Surg. 1987;11:418.
58. Roder JD, Böttcher K, Siewert JR, et al. Prognostic factors in gastric carcinoma. Results of the German Gastric Carcinoma Study 1992. Cancer. 1993;72:2089.
59. Jiang L, Yang KH, Guan QL, et al. Survival and recurrence free benefits with different lymphadenectomy for resectable gastric cancer: a meta-analysis. J Surg Oncol. 2013;107:807.
60. Dent DM, Madden MV, Price SK. Randomized comparison of R1 and R2 gastrectomy for gastric carcinoma. Br J Surg. 1988;75:110.
61. Cuschieri A, Fayers P, Fielding J, et al. Postoperative morbidity and mortality after D1 and D2 resections for gastric cancer: preliminary results of the MRC randomised controlled surgical trial. The Surgical Cooperative Group. Lancet. 1996;347:995.
62. Bonenkamp JJ, Hermans J, Sasako M, et al. Extended lymph-node dissection for gastric cancer. N Engl J Med. 1999;340:908.
63. Degiuli M, Sasako M, Ponti A, et al. Randomized clinical trial comparing survival after D1 or D2 gastrectomy for gastric cancer. Br J Surg. 2014;101:23.
64. Sano T, Sasako M, Yamamoto S, et al. Gastric cancer surgery: morbidity and mortality results from a prospective randomized controlled trial comparing D2 and extended para-aortic lymphadenectomy--Japan Clinical Oncology Group study 9501. J Clin Oncol. 2004;22:2767.
65. Cuschieri A, Weeden S, Fielding J, et al. Patient survival after D1 and D2 resections for gastric cancer: long-term results of the MRC randomised surgical trial. Surgical Co-operative Group. Br J Cancer. 1999;79:1522.
66. Hartgrink HH, van de Velde CJ, Putter H, et al. Extended lymph node dissection for gastric cancer: who may benefit? Final results of the randomized Dutch gastric cancer group trial. J Clin Oncol. 2004;22:2069.
67. Songun I, Putter H, Kranenbarg EM, et al. Surgical treatment of gastric cancer: 15-year follow-up results of the randomised nationwide Dutch D1D2 trial. Lancet Oncol. 2010;11:439.
68. Petrelli NJ. The debate is over; it's time to move on. J Clin Oncol. 2004;22:2041.
69. Sasako M, Sano T, Yamamoto S, et al. D2 lymphadenectomy alone or with para-aortic nodal dissection for gastric cancer. N Engl J Med. 2008;359:453.
70. Kulig J, Popiela T, Kolodziejczyk P, et al. Standard D2 versus extended D2 (D2+) lymphadenectomy for gastric cancer: an interim safety analysis of a multicenter, randomized, clinical trial. Am J Surg. 2007;193:10.
71. Yonemura Y, Wu CC, Fukushima N, et al. Randomized clinical trial of D2 and extended paraaortic lymphadenectomy in patients with gastric cancer. Int J Clin Oncol. 2008;13:132.
72. Chen XZ, Hu JK, Zhou ZG, et al. Meta-analysis of effectiveness and safety of D2 plus para-aortic lymphadenectomy for resectable gastric cancer. J Am Coll Surg. 2010;210:100.

Gastrointestinal Stromal Tumors

Daniel Delitto and Kevin E. Behrns

Introduction

Gastrointestinal stromal tumors (GISTs) represent a distinct group of neoplasms originating in the stromal, or connective tissue, compartment of the gastrointestinal tract. GISTs comprise a recently recognized subgroup of sarcomas, which typically describe malignancies originating in connective tissue. Earlier classification schemes combined GISTs and leiomyomas as one entity. In time, immunohistochemical analysis revealed a lack of smooth muscle expression in the former, setting the stage for subsequent molecular characterization of GISTs. In 1998, this characterization eventually led to the identification of a *c-kit* gain of function mutation, and the widespread use of imatinib, a small molecular c-kit inhibitor of c-kit [1]. This discovery revolutionized the treatment of GIST by introducing effective medical therapy as a viable adjunct to the surgical treatment of GISTs. Indeed, these findings have spawned the description of aberrant growth signaling through constitutively active tyrosine kinase receptors in many tumor types and inhibition of growth signaling continues to hold widespread influence in cancer research. In this review, we will discuss the surgical approach to GISTs, encompassing all relevant aspects from patient presentation through perioperative management.

D. Delitto, M.D.
Department of Surgery, University of Florida, P.O. Box 100286, Gainesville,
FL 32610-0286, USA
e-mail: delitto@ufl.edu

K.E. Behrns, M.D. (✉)
Department of Surgery, University of Florida, P.O. Box 100286, Gainesville,
FL 32610-0286, USA

Department of Surgery, University of Florida, Room 6174, 1600 SW Archer Road,
P.O. Box 100286, Gainesville, FL 32610-0286, USA
e-mail: kevin.behrns@surgery.ufl.edu

© Springer International Publishing Switzerland 2016   25
K.A. Morgan (ed.), *Current Controversies in Cancer Care*
for the Surgeon, DOI 10.1007/978-3-319-16205-8_2

Epidemiology

GISTs represent the most common subtype of sarcoma, accounting for 18 % of sarcomas in a population-based European study [2]. The incidence ranges from 7 to 10 cases per million in Europe and the United States with a prevalence of approximately 130 cases per million population [2–4]. GISTs may arise from any portion of the gastrointestinal tract, although a strong predilection exists for the stomach and small intestine. Pooled population-based cohort analyses indicate the occurrence of approximately 56–60 % of GISTs in the stomach, 30–33 % in the small intestine, 5–10 % in the colon or rectum, and approximately 1 % in the esophagus [5]. Importantly, approximately 23 % of patients present with overt metastatic disease [6].

The incidence of GISTs may display a slight predilection toward men, although the difference is small, and the evidence appears to be inconsistent between populations [5, 7]. A slight racial disparity is evident in the development of GISTs according to a large American population-based investigation, with African Americans exhibiting roughly double the incidence [7]. Median age at the time of diagnosis is 63 years, with less than 0.5 % of patients younger than 20 years of age [5, 7]. The major risk factor for GIST development is a personal history of cancer, present in 34 % of patients, a surprisingly high risk factor [6, 8].

Pathology

Morphologically, GISTs share many features with sarcomas. However, molecular characterization has confirmed GISTs as a separate entity, and specific histopathologic findings are necessary to confirm the diagnosis. Other connective tissue tumors that share characteristics with GISTs include Schwannomas and gangliocytic paragangliomas. However, these neoplasms have distinct immunohistochemistry findings (Table 1), and gangliocytic paragangliomas are almost exclusively found in the duodenum. In particular, the interstitial cells of Cajal (ICC) have been implicated as a common GIST progenitor, marking a striking separation from other stromal tumors in the GI tract. Evidence for an ICC progenitor stems from early immunohistochemical analyses of GIST specimens, which displayed positivity of c-kit and CD34 in both malignant cells and a subset of ICC [9, 10]. Since its discovery in the 1990s, c-kit expression remains the hallmark of GIST diagnosis. c-kit is a receptor tyrosine kinase which dimerizes upon binding to its ligand, stem cell factor (SCF). Subsequent transphosphorylation leads to the induction of multiple, cell pro-survival, proliferative pathways [11–13]. A c-kit gain of function mutation is present in 75–80 % of GISTs, most commonly in the juxtamembrane domain of exon 11 [1, 14].

Table 1 Immunohistochemistry staining characteristics of spindle-cell predominant duodenal tumors

	NSE[a]	Chromogranin	S-100	CK-PAN[b]	DOG-1[c]	CD117 (c-kit)	CD34
Gangliocytic paraganglioma	+ (all 3 cell types)	+ (mostly described in epithelial component)	+ (spindle cell component)	+ 50 % of cases (only epithelioid component)	–	–	–
Schwannoma	+/– (+ in approx 25 % of cases)	–	+ (strong and diffusely positive)	–	–	–	– (rare cases show focal positivity)
GIST	–	–	Mostly – (5 % focal positivity)	–	+ (>90 %)	+ (>90 %)	+ (66 %)

[a]NSE neuron-specific enolase
[b]CK-Pan Pancytokeratin
[c]DOG-1 discovered on GIST

Of the remaining 20–25 % of GISTs without a c-kit mutation, approximately one-third harbor a mutation in the platelet-derived growth factor receptor (PDGFR), another receptor tyrosine kinase with similar growth-promoting properties to c-kit [15, 16]. The remaining GISTs, which do not display mutations in either c-kit or PDGFR, are referred to as wild-type tumors. This nomenclature, however, is slightly inaccurate, as these tumors have a high incidence of other known oncogenic mutations, such as BRAF [17], SDH [18, 19], RAS [20], and NF1 [21]. Thus, GISTs display a unique pattern of oncogenic traits. This knowledge has led to major breakthroughs in their diagnosis and treatment.

Diagnosis

It is important to note that GISTs can grow quite large prior to causing symptoms. For example, an Italian series of 47 consecutive patients diagnosed with GIST correlated symptoms with tumor size. Interestingly, the average size of symptomatic GISTs was 8.9 cm, while the average size of incidentally found GISTs was 2.7 cm [4]. Accordingly, it is estimated that 25 % of GISTs are found incidentally [4, 8, 22]. Symptomatic patients present most frequently with either abdominal discomfort or gastrointestinal bleeding and subsequent anemia [23].

Endoscopic biopsy of the submucosal tumor represents the preferred diagnostic method, which prevents tumor seeding in the abdominal cavity. Histologic diagnosis is of particular benefit if there is any suspicion for other sarcoma subtypes or situations involving a marginally resectable or unresectable tumor to guide chemotherapy. However, if a submucosal lesion in the stomach is easily resectable and has characteristic features of GIST, biopsy is not required prior to resection.

Typically, the diagnosis is made by immunohistochemistry displaying a c-kit positive stromal malignancy. However, it is worthwhile to discuss the differential diagnosis for a c-kit positive lesion. Importantly, metastatic melanoma should always be considered, as they are commonly c-kit positive. Other common malignancies, which stain c-kit positive, include seminomas and small cell lung carcinomas. Additionally, 50 % of angiosarcomas, 50 % of Ewing's sarcomas, and 30 % of neuroblastomas are c-kit positive [24].

The diagnosis may be complicated by the 5 % of GISTs, which stain negative for c-kit. The most important point to remember concerning these situations is that a pathologist experienced in GIST diagnosis must be employed. Multiple additional diagnostic methods have been applied in this situation, including the detection of PDGFR-A [25], BRAF [17], protein kinase C-theta [26], and DOG1 (discovered on GIST1) [27].

Once the diagnosis is made histologically, further imaging is of limited utility. Endoscopic ultrasound (EUS) has been demonstrated to better characterize tumor size and aid in prognostic staging. Additionally, EUS with fine needle aspiration biopsy is a viable, less invasive option for histologic diagnosis, yielding a sensitivity of approximately 84 % [28]. Nodal staging is of limited value as well, as lymphatic spread is not characteristic of a GIST. Further, staging is typically unnecessary for the head, neck, and chest, as extra-abdominal metastases are exceedingly infrequent.

Risk Stratification

Pathologic and clinical features of GISTs affecting prognosis remain controversial. A prognostic nomogram developed at the Memorial Sloan-Kettering Cancer Center from 127 patients has been subsequently validated in two larger cohorts of GIST patients. The results successfully predicted recurrence-free survival and established the current model of risk stratification recommended in GIST. Based on their conclusions, high-risk features include size greater than 3 cm, mitotic rate exceeding five per high-powered field (HPF) and a non-gastric location [29]. Subsequent investigations have confirmed the predictive value of size, mitotic rate, and location on prognosis [30–32]. An example of a widely used risk stratification model employed by the 2008 National Comprehensive Cancer Network (NCCN) guidelines is displayed in Table 2.

Table 2 Risk stratification of primary GISTs

Tumor parameters		Risk for progressive disease[a] (%), based on site of origin			
Mitotic rate	Size (cm)	Stomach	Jejunum/ileum	Duodenum	Rectum
≤5 per 50 HPF	≤2	None (0 %)	None (0 %)	None (0 %)	None (0 %)
	>2, ≤5	Very low (1.9 %)	Low (4.3 %)	Low (8.3 %)	Low (8.5 %)
	>5, ≤10	Low (3.6 %)	Moderate (24 %)	Insufficient data	Insufficient data
	>10	Moderate (10 %)	High (52 %)	High (34 %)	High (57 %)
>5 per HPF	≤2	None[b]	High[b]	Insufficient data	High (54 %)
	>2, ≤5	Moderate (16 %)	High (73 %)	High (50 %)	High (52 %)
	>5, ≤10	High (55 %)	High (85 %)	Insufficient data	Insufficient data
	>10	High (86 %)	High (90 %)	High (86 %)	High (71 %)

Adapted from Miettinen, M., et al. (2005). "Gastrointestinal stromal tumors of the stomach: a clinicopathologic, immunohistochemical, and molecular genetic study of 1765 cases with long-term follow-up." Am J Surg Pathol 29(1): 52–68 and "NCCN Task Force report: update on the management of patients with gastrointestinal stromal tumors." J Natl Compr Canc Netw 8 Suppl 2: S1–41; quiz S42–44
[a]Defined as metastasis or tumor-related death in long-term follow-up of 1055 gastric, 629 small intestinal, 144 duodenal, and 111 rectal GISTS
[b]Denotes small numbers of cases

Medical Management

Prior to the development of imatinib, GISTs were treated with cytotoxic chemotherapy, yielding abysmal results. The median survival for tumors treated with cytotoxic chemotherapy was approximately 14–18 months [33]. As a result, cytotoxic chemotherapy is not recommended currently as a treatment for GIST. Imatinib treatment is now the standard of care, by NCCN recommendations.

The major role for adjuvant imatinib arose from a phase 3 trial, in which 713 patients were randomized postoperatively to receive imatinib versus placebo for 1 year [30]. Ninety-eight percent of patients in the imatinib group experienced 1-year recurrence-free survival compared to only 83 % in the placebo group. Additionally, at median follow-up of 20 months, 30 % of the placebo group had either recurred or died, compared to only 8 % of the imatinib group. Additionally, the benefits of imatinib were especially significant with larger tumors, with thresholds of 6 cm and 10 cm being analyzed [30]. A similar trial examined the duration of imatinib treatment postoperatively, comparing 36 months to 12 months of therapy. The 5-year recurrence-free and overall survivals were 66 and 92 % for 3 years of therapy and 48 and 82 % for 1 year of therapy, respectively [31].

Thus, the NCCN 2012 guidelines state that 1 year of adjuvant imatinib therapy is appropriate in intermediate and high-risk GISTs [34]. Based on the criteria discussed under risk stratification, features justifying adjuvant treatment with imatinib include 5 mitoses/50 HPF, size greater than 3 cm, non-gastric location or tumor rupture [30, 31]. Further, for GISTs at least 5 cm in size, 3 years of adjuvant imatinib is recommended [34].

Additionally, it is pertinent to discuss recommendations for neoadjuvant imatinib, as this directly affects the surgeon's operative planning. Several trials have formed the foundation justifying preoperative administration of imatinib. The first is the RTOG 0132 phase 2 trial, in which 30 patients with primary GIST received 8–12 weeks of neoadjuvant imatinib. A partial response was observed in 7 % of patients, stable disease in 83 % of patients, and 2-year progression-free and overall survival was 83 and 93 %, respectively [35]. A similar trial employed a longer duration of therapy, examining 15 patients receiving 7–9 months of preoperative imatinib. In these patients, a median size reduction of 34 % was observed, and the 3-year progression-free survival rate was 77 % [36]. Of note, all patients in these trials received adjuvant imatinib as well. As insufficient evidence is available to conclude that neoadjuvant therapy leads to superior outcomes, it is currently recognized as a viable modality by the NCCN, but specific therapeutic guidelines have not been established [34].

A recently investigated dilemma facing the surgeon treating GISTs is whether preoperative imatinib can downstage a tumor or offer a less morbid resection. A recent investigation examined this question in 15 patients receiving preoperative imatinib with cytoreductive intent. In this group of patients, three out of four patients initially planned for abdominoperineal resection achieved successful sphincter sparing operations, while the fourth patient had a complete response and underwent no operation. These patients experienced no recurrence at 22 months of follow-up. Additionally, three out of five patients initially planned for total gastrectomy received successful partial gastrectomies. Three initially unresectable GISTs (one duodenal and two gastric GISTs) achieved R0 resections [36]. While small in scope, this investigation establishes a precedent for neoadjuvant imatinib when faced with a highly morbid resection.

Principles of Surgical Management

All extragastric GISTs are considered high risk and currently warrant resection when feasible. Regarding gastric GISTs, the current recommendation is resection if the tumor is at least 2 cm in size [34, 37]. Additionally, high-risk features that are radiographically evident and indications for resection include a heterogeneous mass with irregular borders or cystic components. Importantly, GISTs in locations representing high operative morbidity, such as the gastroesophageal junction, duodenum, and rectum, warrant extensive preoperative multidisciplinary review. The possibility of avoiding a radical resection with neoadjuvant imatinib should be considered.

It is important to note that incidental submucosal tumors less than 1 cm in size are frequently discovered on endoscopy. Although somewhat controversial, routine excision of these lesions is not recommended given their low propensity to progress into clinically significant tumors [38–44].

Current operative recommendations entail segmental resection to negative microscopic margins. Formal oncologic resection of uninvolved tissue and lymph node dissection are unnecessary, as they have shown no clinical benefit [33, 45]. It has even been suggested that re-excision of a microscopically positive margin (R1 resection) imparts little clinical benefit [46]. However, one recommendation, which has remained consistent, is to avoid tumor rupture during surgery. GISTs have the potential to seed intraperitoneal tumors. For this reason, open excisional biopsy should be avoided as well.

In addition to traditional open approaches, laparoscopic resection of gastric GISTs has been consistently associated with low recurrence rates, low morbidity, and shorter hospital stays in multiple series [47–51]. We have included multiple illustrations of our laparoscopic approach, including the typical submucosal appearance and dissection (Figs. 1, 2, 3, and 4).

Follow-up CT should be obtained every 3–6 months postoperatively for the first year [33]. In the event of recurrence, current guidelines recommend an initial trial of imatinib, similar to the treatment of metastatic disease. If no progression is seen after 3–6 months of treatment, reoperation with curative intent may be considered. Unfortunately, outcomes remain poor, as recurrent disease is associated with a 5-year survival of approximately 50 % [46, 52, 53].

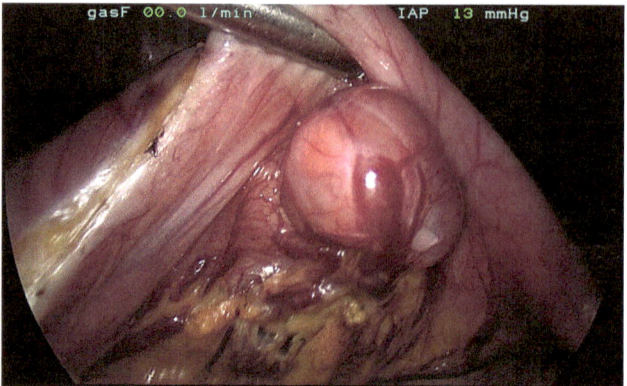

Fig. 1 Typical external appearance of a gastric GIST

Fig. 2 Dissection of GIST
attached at submucosal
layer

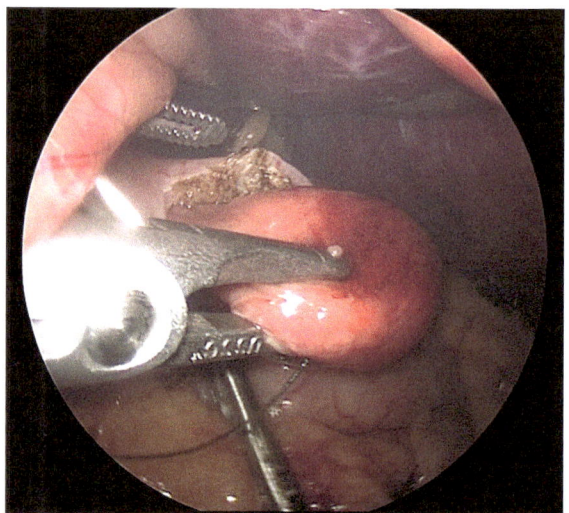

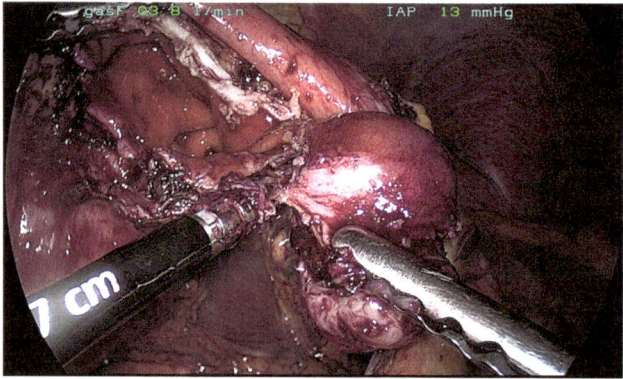

Fig. 3 Completed dissection illustrating the appearance of the tumor in relation to all layers of the
gastric wall

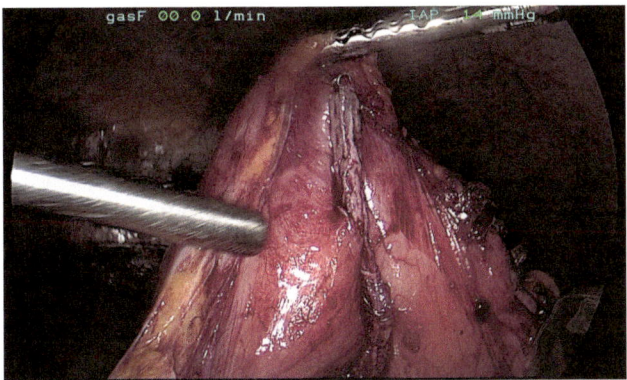

Fig. 4 Primary closure of the gastric defect

Conclusions

In summary, the operative management of GISTs consists of complete resection when possible. Importantly, it is vital that patients have close follow-up with a multidisciplinary team of surgeons, pathologists, and medical oncologists experienced in the management of GISTs. Appropriate interpretation of prognostic pathologic features is essential in guiding the potential clinical benefit of imatinib therapy.

References

1. Hirota S, Isozaki K, Moriyama Y, Hashimoto K, Nishida T, Ishiguro S, et al. Gain-of-function mutations of c-kit in human gastrointestinal stromal tumors. Science. 1998;279(5350): 577–80.
2. Ducimetiere F, Lurkin A, Ranchere-Vince D, Decouvelaere AV, Peoc'h M, Istier L, et al. Incidence of sarcoma histotypes and molecular subtypes in a prospective epidemiological study with central pathology review and molecular testing. PLoS One. 2011;6(8):e20294.
3. Chan KH, Chan CW, Chow WH, Kwan WK, Kong CK, Mak KF, et al. Gastrointestinal stromal tumors in a cohort of Chinese patients in Hong Kong. World J Gastroenterol. 2006; 12(14):2223–8.
4. Nilsson B, Bumming P, Meis-Kindblom JM, Oden A, Dortok A, Gustavsson B, et al. Gastrointestinal stromal tumors: the incidence, prevalence, clinical course, and prognostication in the preimatinib mesylate era – a population-based study in western Sweden. Cancer. 2005;103(4):821–9.
5. Joensuu H, Vehtari A, Riihimaki J, Nishida T, Steigen SE, Brabec P, et al. Risk of recurrence of gastrointestinal stromal tumour after surgery: an analysis of pooled population-based cohorts. Lancet Oncol. 2012;13(3):265–74.
6. Woodall 3rd CE, Brock GN, Fan J, Byam JA, Scoggins CR, McMasters KM, et al. An evaluation of 2537 gastrointestinal stromal tumors for a proposed clinical staging system. Arch Surg. 2009;144(7):670–8.

7. Tran T, Davila JA, El-Serag HB. The epidemiology of malignant gastrointestinal stromal tumors: an analysis of 1,458 cases from 1992 to 2000. Am J Gastroenterol. 2005;100(1):162–8.
8. Mucciarini C, Rossi G, Bertolini F, Valli R, Cirilli C, Rashid I, et al. Incidence and clinico-pathologic features of gastrointestinal stromal tumors. A population-based study. BMC Cancer. 2007;7:230.
9. Kindblom LG, Remotti HE, Aldenborg F, Meis-Kindblom JM. Gastrointestinal pacemaker cell tumor (GIPACT): gastrointestinal stromal tumors show phenotypic characteristics of the interstitial cells of Cajal. Am J Pathol. 1998;152(5):1259–69.
10. Robinson TL, Sircar K, Hewlett BR, Chorneyko K, Riddell RH, Huizinga JD. Gastrointestinal stromal tumors may originate from a subset of CD34-positive interstitial cells of Cajal. Am J Pathol. 2000;156(4):1157–63.
11. Blume-Jensen P, Claesson-Welsh L, Siegbahn A, Zsebo KM, Westermark B, Heldin CH. Activation of the human c-kit product by ligand-induced dimerization mediates circular actin reorganization and chemotaxis. EMBO J. 1991;10(13):4121–8.
12. Zsebo KM, Williams DA, Geissler EN, Broudy VC, Martin FH, Atkins HL, et al. Stem cell factor is encoded at the Sl locus of the mouse and is the ligand for the c-kit tyrosine kinase receptor. Cell. 1990;63(1):213–24.
13. Yuzawa S, Opatowsky Y, Zhang Z, Mandiyan V, Lax I, Schlessinger J. Structural basis for activation of the receptor tyrosine kinase KIT by stem cell factor. Cell. 2007;130(2):323–34.
14. Corless CL, Barnett CM, Heinrich MC. Gastrointestinal stromal tumours: origin and molecu-lar oncology. Nat Rev Cancer. 2011;11(12):865–78.
15. Heinrich MC, Corless CL, Duensing A, McGreevey L, Chen CJ, Joseph N, et al. PDGFRA activating mutations in gastrointestinal stromal tumors. Science. 2003;299(5607):708–10.
16. Hirota S, Ohashi A, Nishida T, Isozaki K, Kinoshita K, Shinomura Y, et al. Gain-of-function mutations of platelet-derived growth factor receptor alpha gene in gastrointestinal stromal tumors. Gastroenterology. 2003;125(3):660–7.
17. Agaram NP, Wong GC, Guo T, Maki RG, Singer S, Dematteo RP, et al. Novel V600E BRAF mutations in imatinib-naive and imatinib-resistant gastrointestinal stromal tumors. Genes Chromosomes Cancer. 2008;47(10):853–9.
18. Janeway KA, Kim SY, Lodish M, Nose V, Rustin P, Gaal J, et al. Defects in succinate dehydro-genase in gastrointestinal stromal tumors lacking KIT and PDGFRA mutations. Proc Natl Acad Sci U S A. 2011;108(1):314–8.
19. Doyle LA, Nelson D, Heinrich MC, Corless CL, Hornick JL. Loss of succinate dehydrogenase subunit B (SDHB) expression is limited to a distinctive subset of gastric wild-type gastrointes-tinal stromal tumours: a comprehensive genotype-phenotype correlation study. Histopathology. 2012;61(5):801–9.
20. Miranda C, Nucifora M, Molinari F, Conca E, Anania MC, Bordoni A, et al. KRAS and BRAF mutations predict primary resistance to imatinib in gastrointestinal stromal tumors. Clin Cancer Res. 2012;18(6):1769–76.
21. Yantiss RK, Rosenberg AE, Sarran L, Besmer P, Antonescu CR. Multiple gastrointestinal stro-mal tumors in type I neurofibromatosis: a pathologic and molecular study. Mod Pathol. 2005;18(4):475–84.
22. Caterino S, Lorenzon L, Petrucciani N, Iannicelli E, Pilozzi E, Romiti A, et al. Gastrointestinal stromal tumors: correlation between symptoms at presentation, tumor location and prognostic factors in 47 consecutive patients. World J Surg Oncol. 2011;9:13.
23. Bumming P, Ahlman H, Andersson J, Meis-Kindblom JM, Kindblom LG, Nilsson B. Population-based study of the diagnosis and treatment of gastrointestinal stromal tumours. Br J Surg. 2006;93(7):836–43.
24. Miettinen M, Lasota J. KIT (CD117): a review on expression in normal and neoplastic tissues, and mutations and their clinicopathologic correlation. Appl Immunohistochem Mol Morphol. 2005;13(3):205–20.
25. Miselli F, Millefanti C, Conca E, Negri T, Piacenza C, Pierotti MA, et al. PDGFRA immunos-taining can help in the diagnosis of gastrointestinal stromal tumors. Am J Surg Pathol. 2008;32(5):738–43.

26. Kim KM, Kang DW, Moon WS, Park JB, Park CK, Sohn JH, et al. PKCtheta expression in gastrointestinal stromal tumor. Mod Pathol. 2006;19(11):1480–6.
27. Miettinen M, Wang ZF, Lasota J. DOG1 antibody in the differential diagnosis of gastrointestinal stromal tumors: a study of 1840 cases. Am J Surg Pathol. 2009;33(9):1401–8.
28. Sepe PS, Moparty B, Pitman MB, Saltzman JR, Brugge WR. EUS-guided FNA for the diagnosis of GI stromal cell tumors: sensitivity and cytologic yield. Gastrointest Endosc. 2009;70(2):254–61.
29. Gold JS, Gonen M, Gutierrez A, Broto JM, Garcia-del-Muro X, Smyrk TC, et al. Development and validation of a prognostic nomogram for recurrence-free survival after complete surgical resection of localised primary gastrointestinal stromal tumour: a retrospective analysis. Lancet Oncol. 2009;10(11):1045–52.
30. Dematteo RP, Ballman KV, Antonescu CR, Maki RG, Pisters PW, Demetri GD, et al. Adjuvant imatinib mesylate after resection of localised, primary gastrointestinal stromal tumour: a randomised, double-blind, placebo-controlled trial. Lancet. 2009;373(9669):1097–104.
31. Joensuu H, Eriksson M, Sundby Hall K, Hartmann JT, Pink D, Schutte J, et al. One vs three years of adjuvant imatinib for operable gastrointestinal stromal tumor: a randomized trial. JAMA. 2012;307(12):1265–72.
32. Joensuu H. Risk stratification of patients diagnosed with gastrointestinal stromal tumor. Hum Pathol. 2008;39(10):1411–9.
33. Demetri GD, von Mehren M, Antonescu CR, DeMatteo RP, Ganjoo KN, Maki RG, et al. NCCN Task Force report: update on the management of patients with gastrointestinal stromal tumors. J Natl Compr Canc Netw. 2010;8 Suppl 2:S1–41. quiz S2-4.
34. von Mehren M, Benjamin RS, Bui MM, Casper ES, Conrad 3rd EU, DeLaney TF, et al. Soft tissue sarcoma, version 2.2012: featured updates to the NCCN guidelines. J Natl Compr Canc Netw. 2012;10(8):951–60.
35. Eisenberg BL, Harris J, Blanke CD, Demetri GD, Heinrich MC, Watson JC, et al. Phase II trial of neoadjuvant/adjuvant imatinib mesylate (IM) for advanced primary and metastatic/recurrent operable gastrointestinal stromal tumor (GIST): early results of RTOG 0132/ACRIN 6665. J Surg Oncol. 2009;99(1):42–7.
36. Fiore M, Palassini E, Fumagalli E, Pilotti S, Tamborini E, Stacchiotti S, et al. Preoperative imatinib mesylate for unresectable or locally advanced primary gastrointestinal stromal tumors (GIST). Eur J Surg Oncol. 2009;35(7):739–45.
37. Sepe PS, Brugge WR. A guide for the diagnosis and management of gastrointestinal stromal cell tumors. Nat Rev Gastroenterol Hepatol. 2009;6(6):363–71.
38. Agaimy A, Wunsch PH, Dirnhofer S, Bihl MP, Terracciano LM, Tornillo L. Microscopic gastrointestinal stromal tumors in esophageal and intestinal surgical resection specimens: a clinicopathologic, immunohistochemical, and molecular study of 19 lesions. Am J Surg Pathol. 2008;32(6):867–73.
39. Rossi S, Gasparotto D, Toffolatti L, Pastrello C, Gallina G, Marzotto A, et al. Molecular and clinicopathologic characterization of gastrointestinal stromal tumors (GISTs) of small size. Am J Surg Pathol. 2010;34(10):1480–91.
40. Chetty R. Small and microscopically detected gastrointestinal stromal tumours: an overview. Pathology. 2008;40(1):9–12.
41. Agaimy A, Wunsch PH, Hofstaedter F, Blaszyk H, Rummele P, Gaumann A, et al. Minute gastric sclerosing stromal tumors (GIST tumorlets) are common in adults and frequently show c-KIT mutations. Am J Surg Pathol. 2007;31(1):113–20.
42. Abraham SC, Krasinskas AM, Hofstetter WL, Swisher SG, Wu TT. "Seedling" mesenchymal tumors (gastrointestinal stromal tumors and leiomyomas) are common incidental tumors of the esophagogastric junction. Am J Surg Pathol. 2007;31(11):1629–35.
43. Kawanowa K, Sakuma Y, Sakurai S, Hishima T, Iwasaki Y, Saito K, et al. High incidence of microscopic gastrointestinal stromal tumors in the stomach. Hum Pathol. 2006;37(12):1527–35.
44. Lok KH, Lai L, Yiu HL, Szeto ML, Leung SK. Endosonographic surveillance of small gastrointestinal tumors originating from muscularis propria. J Gastrointestin Liver Dis. 2009;18(2):177–80.

45. Fong Y, Coit DG, Woodruff JM, Brennan MF. Lymph node metastasis from soft tissue sarcoma in adults. Analysis of data from a prospective database of 1772 sarcoma patients. Ann Surg. 1993;217(1):72–7.
46. DeMatteo RP, Lewis JJ, Leung D, Mudan SS, Woodruff JM, Brennan MF. Two hundred gastrointestinal stromal tumors: recurrence patterns and prognostic factors for survival. Ann Surg. 2000;231(1):51–8.
47. Novitsky YW, Kercher KW, Sing RF, Heniford BT. Long-term outcomes of laparoscopic resection of gastric gastrointestinal stromal tumors. Ann Surg. 2006;243(6):738–45. discussion 45–7.
48. Otani Y, Furukawa T, Yoshida M, Saikawa Y, Wada N, Ueda M, et al. Operative indications for relatively small (2-5 cm) gastrointestinal stromal tumor of the stomach based on analysis of 60 operated cases. Surgery. 2006;139(4):484–92.
49. Nakamori M, Iwahashi M, Nakamura M, Tabuse K, Mori K, Taniguchi K, et al. Laparoscopic resection for gastrointestinal stromal tumors of the stomach. Am J Surg. 2008;196(3):425–9.
50. Nishimura J, Nakajima K, Omori T, Takahashi T, Nishitani A, Ito T, et al. Surgical strategy for gastric gastrointestinal stromal tumors: laparoscopic vs. open resection. Surg Endosc. 2007;21(6):875–8.
51. Huguet KL, Rush Jr RM, Tessier DJ, Schlinkert RT, Hinder RA, Grinberg GG, et al. Laparoscopic gastric gastrointestinal stromal tumor resection: the mayo clinic experience. Arch Surg. 2008;143(6):587–90. discussion 91.
52. Eisenberg BL, Judson I. Surgery and imatinib in the management of GIST: emerging approaches to adjuvant and neoadjuvant therapy. Ann Surg Oncol. 2004;11(5):465–75.
53. Gold JS, Dematteo RP. Combined surgical and molecular therapy: the gastrointestinal stromal tumor model. Ann Surg. 2006;244(2):176–84.

Gastrointestinal Neuroendocrine Tumors: Optimal Outcomes and Surgical Management

Travis Spaulding and Robert C.G. Martin II

Introduction

Neuroendocrine tumors (NETs) are a specific type of neoplasm arising in tissues of neural crest origin. They commonly arise in the gastrointestinal tract because of the high density of neuroendocrine cells, and are found in the foregut (stomach, duodenum, pancreas), midgut (jejunum, ileum, appendix, proximal colon), and hindgut (distal colon, rectum) [1, 2]. NETs are commonly termed "carcinoid" tumors if they are found to be of low grade on histology. The prognosis for NETs is variable, dependent upon tumor biology and origin. This chapter reviews specific features of NETs in each GI segment, with particular focus on factors predicting prognosis and surgical decision-making.

General Considerations

NETs are found in females more often than males, with reported ratios ranging from 2.65 females:2.24 males per 100,000 in Switzerland to 3.98 white females:2.47 white males per 100,000 in the United States [3]. They are often found incidentally during imaging or endoscopy for other clinical diagnoses as they are commonly not large enough at diagnosis to be symptomatic. NETs are increasingly discovered, particularly in the past decade, likely due to increased clinical utilization and technological sophistication of CT, MRI, and functional imaging as well as the higher prevalence of endoscopic procedures [4]. NETs usually occur sporadically, but can arise in the setting of multiple endocrine neoplasia type 1 (MEN1) syndrome.

T. Spaulding, B.S. • R.C.G. Martin II, M.D., Ph.D., F.A.C.S. (✉)
Division of Surgical Oncology, Department of Surgery, University of Louisville,
315 E. Broadway, #312, Louisville, KY 40202, USA
e-mail: robert.martin@louisville.edu

© Springer International Publishing Switzerland 2016
K.A. Morgan (ed.), *Current Controversies in Cancer Care for the Surgeon*, DOI 10.1007/978-3-319-16205-8_3

Table 1 Grading neuroendocrine tumors based on mitotic count and Ki-67 index

Grade	Mitotic count (10HPF)[a]	Ki-67 index (%)
G1	<2	≤2
G2	2–20	3–20
G3	>20	>20

[a]10HPF: high power field-2 mm2, at least 40 fields (at 40× magnification) evaluated in areas of highest mitotic density bMIB1 antibody; % of 2000 tumor cells in areas of highest nuclear labeling

Tumor grade is important when determining a patient's prognosis or risk of recurrence of NETs [5–7]. The World Health Organization (WHO) classification system for gastrointestinal NETs is commonly used to assess NETs histologically [8]. Under this system, categories 1 and 2 include well-differentiated carcinoids and tumors (WDECs/WDETs), of which WDETs include benign tumors or tumors with "slow behavioral characteristics." NETs in category 3 are poorly differentiated, and category 4 neuroendocrine neoplasms have mixed exocrine and endocrine components, with at least 30 % of each as part of the neoplasm. Category 5 is reserved for all other endocrine cell lesions that are not necessarily transformed into neoplasms [5–7]. Grading of NETs is also done via mitotic count (per10hpf) and Ki-67 index, which represents the proliferative potential of a neoplastic lesion. Tumor grading based on these factors is summarized in Table 1.

Imaging

Radiographic imaging is crucial in the evaluation of NETs and in determining optimal surgical management. Contrast-enhanced CT and MRI have the most clinical utility in assessing the primary tumor and the extent of malignant disease, given the excellent sensitivity and specificity of these tests.

Functional imaging, most notably Somatostatin Receptor Scintigraphy (SRS, Octreotide scan) is also utilized, but has lower accuracy compared to multiphase CT and dynamic MRI. In SRS, a radiolabeled somatostatin analog (classically Indium-111-DTPA octreotide) is injected intravenously and localizes in tissues dense with somatostatin receptors (SSTRs), specifically SSTR2 [9]. ^{68}Ga-labeled somatostatin analogs have also become increasingly beneficial in clinical practice. The half-life for these analogs is only 1 h, so imaging studies can be completed in 2–3 h, compared to between 24 and 48 h for SRS [12]. Additionally, less than half of the dose compared to that required for Indium-111-DTPA octreotide is needed, reducing patient risk [13]. Combination of single photon emission CT (SPECT) and SRS to give fusion images can enable clinicians to correlate SSTR activity with anatomical position [10].

SRS can also be useful in treatment planning and in therapy. Gastrointestinal NETs often have a high affinity for somatostatin and its analogs because of high expression of SSTRs. This high expression can be confirmed with SRS, which can be helpful in deciding on somatostatin analog therapy. Somatostatin analogs are used for therapy when surgery is not possible or distant metastases render it ineffective. Administration of this therapy to patients has become less cumbersome as slow depot injections have been developed for octreotide (octreotide long-acting repeatable or LAR) and lanreotide (lanreotide slow release or SR) [15]. The tumor static effects of somatostatin analogs entail a variety of mechanisms, including the inhibitory action of activated SSTR2 and SSTR5 on the mitotic cycle in neoplastic lesions [16]. Additionally, somatostatin analogs seem to have an anti-angiogenesis effect on neoplastic lesions, inhibiting tumor growth via inhibition of vascular endothelial growth factor 1 [17]. Peptide receptor radionuclide therapy (PRRT) is the use of radioactive isotopes bound to somatostatin analogs like octreotide or lanreotide to irradiate neuroendocrine neoplastic tissue [14].

Positron emission tomography (PET) is increasingly being utilized in NET diagnosis. Fluorine-18 (^{18}F)-fluorodeoxyglucose (F-FDG) PET may be more sensitive than SRS for aggressive tumors with proliferative index >15 [10]. F-FDG PET may also have prognostic utility with a maximum standardized uptake value (SUV_{max}) >3 predictive of progression-free survival [11].

Foregut

Foregut carcinoids include NETs of the stomach, duodenum, and pancreas (PNETs). In general, foregut carcinoids appear trabecular histologically and argyrophil silver staining is employed for microscopic differentiation. Each of the foregut NETs has individual characteristics, outcomes, and surgical options worth considering.

Stomach

Unlike most other GI NETs, gastric carcinoids often occur in association with another disease process, rather than sporadically. These tumors are traditionally divided into three types, two of which are associated with concurrent medical conditions. including chronic atrophic gastritis, pernicious anemia (type 1), MEN1, and Zollinger-Ellison Syndrome (ZES) (type 2). Chronic atrophic gastritis is a condition where gastric parietal cells do not secrete adequate amounts of hydrochloric acid (HCl) or intrinsic factor, leading to decreased absorption of vitamin B_{12} in the terminal ileum and a resulting pernicious anemia [18]. The achlohydria stimulates gastrin release from G cells in the antrum, initiating a trophic effect on gastric enterochromaffin-like (ECL) cells, the most common gastric neuroendocrine cell type, which become hyperplastic and potentially neoplastic gastric carcinoids [19]. Type 2 gastric carcinoids are uncommon, often associated with MEN1 or ZES, conditions in which G cells in the duodenum or pancreas become hyperplastic and

Table 2 Recommended surgical management of gastric carcinoid tumors

Comparison of the three types of gastric carcinoid tumors

	Type I	Type II	Type III
Frequency	70–80 %	5–10 %	15–20 %
Associated conditions	Pernicious anemia	ZES, MEN1	None (most are sporadic)
Gastrin level	Increase	Large increase	No change
Tumor characteristics	Multicentric, <2 cm	Multicentric, <2 cm	Solitary, >2 cm
Metastatic potential	<5 %	7–12 %	>50 %
Treatment	Endoscopic resection and surveillance[a]	Endoscopic resection and surveillance[a], gastrinoma resection	Formal surgical resection

[a]Exception: size >2 cm, inability to be removed endoscopically, concomitant adenocarcinoma

secrete high levels of gastrin (gastrinoma). The resulting hypergastrinemia leads to ECL cell hyperplasia, which can progress to a potentially neoplastic lesion [20]. Type 3 gastric carcinoids, on the contrary, arise sporadically and are not associated with elevated gastrin levels. Type 3 tumors are larger, more invasive, and have a greater metastatic potential (>50 %) when compared to types 1 and 2 (Table 2).

Type 1 gastric carcinoids can traditionally be treated endoscopically. In some cases, mitigation of hypergastrinemia is achieved by the removal of gastric G cells via antrectomy, but 14 % of patients may still see a progression in tumor growth [21]. In general, because of the low metastatic potential of type 1 (and 2) gastric carcinoids, prognosis is good. For type 2 gastric carcinoids, management is very similar to type 1 unless the patient has MEN1 syndrome, in which case surgical removal of the gastrinoma is indicated. Because MEN1 syndrome is a condition of neoplastic endocrine tissue, these gastrinomas are often diffuse and sometimes require radical resection of gastric and duodenal G cells [22]. Type 3 gastric carcinoids are larger and more invasive in nature with more metastatic potential, and therefore require a formal oncologic resection with regional lymphadenectomy for their treatment [20].

Duodenum

Duodenal carcinoids are traditionally limited to mucosal and submucosal tissue and do not include duodenal G cell gastrinomas, which are most commonly found in the duodenum but are classified with pancreatic neuroendocrine tumors. Unlike gastric carcinoids, duodenal NET prognosis and surgical treatment options are related almost exclusively to size. Tumors smaller than 1 cm are traditionally treated via endoscopic resection [23], while tumors measuring between 1 and 2 cm are subject to transduodenal excision [24].

For duodenal carcinoids greater than 2 cm in size, more aggressive surgical treatment is indicated but the precise procedure has not been made clear. At a minimum duodenal segmental resection with lymph node dissection should be performed in order to obtain complete resection of the primary tumor and to provide adequate lymph node harvest for staging (defined as at least 12 lymph nodes). Some have reported that partial gastrectomy maybe is necessary [25], but this should only be performed to obtain negative margins. The extent of surgical resection should be determined by tumor grade, size, and location in that order. An important distinction should be made for tumors originating from the ampulla of Vater, as these lesions can have nodal metastases at a very small size. For mobile, superficial lesions where negative margins are obtainable, ampullectomy can be performed; otherwise, pancreatoduodenectomy is indicated [26].

Pancreas

The inherentendocrine function of the pancreas makes it a popular site for neuroendocrine tumors, called pancreatic NETs (PNETs). Essentially any hormone-secreting cell of the pancreas can become neoplastic, the most common being insulinomas, gastrinomas, glucagonomas, VIPomas, and somatostatinomas. PNETs are referred to as functional when they are associated with a clinical diathesis as a result of their hormonal hypersecretion, or nonfunctional when no clinical syndrome is apparent. Nonfunctional PNETs still may hypersecrete enteric hormones including chromogranin A, synaptophysin, and pancreatic polypeptide. While the majority of PNETs are sporadic in nature, some conditions are associated with a higher incidence, including ZES, MEN1, von Hippel-Lindau disease (VHL), neurofibromatosis 1 (NF1), and tuberous sclerosis [27].

Insulinoma

Insulinomas are the most common type of functional PNET. Symptoms of insulinoma are related to the hypersecretion of insulin, leading to episodes of hypoglycemia, neuroglycopenia, diaphoresis, tremor, and palpitations. Whipples triad of low blood glucose, symptoms of hypoglycemia, and relief of symptoms with treatment of hypoglycemia are classically suggestive of disease. Diagnosis can be confirmed with a monitored fast (up to 72 h), documenting high insulin levels in the setting of hypoglycemia (a high insulin:glucose ratio) as well as elevated C-peptide levels and negative urine test for sulfonylureas to rule out exogenous insulin administration [28]. Preoperative analysis and localization can be difficult in insulinomas because they are small and lack the high density of somatostatin receptor type 2 (SSTR2), rendering SRS less clinically useful. Instead, pancreatic protocol CT combined with an endoscopic ultrasound (EUS) has up to 90 % sensitivity in localizing insulinomas [29].

Surgical removal is the best treatment option for insulinomas. Most insulinomas are benign (90 %), solitary, and small, making ablation and enucleation therapies ideal. Case studies have shown patients with severe hypoglycemic episodes have uneventful postoperative recoveries and total resolution of their hypoglycemic symptoms [30, 31].

Gastrinoma

Gastrinoma, commonly referred to as Zollinger Ellison Syndrome (ZES), is the second most common sporadic PNET but the most common PNET for patients with MEN1. Gastrinomas are often malignant on presentation, and are typically multiple in MEN. Patients with recurrent, diffuse, or severe peptic ulcer disease should be evaluated for an underlying gastrinoma. Diagnosis is classically made if IV secretin is administered and serum gastrin levels rise to >200 pg/mL above baseline [32].

ZES is also diagnosed with elevated gastrin levels (>100 pg/mL) in the setting of a basal acid output of >15 mEq/h.

Before surgical intervention, acid secretion is often controlled with proton pump inhibitors. For gastrinoma localization, SRS in combination with CT or MRI offers 80 % sensitivity and 100 % specificity. For patients with very small gastrinomas in the pancreas, EUS is an alternative if SRS with CT or MRI is inconclusive. Most gastrinomas (83 %) are located in the gastrinoma triangle, along the first three portions of the duodenum and the head of the pancreas [33]. These tumors are most commonly in the duodenum and are traditionally small. One study documented 64 cases of duodenal gastrinoma, 39 of which (61.9 %) measured <1 cm [34].

Surgical procedure depends on location and size of the gastrinoma. Gastrinomas located in the head of the pancreas can be traditionally enucleated, while those in the body or tail undergo distal pancreatectomy [32]. Duodenotomy or duodenal transillumination with intraoperative endoscopy to explore for tumors is recommended for both pancreatic and duodenal gastrinomas, particularly in MEN, because of small size and this common location. One study compared a group of patients with and without routine duodenotomy and documented that 68 % of patients undergoing duodenotomy had a survival rate of 52 %, compared to patients without a duodenotomy with 26 % survival [35].

Management of gastrinoma in the setting of MEN1 has historically been controversial, given its diffuse nature and proclivity for recurrence. Current recommended management strategy includes resection of disease to prevent development of distant (hepatic) metastases and to prolong expected survival.

Nonfunctional PNET

Overall nonfunctional PNETs are the most common neuroendocrine tumors of the pancreas. Although sporadic or nonfunctioning PNETs account for <2 % of pancreatic tumors, their incidence is increasing over the past decade, seemingly due to increased utilization and quality of axial imaging [36, 37]. Management of the incidentally discovered, asymptomatic PNET less than 2 cm in size is controversial given the unknown and variable malignant potential, with some advocating surveillance and others advocating resection citing malignant behavior even in small tumors. Nonfunctional PNETs demonstrate significant cytological and morphological heterogeneity. They also demonstrate significant prognostic variability making treatment decisions and clinical pathways challenging. Most studies agree that the presence of distant metastasis is the single most important adverse prognostic factor. After that, it has been validated by various authors that in locoregional disease, the strongest predictors for survival are disease stage and tumor grade. In general, morphologic examination is performed to distinguish well-differentiated, low-grade tumors from poorly differentiated, high-grade tumors [38]. A recent international cohort study on PNETs reported a 10-year survival rate of nearly 90 % after resection of G1 tumors compared to less than 25 % for G3 tumors [39].

Proliferation is determined by measuring the number of mitoses per microscopic high power field and Ki-67 index [36, 41, 42]. The latest iteration of the WHO classification includes Ki-67 index reporting for grade [40]. The Ki-67 index is related to the malignant potential and clinical behavior of PNETs and may be an important prognostic indicator, predicting overall and disease-free survival [40, 43–45]. In addition, an adequate lymph node evaluation, defined as 12 or more lymph nodes, is essential to staging and prognostication.

Current medical therapies for pancreatic neuroendocrine tumors are limited to the unresectable (T4) or metastatic disease, with no demonstrated benefit for adjuvant therapy after surgical resection. While somatostatin analog therapy is established for midgut NET [46] improving progression-free survival, it is not effective for PNETs [47, 48]. Cytotoxic chemotherapies, classically streptozocin, fluorouracil, and doxorubicin or more recently temozolimide and capecitabine combinations, have traditionally been the mainstay of treatment for advanced PNETs. In 2011, two randomized controlled trials of biologic therapies were published which changed the chemotherapeutic landscape for NETs. Use of sunitinib (a multitargeted receptor tyrosine kinase inhibitor) was shown to effect more than a doubling in progression-free survival (11.4 months vs. 5.5 months, $P < 0.001$) and an increase in overall survival. Similarly, the mammalian target of rapamycin (mTOR) inhibitor everolimus more than doubled the progression-free survival from 4.6 months to 11.0 months [49, 50]. While PNETs can present with advanced disease, the natural history of disease is rather indolent, laying the groundwork for innovative therapies for this challenging disease.

Hepatic resection for liver metastases where complete resection, or at least greater than 90 % cytoreduction, can be achieved is advocated in selected patients with metastatic PNETs. In addition, locally ablative therapies have been utilized to treat hepatic metastases with clinical success. Liver transplantation is undertaken for metastatic PNETs only in highly selective cases with very favorable tumor biology (low mitotic count, low Ki-67 index, well-differentiated histology) where all other medical therapies have failed.

Midgut

Midgut carcinoids include those found in the jejunum, ileum, appendix, cecum, and proximal colon. Histologically, midgut carcinoids appear as a solid mass of cells and stain with argentaffin silver. Secretory products from midgut carcinoids include serotonin, prostaglandins, and polypeptides. Hypersecretion of serotonin and kallikrein, in particular, are known to lead to carcinoid syndrome if liver function is decreased and these hormonal products are not cleared from the portal system and circulate systemically, usually because of carcinoid metastases to the liver. Elevated levels of 5-HIAA, a metabolite of serotonin, in the urine is diagnostic for carcinoid syndrome. The potential of liver metastases among midgut carcinoids depends on location, ranging from 2 % (appendix), to 35 % (small bowel), to 60 % (ascending colon).

Small Bowel (Jejunum, Ileum)

While NETs are rare types of neoplasms in other parts of the GI tract (i.e., 3 % in the pancreas), NETs make up one-third of all small bowel neoplasms. They are almost always found within 60 cm of the ileocecal valve in the ileum, arising from serotonin-secreting enterochromafin cells [51]. They can metastasize to lymph nodes early, despite a small size. Patients presenting with small bowel carcinoids are usually in their 6th or 7th decade of life and present with abdominal pain and/or small bowel obstruction [52].

Prognosis for patients with small bowel carcinoids depends on a number of factors. Age >65, tumor size >2 cm, and depth of invasion beyond the muscularis propria are predictors of poor prognosis [53]. Surgical resection is indicated for primary carcinoids of the small bowel, with en bloc lymphadenectomy. If the tumor has metastasized or if carcinoid syndrome is evident, preoperative and intraoperative octreotide treatment is indicated. Octreotide administration prevents carcinoid crisis (extreme hypotensive episode) during surgical resection by mitigating the effects of hormonal release [54]. Postoperatively, octreotide long-acting repeatable (LAR) is indicated in patients with metastatic disease [55]. The presence of metastatic disease is a primary determinant of long-term prognosis, as 5 years overall survival without metastatic disease approaches 60 %, but is as low as 30 % in the presence of liver metastases [56].

Appendix

Incidence of appendiceal carcinoids ranges from 16 to 45 % of GI carcinoids [57]. The majority are asymptomatic and are located in the distal 1/3 of the appendix. Metastases are rare, especially with small tumors <2 cm, so carcinoid syndrome occurs in only 10 % of cases. A large tumor or tumor located in the proximal appendix may be symptomatic, leading to carcinoid syndrome, appendicitis, and/or possible bowel obstruction.

Table 3 Metastatic potential of appendiceal carcinoid tumors, based on tumor biology

Metastatic potential of appendiceal carcinoid tumors by tumor biology	
Histologic differentiation	Metastasis (%)
Well	2
Moderate	50
Poor	80

Surgical resection is dependent upon tumor grade, size, and location. A well-differentiated appendiceal carcinoid located away from the base of the appendix can be removed with a simple appendectomy. If the carcinoid is moderately or poorly differentiated, a right hemi-colectomy is instead indicated, due to the increased risk of lymphatic involvement or metastatic disease with more aggressive tumor biology (Table 3). A right hemi-colectomy is also indicated in specific circumstances, i.e., if the carcinoid involves the base of the appendix or shows mesenteric invasion. Meso-appendiceal invasion, regardless of tumor size, should also be surgically managed with a right hemi-colectomy, although studies have shown that recurrence of carcinoid tumors with meso-appendiceal invasion, even if small, is unlikely with appendectomy alone [58].

Size, depth of invasion, lymph node involvement, and metastases are all significant predictors of prognosis in appendiceal carcinoids [53]. Size is a clear indicator of prognosis, with no tumors being associated with lymph node involvement in appendiceal carcinoids <2 cm, while the incidence rose to 21 % in tumors measuring between 2 and 3 cm and to 44 % in tumors >3 cm [59].

Colon

While the colon is traditionally divided into both midgut and hindgut portions, the majority of colon carcinoids are found in the proximal colon (cecum) in the 7th decade of life. These tumors become large before characteristic symptoms such as abdominal pain, anorexia, and weight loss present, which increase their metastatic potential and worsens prognosis. In previous studies, the average colon carcinoid size at diagnosis was 5 cm, with two-thirds of patients having local nodal or distant metastases [53]. Multivariate analysis of this Surveillance, Epidemiology, and End Result (SEER) dataset between 1974 and 2004 again found tumor size, depth of invasion, lymph node involvement, and metastases as significant predictors of prognosis [53].

Endoscopic or segmental resection is preferred in treatment of small, localized colon carcinoids. Significant nodal and/or distal metastases presents a difficult surgical case but a right hemi-colectomy for cecal carcinoids has been shown effective. In a recent study involving 114 patients with colorectal carcinoids, 53.3 % of patients had local nodal and 26.7 % had distant metastases. After a median follow-up of 4.2 years, there was only one noncarcinoid-related death, with eleven patients disease-free as of their last follow-up visit [60].

Hindgut

Hindgut carcinoids include those of the distal colon and rectum. In general, hindgut carcinoids have mixed histology with variable silver staining. Only 10 % of rectal carcinoids <2 cm in size demonstrate metastases to the liver and there is little evidence of serotonin secretion, so carcinoid syndrome is rare. Because carcinoid tumors in the distal colon are very rare, this section will focus mainly on rectal carcinoids.

Rectum

Rectal carcinoids are usually small and asymptomatic, found incidentally during endoscopy, and are located between 4 and 13 cm from the dentate line [61]. Incidence of rectal carcinoids has increased over the past several decades, from 0.2 per 100,000 population in 1974–0.86 in 2004 [4]. While metastases to the liver are rare, locoregional nodal spread from rectal carcinoids is common. Size >10 mm and lymphovascular invasion are predictive of local nodal and distant metastases [62].

Management of rectal carcinoids is correlated with tumor biology and size. Small (<10 mm), well-differentiated lesions are amenable to endoscopic resection [63–65].

Surgical resection with regional lymphadenectomy is indicated for moderately and poorly differentiated rectal carcinoids or those greater than 20 mm in size [62]. Management of tumors 10–20 mm in size is controversial, with tumor grade and patient characteristics playing a differential role.

Follow-up after procedures for rectal carcinoids are dependent on tumor size and biology. For tumors <10 mm and low Ki-67 index (G1, G2), patient may not require any specific follow-up. A small tumor with high-grade features (G3) requires annual follow-up with endoscopic ultrasound (EUS), colonoscopy, and MRI. For rectal carcinoids 10–20 mm in size, regardless of grade, the same annual follow-up is recommended. For tumors >2 cm, G1–G2 carcinoids should receive annual follow-up and G3 carcinoids should receive follow-up every 4–6 months [66].

Conclusion

The initial surgical management of gastrointestinal neuroendocrine tumors is based primarily on four factors: size of primary tumor, tumor grade, stage by axial imaging, and surgical fitness of the patient. The prognostic importance of tumor grade including mitotic count and Ki-67 index is emphasized. Appropriate management of NETs includes consideration of lymphatic disease. Currently, there is not role for adjuvant hormonal, cytotoxic, or targeted biologic therapies. There are only recommended for advanced, nonsurgical disease.

References

1. Oberndorfer S. Karzinoide tumoren des du¨nndarms. Frankf Z Pathol. 1907;1:426–9.
2. Kloppel G, Anlauf M. Epidemiology, tumour biology and histopathological classification of neuroendocrine tumours of the gastrointestinal tract. Best Pract Res Clin Gastroenterol. 2005;19(4):507–17.
3. Taal BG, Visser O. Epidemiology of neuroendocrine tumours. Neuroendocrinology. 2004;80 Suppl 1:3–7.
4. Yao JC, Hassan M, Phan A, Dagohoy C, Leary C, Mares JE, et al. One hundred years after "carcinoid": epidemiology of and prognostic factors for neuroendocrine tumors in 35,825 cases in the United States. J Clin Oncol. 2008;26(18):3063–72.
5. Rindi G, Kloppel G, Couvelard A, Komminoth P, Korner M, Lopes JM, et al. TNM staging of midgut and hindgut (neuro) endocrine tumors: a consensus proposal including a grading system. Virchows Arch. 2007;451(4):757–62.
6. Rindi G. The ENETS guidelines: the new TNM classification system. Tumori. 2010;96(5): 806–9.
7. Sobin LH, Compton CC. TNM seventh edition: what's new, what's changed: communication from the International Union Against Cancer and the American Joint Committee on Cancer. Cancer. 2010;116(22):5336–9.
8. Solcia E, Klöppel G, Sobin LH. Histological typing of endocrine tumors. WHO international histological classification of tumors. 2nd ed. Berlin: Springer; 2000. p. 56–70.
9. John M, Meyerhof W, Richter D, Waser B, Schaer JC, Scherubl H, et al. Positive somatostatin receptor scintigraphy correlates with the presence of somatostatin receptor subtype 2. Gut. 1996;38(1):33–9.
10. Binderup T, Knigge U, Loft A, Mortensen J, Pfeifer A, Federspiel B, et al. Functional imaging of neuroendocrine tumors: a head-to-head comparison of somatostatin receptor scintigraphy, 123I-MIBG scintigraphy, and 18F-FDG PET. J Nucl Med. 2010;51(5):704–12.
11. Binderup T, Knigge U, Loft A, Federspiel B, Kjaer A. 18F-fluorodeoxyglucose positron emission tomography predicts survival of patients with neuroendocrine tumors. Clin Cancer Res. 2010;16(3):978–85.
12. Oberg K, Castellano D. Current knowledge on diagnosis and staging of neuroendocrine tumors. Cancer Metastasis Rev. 2011;30 Suppl 1:3–7.
13. Pettinato C, Sarnelli A, Di Donna M, Civollani S, Nanni C, Montini G, et al. 68Ga-DOTANOC: biodistribution and dosimetry in patients affected by neuroendocrine tumors. Eur J Nucl Med Mol Imaging. 2008;35(1):72–9.
14. Baldelli R, Barnabei A, Rizza L, Isidori AM, Rota F, Di Giacinto P, et al. Somatostatin analogs therapy in gastroenteropancreatic neuroendocrine tumors: current aspects and new perspectives. Front Endocrinol. 2014;5:7.
15. Oberg K, Kvols L, Caplin M, Delle Fave G, de Herder W, Rindi G, et al. Consensus report on the use of somatostatin analogs for the management of neuroendocrine tumors of the gastroenteropancreatic system. Ann Oncol. 2004;15(6):966–73.
16. Schally AV. Oncological applications of somatostatin analogues. Cancer Res. 1988;48(24 Pt 1):6977–85.
17. Lawnicka H, Stepien H, Wyczolkowska J, Kolago B, Kunert-Radek J, Komorowski J. Effect of somatostatin and octreotide on proliferation and vascular endothelial growth factor secretion from murine endothelial cell line (HECa10) culture. Biochem Biophys Res Commun. 2000;268(2):567–71.
18. Annibale B, Lahner E, Fave GD. Diagnosis and management of pernicious anemia. Curr Gastroenterol Rep. 2011;13(6):518–24.
19. Lahner E, Norman GL, Severi C, Encabo S, Shums Z, Vannella L, et al. Reassessment of intrinsic factor and parietal cell autoantibodies in atrophic gastritis with respect to cobalamin deficiency. Am J Gastroenterol. 2009;104(8):2071–9.

20. Borch K, Ahren B, Ahlman H, Falkmer S, Granerus G, Grimelius L. Gastric carcinoids: biologic behavior and prognosis after differentiated treatment in relation to type. Ann Surg. 2005;242(1):64–73.
21. Jordan Jr PH, Barroso A, Sweeney J. Gastric carcinoids in patients with hypergastrinemia. J Am Coll Surg. 2004;199(4):552–5.
22. Norton JA, Melcher ML, Gibril F, Jensen RT. Gastric carcinoid tumors in multiple endocrine neoplasia-1 patients with Zollinger-Ellison syndrome can be symptomatic, demonstrate aggressive growth, and require surgical treatment. Surgery. 2004;136(6):1267–74.
23. Nikou GC, Toubanakis C, Moulakakis KG, Pavlatos S, Kosmidis C, Mallas E, et al. Carcinoid tumors of the duodenum and the ampulla of Vater: current diagnostic and therapeutic approach in a series of 8 patients. Case series. Int J Surg. 2011;9(3):248–53.
24. Zyromski NJ, Kendrick ML, Nagorney DM, Grant CS, Donohue JH, Farnell MB, et al. Duodenal carcinoid tumors: how aggressive should we be? J Gastrointest Surg. 2001;5(6):588–93.
25. Waisberg J, Joppert-Netto G, Vasconcellos C, Sartini GH, Miranda LS, Franco MI. Carcinoid tumor of the duodenum: a rare tumor at an unusual site. Case series from a single institution. Arq Gastroenterol. 2013;50(1):3–9.
26. Carter JT, Grenert JP, Rubenstein L, Stewart L, Way LW. Neuroendocrine tumors of the ampulla of Vater: biological behavior and surgical management. Arch Surg. 2009;144(6):527–31.
27. Jensen RT, Berna MJ, Bingham DB, Norton JA. Inherited pancreatic endocrine tumor syndromes: advances in molecular pathogenesis, diagnosis, management, and controversies. Cancer. 2008;113(7 Suppl):1807–43.
28. Okabayashi T, Shima Y, Sumiyoshi T, Kozuki A, Ito S, Ogawa Y, et al. Diagnosis and management of Insulinomas. World J Gastroenterol. 2013;19(6):829–37.
29. Anderson MA, Carpenter S, Thompson NW, Nostrant TT, Elta GH, Scheiman JM. Endoscopic ultrasound is highly accurate and directs management in patients with neuroendocrine tumors of the pancreas. Am J Gastroenterol. 2000;95(9):2271–7.
30. Jurgensen C, Schuppan D, Neser F, Ernstberger J, Junghans U, Stolzel U. EUS-guided alcohol ablation of an Insulinomas. Gastrointest Endosc. 2006;63(7):1059–62.
31. Limmer S, Huppert PE, Juette V, Lenhart A, Welte M, Wietholtz H. Radiofrequency ablation of solitary pancreatic Insulinomas in a patient with episodes of severe hypoglycemia. Eur J Gastroenterol Hepatol. 2009;21(9):1097–101.
32. Huang LC, Poultsides GA, Norton JA. Surgical management of neuroendocrine tumors of the gastrointestinal tract. Oncology. 2011;25(9):794–803.
33. Passaro Jr E, Howard TJ, Sawicki MP, Watt PC, Stabile BE. The origin of sporadic gastrinomas within the gastrinoma triangle: a theory. Arch Surg. 1998;133(1):13–6. discussion 7.
34. Zogakis TG, Gibril F, Libutti SK, Norton JA, White DE, Jensen RT, et al. Management and outcome of patients with sporadic gastrinoma arising in the duodenum. Ann Surg. 2003;238(1):42–8.
35. Norton JA, Alexander HR, Fraker DL, Venzon DJ, Gibril F, Jensen RT. Does the use of routine duodenotomy (DUODX) affect rate of cure, development of liver metastases, or survival in patients with Zollinger-Ellison syndrome? Ann Surg. 2004;239(5):617–25. discussion 26.
36. Klimstra DS, Arnold R, Capella C, et al. Tumors of the endocrine pancreas. In: Bosman FT, Carneiro F, Hruban RH, Theise ND, editors. World Health Organization classification of tumors, Pathology and genetics of tumors of the digestive system. Lyon, France: IARC Press; 2010. p. 322–6.
37. Hruban RH, Pitman MB, Klimstra DS. Tumors of the pancreas. 6th ed. Washington, DC: Armed Forces Institute of Pathology; 2007. p. 251–304.
38. Capelli P, Martignoni G, Pedica F, et al. Endocrine neoplasms of the pancreas: pathologic and genetic features. Arch Pathol Lab Med. 2009;133:350–64.
39. Chatzipantelis P, Konstantinou P, Kaklamanos M, Apostolou G, Salla C. The role of cytomorphology and proliferative activity in predicting biologic behavior of pancreatic neuroendocrine tumors; a study by endoscopic ultrasound-guided fine-needle aspiration cytology. Cancer. 2009;117:211–6.

40. Asa SL. Pancreatic endocrine tumors. Mod Pathol. 2011;24 suppl 2:S66–77.
41. Rindi G, Kloppel G, Alhman H, All Other Frascati Consensus Conference Participants; European Neuroendocrine Tumor Society (ENETS), et al. TNM staging of foregut (neuro) endocrine tumors: a consensus proposal including a grading system. Virchows Arch. 2006;449:395–401.
42. Verbeke CS. Endocrine tumours of the pancreas. Histopathology. 2010;56:669–82.
43. Klimstra DS, Modlin IR, Coppola D, Lloyd RV, Suster S. The pathologic classification of neuroendocrine tumors: a review of nomenclature, grading, and staging systems. Pancreas. 2010;39:707–12.
44. Adsay V. Ki67 labeling index in neuroendocrine tumors of the gastrointestinal tract and pancreatobiliary tract: to count or not to count is not the question, but rather how to count. Am J Surg Pathol. 2012;36:1743–6.
45. Piani C, Franchi GM, Cappelletti C, et al. Cytological Ki-67 in pancreatic neuroendocrine tumors: an opportunity for pre-operative grading. Endocr Relat Cancer. 2008;15:175–81.
46. Gerdes J, Lemke H, Baisch H, Wacker HH, Schwab U, Stein H. Cell cycle analysis of a cell proliferation-associated human nuclear antigen defined by the monoclonal antibody Ki-67. J Immunol. 1984;133:1710–5.
47. Tang LH, Gonen M, Hedvat C, Modlin IM, Klimstra DS. Objective quantification of the Ki67 proliferation index in neuroendocrine tumors of the gastropancreatic system: a comparison of digital image analysis with manual methods. Am J Surg Pathol. 2012;36:1761–70.
48. Remes SM, Tuominen VJ, Helin H, Isola J, Arola J. Grading of neuroendocrine tumors with Ki-67 requires high-quality assessment practices. Am J Surg Pathol. 2012;36:1359–63.
49. Falconi M, Bartsch DK, Kriksson G, Barcelona Consensus Conference participants, et al. ENETS Consensus Guidelines for the management of patients with digestive neuroendocrine neoplasms of the digestive system: well-differentiated pancreatic non-functioning tumors. Neuroendocrinology. 2012;95:120–34.
50. Pavel M, Baudin E, Couvelard A, Barcelona Consensus Conference Participants, et al. ENETS Consensus Guidelines for the management of patients with liver and other distant metastases from neuroendocrine neoplasms of foregut, midgut, hindgut, and unknown primary. Neuroendocrinology. 2012;95:157–76.
51. Reynolds I, Healy P, McNamara DA. Malignant tumours of the small intestine. Surgeon. 2014.
52. Rodrigues G, Prabhu R, Ravi B. Small bowel carcinoid: a rare cause of bowel obstruction. BMJ Case Rep. 2013. doi: 10.1136/bcr-2013-200875.
53. Landry CS, Brock G, Scoggins CR, McMasters KM, Martin 2nd RC. A proposed staging system for gastric carcinoid tumors based on an analysis of 1,543 patients. Ann Surg Oncol. 2009;16(1):51–60.
54. O'Toole D, Ducreux M, Bommelaer G, Wemeau JL, Bouche O, Catus F, et al. Treatment of carcinoid syndrome: a prospective crossover evaluation of lanreotide versus octreotide in terms of efficacy, patient acceptability, and tolerance. Cancer. 2000;88(4):770–6.
55. Shen C, Shih YC, Xu Y, Yao JC. Octreotide long-acting repeatable use among elderly patients with carcinoid syndrome and survival outcomes: a population-based analysis. Cancer. 2014;120(13):2039–49.
56. Bilimoria KY, Bentrem DJ, Wayne JD, Ko CY, Bennett CL, Talamonti MS. Small bowel cancer in the United States: changes in epidemiology, treatment, and survival over the last 20 years. Ann Surg. 2009;249(1):63–71.
57. Maggard MA, O'Connell JB, Ko CY. Updated population-based review of carcinoid tumors. Ann Surg. 2004;240(1):117–22.
58. Kulke MH, Mayer RJ. Carcinoid tumors. N Engl J Med. 1999;340(11):858–68.
59. Moertel CG, Weiland LH, Nagorney DM, Dockerty MB. Carcinoid tumor of the appendix: treatment and prognosis. N Engl J Med. 1987;317(27):1699–701.
60. Murray SE, Lloyd RV, Sippel RS, Chen H. Clinicopathologic characteristics of colonic carcinoid tumors. J Surg Res. 2013;184(1):183–8.

61. Peralta EA. Rare anorectal neoplasms: gastrointestinal stromal tumor, carcinoid, and lymphoma. Clin Colon Rectal Surg. 2009;22(2):107–14.
62. Shields CJ, Tiret E, Winter DC, International Rectal Carcinoid Study Group. Carcinoid tumors of the rectum: a multi-institutional international collaboration. Ann Surg. 2010;252(5):750–5.
63. Ono A, Fujii T, Saito Y, Matsuda T, Lee DT, Gotoda T, et al. Endoscopic submucosal resection of rectal carcinoid tumors with a ligation device. Gastrointest Endosc. 2003;57(4):583–7.
64. Kwaan MR, Goldberg JE, Bleday R. Rectal carcinoid tumors: review of results after endoscopic and surgical therapy. Arch Surg. 2008;143(5):471–5.
65. Park HW, Byeon JS, Park YS, Yang DH, Yoon SM, Kim KJ, et al. Endoscopic submucosal dissection for treatment of rectal carcinoid tumors. Gastrointest Endosc. 2010;72(1):143–9.
66. Caplin M, Sundin A, Nillson O, Baum RP, Klose KJ, Kelestimur F, et al. ENETS Consensus Guidelines for the management of patients with digestive neuroendocrine neoplasms: colorectal neuroendocrine neoplasms. Neuroendocrinology. 2012;95(2):88–97.

Current Controversies in the Management of Colon and Rectal Cancer

Pinckney J. Maxwell IV and E. Ramsay Camp

Initial Presentation

Colorectal cancer is the third most common cancer in men and women, after prostate and lung/bronchus in men and breast and lung/bronchus in women [1]. The American Cancer Society (ACS) expects an estimated 136,830 new diagnoses of colon and rectal cancer in 2014. Symptoms of colorectal cancer include bleeding, changes in bowel habits, obstruction, abdominal pain, and malaise. Frequently, anemia may be the only sign a patient exhibits. Patients with symptoms suspicious for colorectal cancer should undergo a complete colonoscopic evaluation. Importantly, a potential anorectal source of bleeding such as hemorrhoids should not preclude a complete colonic examination.

Colorectal Cancer Screening

Patients with no personal history of colorectal polyps or cancers, no personal history of inflammatory bowel disease (IBD), no symptoms suspicious for colorectal cancer, no family history of colorectal polyps or cancers, and no evidence of a familial or genetic syndrome can be screened as average risk. Two main categories of screening tests include those that detect adenomatous polyps and cancer (flexible sigmoidoscopy, colonoscopy, double-contrast barium enema, and CT colonography) and those

P.J. Maxwell IV, M.D., F.A.C.S. • E.R. Camp, M.D., M.S.C.R., F.A.C.S. (✉)
Department of Surgery, Medical University of South Carolina,
25 Courtenay Drive, Suite 7100A, Charleston, SC 29425, USA

The Ralph H. Johnson VA Medical Center, Charleston, SC 29425, USA
e-mail: campe@musc.edu

© Springer International Publishing Switzerland 2016
K.A. Morgan (ed.), *Current Controversies in Cancer Care
for the Surgeon*, DOI 10.1007/978-3-319-16205-8_4

that primarily detect cancer (fecal occult blood testing, fecal immunohistochemical testing, and stool DNA testing). The goal of screening is to reduce mortality by reducing the incidence of advanced disease. Testing for polyps and cancer is generally procedure related, while testing only for cancers can occur with stool studies alone. Assessing stool samples only has the potential to increase the ease, availability, and performance of colorectal cancer screening.

Regardless of the method employed, testing in the average risk, asymptomatic patient should begin at age 50. A total colonoscopy is only required every 10 years, but it requires an oral bowel prep and carries the small risk of perforation of less than 1 out of 1000 [2]. Alternatively, flexible sigmoidoscopy (FS) is required every 5 years when combined with fecal occult blood testing (FOBT) annually. The testing is more frequent, but requires only enemas for preparation and carries a lower risk of perforation. Air-contrast barium enemas can be used for screening every 5 years but also requires an oral bowel prep and are only diagnostic without the ability to remove polyps. CT colonography continues to evolve as a method for screening every 5 years and has the potential for more accessible screening; however, there are limitations on the identification of polyps less than 1 cm. Similar to the air-contrast enema, CT colonography also requires oral bowel preparation and is only diagnostic. FOBT and fecal immunohistochemical testing (FIT) require annual testing. The interval for stool DNA testing is uncertain, and this procedure tests only for a limited number of mutations. The most complete screening test, allowing removal of precancerous lesions if identified, remains the total colonoscopy.

Screening the High-Risk Patient

High-risk patients include those with a personal history of colorectal polyps or cancers, a family history of colorectal cancer in a first-degree relative, those with Crohn's disease or ulcerative colitis, and those with a personal or family history of familial adenomatous polyposis or hereditary nonpolyposis colon cancer. Screening in these patients has been adjusted for changes in incidence and age of onset of neoplasia (Table 1).

Familial Colorectal Cancer Syndromes

Familial adenomatous polyposis (FAP) is an inherited, non-sex-linked, Mendelian dominant disease that accounts for approximately 1 % of all colorectal cancers. The high penetrance of FAP means that there is a 50 % chance of development within affected families. However, 20 % of FAP patients have no family history, likely representing new and spontaneous mutations. The disorder is due to mutations in either the tumor-suppressor APC gene, which is located on chromosome 5 (5q21-q22), or in the MUTYH gene, which is located on chromosome 1 (1p34.3-p32.1). FAP is characterized by the progressive development of hundreds or thousands of

Table 1 Screening the high-risk patient for colorectal cancer

Risk category	Age to begin	Recomm.	Comment
Personal history of <3 adenomas with low-grade dysplasia	5–10 years after the initial polypectomy	Colonoscopy	Examination interval should be based on other clinical factors such as prior examination findings, family history, or preferences of the endoscopist or patient
Personal history of 3–10 adenomas, or 1 adenoma >1 cm, or any adenoma with villous features or high-grade dysplasia	3 Years after the initial polypectomy	Colonoscopy	Adenomas require compete excision. If the follow-up is normal, the next examination should be in 5 years. More than 10 adenomas should raise the suspicion of a familial syndrome
Personal history of colorectal cancer	1 Year after resection	Colonoscopy	Patients should undergo high-quality preoperative clearing. Follow-up after normal examinations should be extended to 3 years, and then to 5 years
Family history of adenomas or cancer in a first-degree relative <60 years of age or in 2 first-degree relatives at any age	Age 40 years, or 10 years before the youngest case	Colonoscopy	Every 5 years
Family history of adenomas or cancer in a first-degree relative >60 years of age or in 2 second-degree relatives with cancer	Age 40 years	Colonoscopy	Screening should be initiated at an earlier age. Intervals based on findings or by the average risk patient
FAP or suspected FAP	Age 10–12 years	Annual FS, counseling for genetic testing if showing polyps	Colectomy should be considered for positive genetic testing
HNPCC or risk of HNPCC	Age 20–25 years, or 10 years before the youngest case	Colonoscopy, counseling for genetic testing	Every 1–2 years. Genetic testing should be offered to first-degree relatives of persons with a known DNA mismatch repair gene, or with 1 of the first 3 Bethesda criteria
IBD, Crohn's or chronic UC	8 Years after the onset of pancolitis, or 12–15 years after the onset of left-sided colitis	Colonoscopies with random 4-quad biopsies every 10 cm for dysplasia	Screening should be offered every 1–2 years, and patients are best referred to a center with experience in the surveillance and management of IBD

adenomatous polyps located throughout the entire colon. The clinical diagnosis is based on the histologic confirmation of at least 100 adenomas. All patients will eventually develop colorectal cancer. The adenomas generally appear by the mid-20s and cancers generally appear by the late-30s. An attenuated form of FAP is recognized in which fewer adenomas (20–100) are identified. Adenomas and cancers develop somewhat later, at the average ages of 44 and 56, respectively. FAP also exhibits extracolonic manifestations including gastric/duodenal/small bowel polyps, osteomas and desmoids tumors (Gardner's syndrome), eye lesions such as congenital hypertrophy of retinal pigment epithelium (CHRPE), epidermoid cysts, and brain neoplasms (Turcot's syndrome).

Hereditary nonpolyposis colon cancer (HNPCC), also called Lynch syndrome, is an inherited, non-sex-linked, Mendelian dominant disease with virtually complete penetrance. It is the most common genetic form of colorectal cancer and includes 2–4 % of all colorectal cancers [3, 4]. HNPCC is due to a defect in various DNA mismatch repair genes (MLH1, MSH2, MSH6, PMS, PMS2), which leads to microsatellite instability (MSI-H). A number of evidence-based criteria are available for the diagnosis of HNPCC, including the Amsterdam I and II criteria and the Bethesda guidelines (Table 2). According to the EPICOLON study, the revised Bethesda guidelines are the most discriminating set of clinical parameters for diagnosing HNPCC [5].

Table 2 Diagnosis of hereditary nonpolyposis colon cancer

Amsterdam I Criteria, 1990
1. Three or more family members with histologically verified colorectal cancer, one of whom is a first-degree relative (parent, child, sibling) of the other two
2. Two successive affected generations
3. One or more colon cancers diagnosed under age 50 years
4. Familial adenomatous polyposis has been excluded
Amsterdam II Criteria, 1999
1. Three or more family members with histologically verified HNPCC-related cancers (endometrium, ovary, stomach, small intestine, hepatobiliary, upper urinary tract, brain, and skin), one of whom is a first-degree relative (parent, child, sibling) of the other two
2. Two successive affected generations
3. One or more colon cancers diagnosed under age 50 years
4. Familial adenomatous polyposis has been excluded
Revised Bethesda Guidelines, 2002
1. Colorectal cancer diagnosed in a patient who is less than 50 years of age
2. Presence of a synchronous, metachronous colorectal, or other HNPCC-related malignancy, regardless of age
3. Colorectal cancer with the MSI-H histology diagnosed in a patient who is less than 60 years of age
– Presence of carcinoma infiltrating lymphocytes, Crohn's-like lymphocytic reaction, mucinous/signet-ring differentiation, or medullary growth pattern
– No general consensus based on this age
4. Colorectal cancer diagnosed in one or more first-degree relatives with an HNPCC-related neoplasm
– With one or more neoplasm being diagnosed at an age less than 50 years
5. Colorectal cancer diagnosed in two or more first or second-degree relatives with HNPCC-related malignancies, regardless of age

Diagnosis of HNPCC may be established by immunohistochemical (IHC) analysis for mismatch repair (MMR) protein expression, which decrease due to mutation, or with analysis for MSI detection resulting from MMR deficiency [6]. Some controversy exists, however, regarding the application of IHC and MSI testing. The NCCN endorses IHC and MSI testing on all patients diagnosed prior to age 70 in addition to older patients who fulfill the Bethesda criteria. Other institutions routinely test all specimens for both IHC and MSI as supported by the Evaluation of Genomic Applications in the Practice and Prevention (EGAPP) working group at the CDC [7, 8].

HNPCC is subdivided into Lynch syndrome types I and II. Lynch type I refers to site-specific nonpolyposis colon cancer, and Lynch type II (formerly called familial cancer syndrome) refers to cancers that develop in the colon and other organs such as the endometrium, ovaries, stomach, pancreas, and proximal urinary tract and other sites.

Lynch syndrome differs from sporadic colorectal cancer in a number of important ways. It has an autosomal dominant inheritance, a predominance of proximal lesions (75 % are found in the right colon), an excess of multiple primary colorectal cancers (18 %), an early age of onset averaging 44 years, a significantly improved survival rate of right-sided lesions when compared with family members with distal colorectal cancer (53 % vs. 35 % 5-year survival), and an increased risk for developing metachronous lesions (24 %). Patients and family members of those diagnosed with HNPCC or FAP should undergo genetic testing to aid in future diagnosis and treatment options.

Inflammatory Bowel Disease

Both Crohn's disease and ulcerative colitis (UC) confer an increased risk of colorectal cancer, with UC conveying approximately double the risk associated with Crohn's disease. The duration and severity of Crohn's disease and the duration and extent (left-sided colitis versus pancolitis) of UC contribute to cancer risk in inflammatory bowel disease (IBD). Cancer in Crohn's disease generally occurs in a stricture or bypass segment. Importantly, neoplasia in UC does not follow the adenoma–carcinoma sequence of sporadic colorectal cancer. This change has important screening and treatment implications.

Management of the Malignant Polyp

Malignant polyps are defined as polyps identified to have a focus of cancer invading into the submucosa (pT1). Polyps with carcinoma not invading into the submucosa are defined as carcinoma in situ (pTis). Due to the lack of invasion, carcinoma in situ polyps are unable to metastasize to lymph nodes. Polyps with malignant pathology or with a concerning appearance should be endoscopically tattooed within 2 weeks or at the time of polypectomy.

Once a malignant polyp is identified, the decision to proceed with surgical resection is based on histologic features, morphology, and polypectomy margins. Adverse histologic features include grade 3 or 4 and angiolymphatic invasion. Sessile rather than pedunculated morphology predicts worse outcomes in terms of recurrence, mortality, and hematogenous metastasis potentially due to a higher likelihood of positive margins after attempted endoscopic polypectomy [9, 10]. Incompletely resected sessile polyps should be considered for colectomy. There is no clear consensus as to the identification of a positive margin; however, the current definition is the presence of carcinoma within 1–2 mm of the transected margin or at the margin in a cauterized specimen [11]. Positive or unknown margins, fragmented specimens, adverse histologic features, and potentially sessile morphology are indications for laparoscopic or open segmental colectomy with en bloc lymphadenectomy. Prior to resection, all patients should have a complete colonic evaluation to rule out synchronous lesions.

Management of Colon Cancer

Prior to operative intervention, initial management should include a careful history and physical with laboratory testing that includes a carcinoembryonic antigen (CEA) level. A complete evaluation of the colon is essential utilizing colonoscopy with biopsy, or a secondary modality if colonoscopy is incomplete or unavailable. Preoperative staging with CT scans of the chest, abdomen, and pelvis should be performed to assess for local invasion and for metastatic disease.

Surgical Approach to Colon Cancer

The primary therapy for tumors of the colon is operative. The basic principles of surgery for colon cancer include:

1. Exploration: adequate visual, tactile, and potentially intraoperative hepatic ultrasound staging at the time of primary resection.
2. Removal of the entire cancer with enough bowel proximal and distal to encompass the possibility of submucosal lymphatic tumor spread.
3. Removal of regional mesenteric pedicle, including draining lymphatics, based on the predictable lymphatic spread of the disease and the potential for regional mesenteric involvement without concurrent distant involvement.
4. En bloc resection of involved structures (T4 tumors).

Table 3 Pathologic staging systems for colorectal cancer

Pathologic features	Stage	TNM	Dukes	Astler-Coller	5 years survival (%)
Depth of invasion					
Lamina propria, muscularis mucosa		0	T0/Tis	A	>90
Submucosa	I	T1	A	B1	
Muscularis propria	I	T2	A	B1	
Subserosa, pericolic fat	II	T3	B	B1	70–85
Adjacent organs, perforation	II	T4	B	B2	55–65
Lymph nodal involvement					
None		N0			
1–3 Nodes	III	N1	C	C1, C2	45–55
>3 Nodes	III	N2	C	C1, C2	20–30
Distant metastatic disease					
Absent		M0			
Present	IV	M1	D		<5

Segmental colonic resections (right, transverse, left, or sigmoid colectomy) are undertaken based on the tumor location and the related arterial vasculature. These resections define both a convenient anatomic boundary for standard colonic resection and also provide for adequate regional lymph node clearance because the major draining lymphatics follow these blood vessels in the mesentery. The decision for adjuvant chemotherapy and/or radiation therapy is based on pathologic staging. This information also provides prognostic information regarding survival to the patient and family. A number of staging systems have been developed; however, the TNM system is most commonly used in the US (Table 3).

Laparoscopic Surgical Resection

Numerous studies have proven that laparoscopic surgery is appropriate, and perhaps preferred, for colon cancer. The landmark COST trial in 2004 established that laparoscopic resection is equivalent to open resection for colon cancer [12]. The study included 872 patients who were randomly assigned to curative surgery via the open or laparoscopic approach. The results revealed no significant difference in 5-year recurrence or overall survival after a median follow-up of 7 years. In the COLOR trial, 1248 patients were similarly randomly assigned to curative surgery via the open or laparoscopic approach [13]. The results revealed that the surgical approaches were equivalent in terms of disease-free survival with a non-statistically significant absolute difference in 3-year disease-free survival of only 2.0 % favoring the open approach.

Complicated Disease

Colorectal tumors may present with complications including obstruction, perforation, or significant bleeding. These presentations are generally related to more
advanced disease and may preclude a complete staging work-up or potential neoadjuvant therapy. Unless patients are unstable or critically ill, or the tumor is unresectable, the tumor should be resected appropriately.

Surgery for High-Risk Conditions

High-risk conditions for the development of colorectal malignancies include
FAP, HNPCC, and chronic UC. Surgical management may be prophylactic or
possibly therapeutic after a malignancy has been diagnosed. The mainstay of
operative management in FAP and chronic UC is a total proctocolectomy.
Reconstructive options include an ileal pouch-anal anastomosis with or without
temporary diversion, a continent ileostomy (Kock pouch), or an end ileostomy. A
total abdominal colectomy with ileorectal anastomosis may be performed for
temporary preservation of rectal function in selected cases of chronic UC with
rectal sparing and for FAP with few rectal polyps, but this requires aggressive
surveillance of the remaining rectum due to the high risk of malignancy.
Patients with HNPCC should also undergo subtotal colectomy with ileorectal
anastomosis; due to the preponderance of associated gynecologic malignancy,
a total hysterectomy with bilateral salpingoophorectomy should be offered to
women with HNPCC.

Lymph Node Evaluation

Adequate lymph node sampling at the time of resection has important prognostic
and therapeutic implications. Population-based research revealed an association
between examination of ≥ 12 lymph nodes and improvement in survival [14, 15].
Evaluation of the Intergroup Trial INT-0089 revealed an increase in survival for
both node-positive and node-negative patients with an increasing number of lymph
nodes examined [16]. These findings suggest that increased lymph node assessment is related to more accurate pathologic staging and, therefore, more appropriate treatment planning, as well as reflect high-quality surgical resection [17].
However, recent research suggests that the impact of lymph node harvest is more
complex, and the benefit observed is likely multi-factorial. Given the impact of
lymph node harvest on long-term outcomes, node-negative patients with fewer
than 12 nodes evaluated should be considered high risk and be considered for adjuvant chemotherapy.

Management of Rectal Cancer

Rectal cancer is defined as a cancerous mass located within 12 cm of the anal verge as identified by rigid endoscopy [18]. Management of rectal cancers is complex with treatment strategies impacting survival as well as quality of life. Anatomical location of the tumors within the pelvis also presents unique challenges and increases the chance of local recurrence compared with colon cancer.

Surgical resection remains central to the management of rectal cancer; however, most rectal cancers require a multi-disciplinary approach combining surgery with chemotherapy and radiation. For locally advanced rectal cancer (LARC), neoadjuvant chemoradiation therapy has been used effectively with superior results as compared to adjuvant therapy [19]. Even though radical surgery remains the standard of care for LARC patients, select patient groups have been treated successfully with more conservative approaches including observation or local excision alone following neoadjuvant therapy [20].

Initial Evaluation

In the era of neoadjuvant therapy, a critical component in the initial management of patients with rectal cancer is staging of the primary tumor and regional lymph node basin. Similar to colon cancer, the TNM staging system of the primary tumor is based on depth of invasion (T) and regional lymph node invasion (N). Assessing for the presence of a distant metastasis (M) is also performed to determine the appropriate therapy. The radiographic techniques used for initial staging of the primary tumor and regional lymph nodes are either endoscopic ultrasound (EUS) or magnetic resonance imaging (MRI). Endoscopic ultrasound (EUS) accurately predicts the primary (T) stage prior to treatment in 80–95 % of the cases [21]. A recent meta-analysis demonstrated that EUS and MRI were both effective especially for depth of tumor penetration [22]. However, both modalities are less effective for identifying nodal disease. EUS only correctly predicts the nodal (N) stage in approximately 70 % of the cases [22]. Complete colonoscopy is recommended to evaluate for synchronous lesions, and CT scans of the chest, abdomen, and pelvis are used for the evaluation of distant disease. PET CT scans are not routinely incorporated into the initial evaluation.

Surgical Approach to Rectal Cancer

Two different general approaches for rectal tumors are typically performed, including local excision and radical resection. Many factors influence the surgical decision-making process such as pathologic tumor features, patient comorbidities, and the impact on quality of life.

Local excision is an appealing surgical approach, with the advantages of limited morbidity and avoidance of a colostomy. Tumors in the lower or middle thirds of the rectum are accessible by simple transanal excision, but tumors of the upper rectum require the use of transanal endoscopic microsurgery (TEMS) techniques for resection. Local excision is the treatment of choice for a select, small group of all patients diagnosed with rectal cancer (<10 %). Tumors amenable to transanal excision are small (<3 cm), <25 % of the rectal circumference, confined to the mucosa or submucosa (Tis or T1), lack nodal involvement by preoperative imaging, and have favorable pathologic characteristics (well or moderately differentiated with no lymphovascular invasion). Local excision is performed ideally with a >5 mm normal margin and is oriented for pathologic evaluation. However, a major disadvantage is the lack of definitive nodal staging, which may account for the increased rate of local recurrence as compared with radical surgery. Local excision of T2 tumors has resulted in unacceptable high local recurrence rates up to 45 % [23]. Unfortunately, the addition of adjuvant chemoradiation has not improved the oncologic results significantly.

Tumors staged at T2 or greater require a formal resection, and the type of resection depends on tumor location. Upper and middle rectal tumors generally can be managed with a low or very low anterior resection. Lower rectal tumors frequently require a proctectomy with coloanal anastomosis or an abdominoperineal resection (APR). Tumors involving the sphincter mechanism require an APR. A critical component of the proctectomy is a tumor appropriate total mesorectal excision (TME). TME involves sharp dissection between pre-sacral fascia and the fascia propria of the rectum encompassing the entire mesorectum [24]. If successfully performed, TME achieves complete excision of all mesorectal tissue en bloc with the tumor and associated lymph nodes and vasculature. TME should be extended at least 5 cm past the level of the tumor. If correctly maintained, TME increases the likelihood of autonomic nerve preservation.

Another critical component to optimize outcomes is accurate pathologic margin assessment. The goal of resection is to obtain a 5 cm distal margin including TME; however, lower tumors can be successfully managed with less than a 2 cm distal mucosal margin [25]. The circumferential (radial) margin of resection has been recognized as a key pathologic factor in long-term outcomes [26, 27]. A positive CRM has been defined as a tumor within 1 mm of the surgical specimen. The status of the CRM is a strong predictor of local recurrence and long-term survival [9, 10]. In the landmark study by Adam et al., a positive CRM was associated with an 80 % rate of local pelvic recurrence [26].

Neoadjuvant Chemoradiation for Locally Advanced Rectal Cancer

Neoadjuvant chemoradiation therapy (NCR) is an appropriate therapeutic strategy for locally advanced rectal cancer (LARC) defined as primary stage T3 and 4, as well as node (N)-positive cancers. Beneficial treatment results have been demonstrated in many studies including randomized as well as Phase II trials [19, 28].

Table 4 Results from the German Rectal Cancer trial (CAO/ARO/AIO-94)

	Neo-adjuvant CMT (%)	Adjuvant CMT (%)	*P* value
5 Years LR	6	13	0.006
5 Years OS	76	74	0.80
Sphincter preserved	39	19	0.004
Anastomotic stricture	4	12	0.003
Grade ¾ toxicity	27	40	0.001

CMT combined modality therapy, *LR* local recurrence, *OS* overall survival

The benchmark randomized control multi-institutional trial, the German Rectal Cancer trial, randomized LARC patients to receive either standard adjuvant chemoradiation following resection or neoadjuvant chemoradiation followed by resection [19]. This trial highlighted the benefits of preoperative therapy by demonstrating an improved tolerance of prescribed therapy, improved sphincter preservation, and fewer treatment-related complications (Table 4) [19]. Although no overall survival benefit was demonstrated, disease-free survival was significantly improved with neoadjuvant therapy, thus highlighting its critical advantages as compared to adjuvant therapy. One disadvantage of neoadjuvant therapy is the potential to over-treat tumors that are staged inaccurately as more advanced malignancies. If neoadjuvant therapy is not offered, then Stage 2/3 patients should receive adjuvant chemoradiation.

Conservative Management Following Neoadjuvant Chemoradiation

Even though radical surgery remains the standard of care for LARC patients, surgeons have treated select LARC patients with more conservative approaches including observation (wait-and-see) or local excision (LE) alone following neoadjuvant CMT [20, 29–31]. Generally, this experimental approach has been reserved for patients with a complete clinical response to NCR and/or patients whose condition is too poor or who adamantly refuse radical surgery. The landmark investigation by Habr-Gama et al. compared the outcomes of 71 closely observed patients with a complete clinical response versus a similar cohort that had an incomplete clinical response yet had a pathologic complete response on final pathology [20]. In this study, a clinical complete response was defined as a patient who had no evidence of recurrent disease at 12 months following completion of therapy. Long-term overall and disease-free survival did not differ significantly between the 2 groups of patients. Unfortunately, other groups have not demonstrated similar levels of success with a non-operative approach, thus decreasing optimism for this approach.

Similarly, studies evaluating conservative treatment approaches, e.g., LE following CMT for rectal cancer patients undergoing neoadjuvant therapy, have demonstrated

Table 5 The experience with local excision following neoadjuvant chemoradiation for locally advanced rectal cancer

	#Pts	Mean F/U (mo)	pR (%)	LR (%)	Metastasis
Moffitt [31]	26	24	pT0-65	0	0
			pPR-35	1	1
UF [30]	11	55	pT0-73	0	1
			pPR-27	0	0
MDACC [29]	26	46	pT0-54	0	1
			pPR-46	2/12	2
Total	63	42	pT0-62	0	2.5 %
			pPR-38	12.5 %	12.5 %

pT0 complete pathologic response, *pR* partial response

Table 6 Rates of persistent mesorectal disease based on rectal cancer downstaging with neoadjuvant chemoradiation

	MDACC [32] $n=219$ (%)	MSKCC [34] $n=187$ (%)	Wash U./Western PA [33]; $n=644$ (%)	Padova [35] $n=235$ (%)
pT0	9	7	2	2
pT1	20	8	4	15
pT2	23	22	23	17
pT3		37	47	38
pT4		67	48	33

that patients who achieved a pathologic CR had long-term outcomes comparable to radical surgery (Table 5) [30–32]. However, studies of this conservative surgical approach in such highly selected patients raise the following concerns. Those prior investigations (1) have been retrospective, (2) have not assessed the mesorectal lymph nodes and, (3) need longer follow-up time periods. Even with significant downstaging of the primary tumor with NCR, many groups have demonstrated high rates of persistent mesorectal disease (Table 6) [32–35]. Currently, a wait-and-see strategy remains investigational and, therefore, should not be considered the standard of care. In the future, improved staging procedures, as well as improved clinical or molecular predictors, may enhance the success of this conservative approach.

Laparoscopic Rectal Cancer Resection

Similar to laparoscopy for colon cancer, laparoscopy for rectal cancer is gaining acceptance. The randomized CLASSIC trial comparing open to laparoscopic resection provided the strongest evidence supporting laparoscopic rectal cancer resection [36]. In this trial, approximately half of the 794 patients had rectal cancer. No differences were observed, however, between the two treatment groups in terms of overall survival, disease-free survival, and local recurrence. Other prospective studies have demonstrated short-term benefits such as shorter hospital stay, less blood loss, and quicker return of bowel function.

Conclusions

Colorectal cancer is a common, highly treatable and frequently curable malignancy. There are exciting advances in the both the medical management of disease (i.e., neoadjuvant therapies, personalized regimens) and the surgical approaches (i.e., laparoscopic and robotic techniques) that promise to improve our ability to treat CRC.

References

1. Siegel R, Naishadham D, Jemal A. Cancer statistics, 2013. CA Cancer J Clin. 2013;63(1): 11–30.
2. Arora G, Mannalithara A, Singh G, Gerson LB, Triadafilopoulos G. Risk of perforation from a colonoscopy in adults: a large population-based study. Gastrointest Endosc. 2009;69(3 Pt 2): 654–64.
3. Hampel H, Frankel WL, Martin E, Arnold M, Khanduja K, Kuebler P, et al. Feasibility of screening for Lynch syndrome among patients with colorectal cancer. J Clin Oncol. 2008;26(35):5783–8.
4. Lynch HT, de la Chapelle A. Hereditary colorectal cancer. N Engl J Med. 2003;348(10): 919–32.
5. Castellvi-Bel S, Ruiz-Ponte C, Fernandez-Rozadilla C, Abuli A, Munoz J, Bessa X, et al. Seeking genetic susceptibility variants for colorectal cancer: the EPICOLON consortium experience. Mutagenesis. 2012;27(2):153–9.
6. Hendriks YM, de Jong AE, Morreau H, Tops CM, Vasen HF, Wijnen JT, et al. Diagnostic approach and management of Lynch syndrome (hereditary nonpolyposis colorectal carcinoma): a guide for clinicians. CA Cancer J Clin. 2006;56(4):213–25.
7. Evaluation of Genomic Applications in Practice and Prevention Working Group. Recommendations from the EGAPP Working Group: genetic testing strategies in newly diagnosed individuals with colorectal cancer aimed at reducing morbidity and mortality from Lynch syndrome in relatives. Genet Med. 2009;11(1):35–41.
8. Ladabaum U, Wang G, Terdiman J, Blanco A, Kuppermann M, Boland CR, et al. Strategies to identify the Lynch syndrome among patients with colorectal cancer: a cost-effectiveness analysis. Ann Intern Med. 2011;155(2):69–79.
9. Cooper HS. Pathologic issues in the treatment of endoscopically removed malignant colorectal polyps. J Natl Compr Canc Netw. 2007;5(9):991–6.
10. Hassan C, Zullo A, Risio M, Rossini FP, Morini S. Histologic risk factors and clinical outcome in colorectal malignant polyp: a pooled-data analysis. Dis Colon Rectum. 2005;48(8):1588–96.
11. Seitz U, Bohnacker S, Seewald S, Thonke F, Brand B, Braiutigam T, et al. Is endoscopic polypectomy an adequate therapy for malignant colorectal adenomas? Presentation of 114 patients and review of the literature. Dis Colon Rectum. 2004;47(11):1789–96. discussion 96-7.
12. Fleshman J, Sargent DJ, Green E, Anvari M, Stryker SJ, Beart Jr RW, et al. Laparoscopic colectomy for cancer is not inferior to open surgery based on 5-year data from the COST Study Group trial. Ann Surg. 2007;246(4):655–62. discussion 62-4.

13. Colon Cancer Laparoscopic or Open Resection Study Group, Buunen M, Veldkamp R, Hop WC, Kuhry E, Jeekel J, et al. Survival after laparoscopic surgery versus open surgery for colon cancer: long-term outcome of a randomised clinical trial. Lancet Oncol. 2009;10(1):44–52.

14. Bilimoria KY, Palis B, Stewart AK, Bentrem DJ, Freel AC, Sigurdson ER, et al. Impact of tumor location on nodal evaluation for colon cancer. Dis Colon Rectum. 2008;51(2):154–61.

15. Lykke J, Roikjaer O, Jess P, Danish Colorectal Cancer Group. The relation between lymph node status and survival in Stage I-III colon cancer: results from a prospective nationwide cohort study. Colorectal Dis. 2013;15(5):559–65.

16. Le Voyer TE, Sigurdson ER, Hanlon AL, Mayer RJ, Macdonald JS, Catalano PJ, et al. Colon cancer survival is associated with increasing number of lymph nodes analyzed: a secondary survey of intergroup trial INT-0089. J Clin Oncol. 2003;21(15):2912–9.

17. Parsons HM, Tuttle TM, Kuntz KM, Begun JW, McGovern PM, Virnig BA. Association between lymph node evaluation for colon cancer and node positivity over the past 20 years. JAMA. 2011;306(10):1089–97.

18. Nelson H, Petrelli N, Carlin A, Couture J, Fleshman J, Guillem J, et al. Guidelines 2000 for colon and rectal cancer surgery. J Natl Cancer Inst. 2001;93(8):583–96.

19. Sauer R, Becker H, Hohenberger W, Rodel C, Wittekind C, Fietkau R, et al. Preoperative versus postoperative chemoradiotherapy for rectal cancer. N Engl J Med. 2004;351(17):1731–40.

20. Habr-Gama A, Perez RO, Nadalin W, Sabbaga J, Ribeiro Jr U, Silva e Sousa Jr AH, et al. Operative versus nonoperative treatment for stage 0 distal rectal cancer following chemoradiation therapy: long-term results. Ann Surg. 2004;240(4):711–7. discussion 7–8.

21. Meyenberger C, Huch Boni RA, Bertschinger P, Zala GF, Klotz HP, Krestin GP. Endoscopic ultrasound and endorectal magnetic resonance imaging: a prospective, comparative study for preoperative staging and follow-up of rectal cancer. Endoscopy. 1995;27(7):469–79.

22. Bipat S, Glas AS, Slors FJ, Zwinderman AH, Bossuyt PM, Stoker J. Rectal cancer: local staging and assessment of lymph node involvement with endoluminal US, CT, and MR imaging – a meta-analysis. Radiology. 2004;232(3):773–83.

23. Sengupta S, Tjandra JJ. Local excision of rectal cancer: what is the evidence? Dis Colon Rectum. 2001;44(9):1345–61.

24. Scott N, Jackson P, al-Jaberi T, Dixon MF, Quirke P, Finan PJ. Total mesorectal excision and local recurrence: a study of tumour spread in the mesorectum distal to rectal cancer. Br J Surg. 1995;82(8):1031–3.

25. Bujko K, Rutkowski A, Chang GJ, Michalski W, Chmielik E, Kusnierz J. Is the 1-cm rule of distal bowel resection margin in rectal cancer based on clinical evidence? A systematic review. Indian J Surg Oncol. 2012;3(2):139–46.

26. Adam IJ, Mohamdee MO, Martin IG, Scott N, Finan PJ, Johnston D, et al. Role of circumferential margin involvement in the local recurrence of rectal cancer. Lancet. 1994;344(8924):707–11.

27. Birbeck KF, Macklin CP, Tiffin NJ, Parsons W, Dixon MF, Mapstone NP, et al. Rates of circumferential resection margin involvement vary between surgeons and predict outcomes in rectal cancer surgery. Ann Surg. 2002;235(4):449–57.

28. Glynne-Jones R, Harrison M, Hughes R. Challenges in the neoadjuvant treatment of rectal cancer: balancing the risk of recurrence and quality of life. Cancer Radiother. 2013; 17(7):675–85.

29. Bonnen M, Crane C, Vauthey JN, Skibber J, Delclos ME, Rodriguez-Bigas M, et al. Long-term results using local excision after preoperative chemoradiation among selected T3 rectal cancer patients. Int J Radiat Oncol Biol Phys. 2004;60(4):1098–105.

30. Schell SR, Zlotecki RA, Mendenhall WM, Marsh RW, Vauthey JN, Copeland 3rd EM. Transanal excision of locally advanced rectal cancers downstaged using neoadjuvant chemoradiotherapy. J Am Coll Surg. 2002;194(5):584–90. discussion 90–1.

31. Nair RM, Siegel EM, Chen DT, Fulp WJ, Yeatman TJ, Malafa MP, et al. Long-term results of transanal excision after neoadjuvant chemoradiation for T2 and T3 adenocarcinomas of the rectum. J Gastrointest Surg. 2008;12(10):1797–805. discussion 805–6.

32. Bedrosian I, Rodriguez-Bigas MA, Feig B, Hunt KK, Ellis L, Curley SA, et al. Predicting the node-negative mesorectum after preoperative chemoradiation for locally advanced rectal carcinoma. J Gastrointest Surg. 2004;8(1):56–62. discussion 3.
33. Read TE, Andujar JE, Caushaj PF, Johnston DR, Dietz DW, Myerson RJ, et al. Neoadjuvant therapy for rectal cancer: histologic response of the primary tumor predicts nodal status. Dis Colon Rectum. 2004;47(6):825–31.
34. Stipa F, Zernecke A, Moore HG, Minsky BD, Wong WD, Weiser M, et al. Residual mesorectal lymph node involvement following neoadjuvant combined-modality therapy: rationale for radical resection? Ann Surg Oncol. 2004;11(2):187–91.
35. Pucciarelli S, Capirci C, Emanuele U, Toppan P, Friso ML, Pennelli GM, et al. Relationship between pathologic T-stage and nodal metastasis after preoperative chemoradiotherapy for locally advanced rectal cancer. Ann Surg Oncol. 2005;12(2):111–6.
36. Jayne DG, Guillou PJ, Thorpe H, Quirke P, Copeland J, Smith AM, et al. Randomized trial of laparoscopic-assisted resection of colorectal carcinoma: 3-year results of the UK MRC CLASICC Trial Group. J Clin Oncol. 2007;25(21):3061–8.

Modern Locoregional Treatment of Colorectal Cancer Liver Metastases

Julie N. Leal and Michael I. D'Angelica

Introduction

Colorectal cancer (CRC) is the third most common malignancy in the USA. In 2012, over 140,000 new cases were diagnosed and over 55, 000 deaths were directly attributed to CRC [1, 2]. Up to 20 % of patients with CRC have metastatic disease at the time of primary diagnosis and as many as 50 % subsequently develop metastatic spread during the course of follow-up. The liver is the most common location of metastases. Approximately 80 % of all patients with metastatic CRC have some form of liver involvement, either alone (40 %) or in conjunction with other extrahepatic sites (60 %) [3–5]. In the setting of colorectal cancer liver metastases (CRLM) the only treatment with curative potential is complete resection. Unfortunately, at the time of diagnosis it is estimated that only 15–20 % of patients have disease that is amenable to resection [6]. In patients with resected liver only metastases, 5 and 10-year overall survivals (OS) range between 25 % and 74 %, and 9–50 %, respectively [7–10]. Conversely, median survival in patients with potentially resectable CRLM who remain untreated varies between 6 and 12 months, and survival past 3 years is rare [11, 12]. Furthermore, in patients with unresectable CRLM treatment with modern chemotherapy is associated with median OS of up to 21 months;

J.N. Leal, M.D., F.R.C.S.C.
Division of Hepatopancreatobiliary Surgery, Department of Surgery, Memorial Sloan Kettering Cancer Center, Weill School of Medicine, Cornell University, New York, NY USA

2003 Santa Cruz Ave, Menlo Park, CA 94025, USA
e-mail: julienleal2014@gmail.com

M.I. D'Angelica, M.D., F.A.C.S. (✉)
Department of Surgery, Memorial Sloan Kettering Cancer Center, Weill School of Medicine, Cornell University, 1275 York Avenue, Bobst Building, 8th Floor, Rm C-898, New York, NY 10065, USA
e-mail: dangelim@mskcc.org

© Springer International Publishing Switzerland 2016
K.A. Morgan (ed.), *Current Controversies in Cancer Care for the Surgeon*, DOI 10.1007/978-3-319-16205-8_5

however, chemotherapy alone is uncommonly associated with 5 year survival (2–5 %) and to date has not been associated with durable cure [13].

Complete resection of CRLM's is paramount to achieving long-term survival. To date, however, a globally accepted definition of "resectability" is lacking. Historically, the number, distribution, and size of metastases dictated surgical eligibility. More recently, refinements in surgical techniques, and development of surgical adjuncts, such as portal vein embolization and ablative therapies, have resulted in a shift towards surgical treatment of more extensive disease irrespective of absolute tumor size and/or number [3, 8, 14]. This increasingly aggressive approach to surgical extirpation of CRLMs appears to be safe and when performed at experienced centers it is associated with surgical morbidity of 20–30 %, and mortality rates of <3 %. In terms of oncologic outcomes, disease recurrence following resection of more extensive CRLM is high and can be seen in up to 90 % of cases. Although OS in this higher risk group is not equivalent to that observed in patients undergoing resection based on more restrictive definitions, associated prolonged survival is longer than that seen with nonsurgical therapies [8, 15–18]. In 2013, an expert consensus group revised the working definition of resectability stating that CRLM can be considered technically resectable if all lesions can be removed with negative margins, leaving at least two contiguous disease-free segments with adequate vascular inflow/outflow and biliary drainage, and an overall future liver remnant (FLR) volume of 20–30 % [19]. This most recent definition highlights the focus on the size and functionality of the FLR rather than the overall degree of tumor burden and underlying tumor biology. This current definition relies too heavily on technical resectability alone, essentially ignoring tumor biology and the very high recurrence rates among patients with extensive CRLM.

Previously, treatment options for patients with unresectable CRLM were few and primarily palliative in intent. Early studies of 5-fluorouracil (5-FU) based chemotherapy alone were associated with minimal intrahepatic tumoricidal effects and subsequent poor response rates (RR < 20 %) [6]. More recently, modern combination chemotherapy regimens including 5-FU, leucovorin, oxaliplatin and/or irinotecan used in the first-line setting have been associated with significantly improved RR (up to 50 %). Depending on the chemotherapy regimen, improvements in RR have been associated with conversion to complete resection in 10–30 % of initially unresectable patients [20–23]. In addition to improvements in chemotherapy, development of targeted therapies, and application of novel locoregional treatments, offer higher response rates and the improved potential for down-staging of disease and increasing conversion rates.

Complete resection of CRLM offers the greatest potential for long-term survival and is the only treatment associated with the possibility of cure. Recent advances in the management of CRLM have focused on developing measures to improve not only the safety and efficacy of surgery for those patients with resectable CRLM but also to increase the number of patients eligible for resection. Over the past decade the armamentarium of diagnostic, treatment, and surveillance options for CRLM has expanded significantly and will continue to do so in the future. It is therefore incumbent upon the clinician to remain apprised of current treatment standards as well as debates surrounding optimal implementation of newer therapies.

Clinical Presentation

CRLM may present in either a synchronous or metachronous fashion. Synchronous CRLM are defined, somewhat arbitrarily, as metastases detected within 12 months of the primary CRC diagnosis and account for 25–30 % of all CRLM [24]. Typically, these metastases are asymptomatic and may be identified at the time of staging investigations for the primary tumor, intraoperatively at the time of primary resection, or during routine postoperative disease surveillance [25]. In a minority of patients, radiologic investigation for nonspecific symptomatology such as fatigue, weight loss, anorexia, abdominal discomfort, bloating, and/or flank pain leads to the incidental diagnosis of CRLM prior to the primary CRC. Presence of a palpable liver mass, hepatomegaly, jaundice, or clinical evidence of liver insufficiency is currently uncommon but if found associated with a poor outcome. Given the routine use of cross-sectional imaging in CRC patients, physical examination is usually non-contributory.

Metachronous CRLM account for two thirds of all CRLM. Clinical presentation in this subset of patients varies depending on the population in which they are detected. In patients participating in active surveillance programs following resection of the primary tumor, CRLM are typically identified on follow-up cross-sectional imaging or in the setting of a rising tumor marker (CEA) without specific symptoms. Alternatively, in the absence of surveillance, presentation in this cohort is often later and associated with the onset of nonspecific signs and/or symptoms mentioned above. Therapeutic options for CRLM are predicated on both patient and tumor factors, as such, all patients with potential CRLM warrant thorough evaluation aimed at providing an accurate diagnosis, determining extent of disease, and assessing overall functional status.

Evaluation of Disease

Resectability Versus Operability

Determining patients in whom surgical resection will provide significant benefit is dependent upon fastidious evaluation, not only of technical resectability, but also of operability. Assessment of operability includes characterization of overall health status and evaluation of biologic disease behavior. Patient related factors such as severe comorbid disease and/or poor functional status increase the risk of perioperative complication and mortality, and in some patients may be prohibitive [26]. Disease biology is a critical component of the assessment of operability. Short disease-free interval (time from primary CRC to CRLM), rapid disease progression, and/or progression of disease while on therapy can be used clinically as surrogates of aggressive cancer biology. Although these are not absolute contraindications to resection they portend worse outcomes following surgery such that alternative approaches to management may be considered [19]. In those patients deemed to be operable, a thorough evaluation of technical resectability by a hepatobiliary surgeon is essential and should include assessment of tumor burden within the liver, evaluation of the future liver remnant (FLR), and search for evidence of extrahepatic disease (EHD).

Table 1 Comparison of common imaging modalities used for the detection and characterization of colorectal liver metastases

Modality	Advantages	Limitations	Sensitivity (%)
CT	– Widespread availability	– poor detection and characterization of lesions <10 mm	70–85
	– Relatively low cost	– reduced sensitivity in setting of chemotherapy induced liver injury (steatosis)	
	– Rapid image acquisition	– requires iodinated contrast	
	– Evaluation of EHD	– contraindicated in patients with renal dysfunction/ failure	
	– Volume assessment of FLR	– radiation exposure	
	– Vascular mapping (CTA)		
	– Therapeutic monitoring		
MRI	– improved detection/ characterization of:	– limited availability	91–97
	– small lesions (<10 mm)	– image acquisition time consuming requiring significant patient compliance	
	– lesions in the setting of chemotherapy induced liver injury (steatosis)	– expensive	
	– no radiation exposure	– contraindicated in setting of certain medical implants (PM, stents etc.)	
FDG PET	– Evaluation of EHD	– limited availability	78–95
	– surveillance for recurrence	– high false positive rates, leading to unnecessary work-up	
	– increased sensitivity/ specificity when combined with CT	– expensive	
		– poor detection following chemotherapy	
		– poor detection of lesions <10 mm	

EHD = extrahepatic disease, FLR = future liver remnant, CTA = CT angiography

Radiologic Assessment

Evaluation of local tumor burden is essential to the assessment of potential surgical candidates. This includes identification of the number of segments involved, the relation of tumor(s) to vascular inflow/outflow and major bile ducts, and estimation of the FLR. Each major imaging modality has inherent benefits and limitations (Table 1), and at present there is no agreed upon gold standard for identifying CRLM

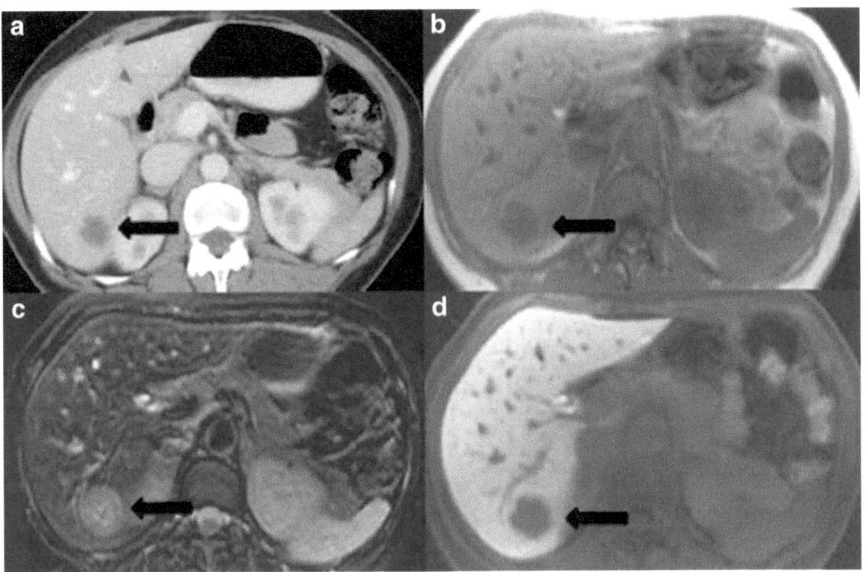

Fig. 1 Comparison of radiographic imaging modalities for colorectal cancer liver metastases with, (**a**) dynamic contrast enhanced CT-portovenous phase, (**b**) T1-weighted MRI, (**c**) T2-weighted MRI with fat suppression, (**d**) T1 weighted MRI post contrast with liver-specific contrast media (EOVIST™) on delayed hepatobiliary phase (⬅ tumor)

or critical anatomic structures. Selection of imaging technique(s) is typically dependent on individual and institution biases. In the past trans-abdominal ultrasound (US) was used extensively to image the liver, however, the sensitivity of this modality for the characterization of CRLM is low, reportedly failing to detect up to 50 % of lesions [27]. Consequently, trans-abdominal US is not recommended for assessment of resectability. To overcome some of the limitations of standard US in defining CRLM, addition of microbubble contrast media has been suggested. Current studies suggest contrast enhanced ultrasound (CEUS) performs similar to CT and contrast enhanced magnetic resonance imaging in identification and characterization of liver lesions [28]. Although uncommon, CEUS has been used intraoperatively to assess tumor burden with some success [29]. At present, the role of CEUS in the management of CRLM is not well defined and in the USA its clinical use has been hampered by a lack of regulatory approval of microbubble contrast media.

Dynamic contrast enhanced computerized tomography refers to CT imaging of the liver in which images are obtained in three phases (triphasic); non-contrast, arterial, and portovenous. CRLM are typically hypoattenuating compared to the background liver parenchyma, and are best visualized during the portovenous phase (Fig. 1a). Sensitivity of modern thin slice, triphasic, contrast enhanced CT for the detection of CRLM ranges from 80 to 90 % and is significantly higher than standard contrast enhanced CT (sensitivity 60–75 %) [25]. These performance characteristics, in conjunction with widespread availability and relative cost-effectiveness, have led dynamic CT to be the most common radiology investigation for evaluation of CRLM [30]. However, CT is limited in its ability to identify and characterize smaller liver lesions, specifically those lesions <10 mm. Wiering et al. noted that despite CT being 97 % successful in detecting lesions >20 mm and 72 % successful for lesions 10–20 mm, CT performed poorly for lesions <10 mm, with a success rate of only 16 % [31]. Furthermore, previous treatment with cytotoxic chemotherapy may lead to steatosis of the underlying liver parenchyma and a subsequent decrease in the ability to discriminate between CRLM and normal liver. This phenomenon significantly decreases the sensitivity of CT to detect CRLM [32]. This has been observed in multiple studies. A recently published meta-analysis suggests pooled sensitivity estimates for CT following chemotherapy to be 69.9 % (65.6–73.9 %) compared to 80.5 % (67.0–89.4 %) in chemotherapy naïve patients [33]. Despite these limitations, CT remains the most common initial radiology investigation for evaluation of CRLM [30], with reservation of alternative investigations for "problem-solving" in the setting of lesions too small to characterize on CT or in chemotherapy treated patients.

Magnetic resonance imaging (MRI) provides exquisite soft tissue resolution when compared to other imaging modalities. As a consequence MRI offers several advantages in terms of detection and characterization of smaller lesions, and evaluation of the liver in the setting of previous chemotherapy or other underlying parenchymal abnormalities. CRLM appear hypointense to isointense on T1-weighted images, and isointense to hyperintense on T2-weighted images (Fig. 1b/c). Overall, the sensitivity of contrast enhanced MRI to detect CRLM is reported to range from 91 to 97 % [34] and the accuracy in stratifying too small to characterize lesions (<10 mm) as benign or malignant is over 90 %. Furthermore, specificity of liver MRI for the diagnosis of malignant lesions far exceeds that of CT (97.5 % versus 77.3 %) [35]. Use of chemotherapy can lead to steatosis and increasing amounts of fat within the liver which makes CRLM more difficult to detect. MRI is advantageous in this setting as images can be reformatted using "fat-suppression" techniques leading to improved detection of CRLM when compared to other imaging modalities. Meta-analyses of studies of patients with CRLM previously treated with chemotherapy suggest a sensitivity of liver MRI of 85.7 % (69.7–94.0 %), which is significantly improved over other imaging techniques [33]. Development of newer tissue-specific contrast agents such as gadozetate (Gd-EOB-DTPA; Eovist), that are taken up by hepatocytes can further improve the performance of MRI in identifying and characterizing CRLM (Fig. 1d) [36]. Additionally, diffusion weighted MRI (DWI), which relies on the differential proton diffusion characteristics between benign and malignant tissue, is another modification of standard MRI that may improve evaluation the liver for CRLM [37] The major limitations of MRI evaluation is the requirement for substantial patient compliance to minimize motion artifact, poor assessment of disease outside the liver, high cost, and limited availability, as such it is not the ideal initial investigation in the setting of CRLM. However, evidence suggests that available MRI techniques allow better characterization of small (<10 mm) CRLM and improve detection rates in the setting of previous chemotherapy. It is this subset of patients for whom use of MRI is likely warranted.

Over the last two decades novel functional imaging techniques such as positron emission tomography using the radiolabelled 18-fluoro-deoxyglucose (FDG-PET) have proven useful in the detection of cancer. Images associated with FDG PET are dependent on the degree of uptake and accumulation of radiolabeled tracer. Cells that are highly active metabolically, such as cancer cells, tend to take up and hold onto greater amounts of radiotracer when compared to less active cells. Visualized foci of increased uptake are quantified using the standardized uptake value (SUV = activity per unit volume/injected activity per body weight). To date, FDG PET has been extensively evaluated in the setting of CRLM. Multiple meta-analysis and systematic reviews of trials regarding the diagnostic performance of FDG PET have been published [38–41] and suggest overall sensitivity of the test for the detection of CRLM to be significantly improved over MRI and CT (94.1 % versus 88.2 % and 83.6 %, respectively) [41]. However, much criticism exists regarding the implication of these findings and many suggest these studies are hampered by inappropriate comparison groups with poor quality imaging, thus FDG PET is typically reserved for problem-solving and/or evaluation for extrahepatic disease. Although FDG PET performs very well as a diagnostic test, it lacks spatial resolution of anatomic details, and evaluation of technical resectability is not feasible. Fusion of FDG PET with high quality CT (PET-CT) is an attempt to combat this limitation and is rapidly replacing stand alone PET scanning. Overall, the combined PET-CT allows for highly sensitive detection of CRLM and impressive tumor localization [30]. FDG PET is advantageous in that the entire body is imaged and its use as a component of the preoperative extent of disease work up for patients with CRLM and concern for EHD has been evaluated. Earlier studies evaluating PET-CT in this setting suggested improved evaluation of tumor burden and a subsequent reduction in futile laparotomy of up to 20 % [42] Based on this, it was concluded that routine use of preoperative staging PET-CT was essential to avoid unnecessary surgery. However, most recently, a randomized control trial of preoperative PET-CT versus no PET-CT in patients with initially resectable CRLM was conducted and the impact on surgical management was assessed [43]. In the 263 patients undergoing PET-CT in this trial, overall surgical plan was changed (canceled, more extensive liver resection, or more extensive extrahepatic resection) in only 23 (8.7 %) patients. More importantly, of these changes in management only 9 (2.7 %) patients avoided futile laparotomy, which is in stark contrast to the 20 % previously reported [42]. Major limitations to FDG-PET and PET-CT include limited accessibility, high cost, and poor diagnostic sensitivity for lesions <10 mm and in the setting of previous chemotherapy [33]. These limitations in conjunction with the best available evidence suggest that standardized use of PET-CT as a staging tool in patients with CRLM rarely results in clinically significant changes in management plans and is not cost-effective. PET-CT use should be reserved for cases in which diagnostic uncertainty regarding the presence or absence of EHD exists.

Radiographic imaging plays an integral role in the detection and characterization of CRLM as well as identification of EHD. To date, no gold standard imaging modality for evaluation of patients with CRLM has been defined. Based on currently available evidence, and cost-effectiveness, a reasonable algorithm for investigation of CRLM would include; initial dynamic CT (in most patients this will be adequate to determine technical resectability and extent of disease), if lesions are seen on CT that are too small to characterize (<10 mm) or if there is evidence of significant chemotherapy induced parenchyma injury, MRI should be performed. PET-CT is expensive and unnecessary in most patients. Its use should be reserved for those difficult cases in which delineation of potential EHD is necessary.

Evaluation of the Future Liver Remnant

FLR refers to the portion of liver that will remain in situ following hepatic resection and is one of the major determinants of technical resectability and postoperative morbidity. Evaluation of both quantity (volume) and quality (uptake/excretion/synthetic function) of the FLR is important in order to determine risk of postoperative liver insufficiency [19]. FLR volume is primarily determined using preoperative cross sectional imaging. Using available imaging and standard radiologic software, the proposed line of transection is drawn and the remnant volume of liver is subsequently calculated. Typically, FLR is measured as a proportion of total liver volume (TLV) and expressed as a percentage. It may also be evaluated and expressed as a ratio of FLR to body weight (BW) [44] Any cysts, tumors, and/or zones of previous ablation are outlined and excluded from the final measured volumes. Adequate FLR volume is essential to minimize the risk of postoperative liver insufficiency. However, the absolute volume of FLR required is dependent on the status of the underlying liver parenchyma. Multiple methods for evaluating hepatic reserve/function and predicting outcome exist. In North America clinicians tend to rely heavily on single laboratory values (total bilirubin) and or clinical scoring systems (Child-Pugh, MELD) [45] to estimate degree of liver dysfunction and potential risk. On the other hand, in the East, indocyanine green clearance tests measuring hepatic perfusion and excretory function are a common means of assessing liver function [46]. Accepted minimal FLR is contingent on both volume and function. Although data are limited, generally accepted minimal static FLR values for normal liver, chemotherapy treated liver, and cirrhotic liver are; >20 %, >30 % and >40 %, respectively [47]. Based on thorough evaluation FLR may be considered adequate, borderline, or insufficient for safe resection. In the foremost group surgical resection may be pursued without further intervention. In patients with borderline and insufficient FLR techniques have been developed to induce hypertrophy of the remnant liver such that resection may be achievable.

Strategies to Increase Future Liver Remnant Volume

Laboratory studies conducted as early as the 1920s indicated that interruption of the portal venous flow to the liver resulted in atrophy of the ipsilateral segment and compensatory hypertrophy of the contralateral side [48]. This translated into the clinical hypothesis that in patients requiring major hepatic resection, where FLR

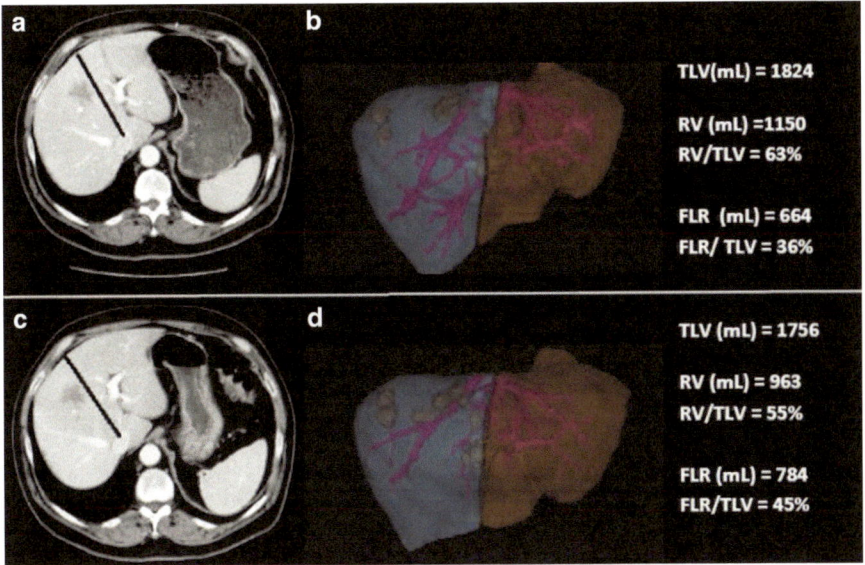

Fig. 2 CT imaging and volumetric rendering of the liver; (**a**) before portal vein embolization and, (**b**) after portal vein embolization (▬▬▬ line of proposed parenchymal transection, TLV = total liver volume, RV = resection volume, FLR = future liver remnant)

would be inadequate, diversion of portal blood flow from the portion of liver to be resected could result in hypertrophy of the FLR and subsequently allow safer resection of larger volumes of liver.

The most common method to achieve cessation of portal flow is percutaneous embolization. In the early 1980s proof of concept studies by Kinochita et al. [49] described perioperative portal vein embolization (PVE) in humans. Later PVE was used on a larger scale clinically with success in the setting of major resection for hilar cholangiocarcinoma and other primary hepatic malignancies [50]. In 2003, Belghiti et al. published a prospective trial of right hepatectomy with and without preoperative PVE. Subgroup analysis of patients with and without chronic liver disease (CLD) revealed that although hypertrophy of the FLR occurs in both groups, clinical benefit in terms of reduced overall morbidity and liver insufficiency was only observed in patients with CLD, no benefit of PVE was observed in the patients with normal underlying liver parenchyma [51]. To date no other prospective trial of PVE has been completed and present indications for preoperative PVE include any hepatic resection in which concern exists regarding the adequacy of the FLR. It is generally accepted that in order to minimize the risk of perioperative liver insufficiency PVE should be considered if the post-resectional liver volume is estimated to be ≤20 % [19, 52]. PVE is most commonly completed via percutaneous transhepatic route. Open techniques have also been described with access to the portal vein via iliocolic branches; although equally as effective in inducing hypertrophy, this requires mini-laparotomy and is rarely utilized [50]. Typically, 4 weeks following the procedure, adequacy of PVE is assessed with repeat cross section imaging and liver volumetry. Figure 2 illustrates CT images and volumetric rendering of the liver prior to and following PVE. In a recent meta-analysis typical absolute volume changes observed with PVE ranged from 8 to 27 % [52]. Traditionally, static measurements of the FLR (sFLR) volume have been used in the prediction of postoperative liver insufficiency. More recently, however, it has been suggested that it is not only the absolute sFLR volume (i.e., >20 % sFLR in normal liver) but also the degree of hypertrophy (DH) [53] and the kinetic growth rate (KGR) [54] of the FLR following PVE that are important in assessment of the adequacy of the FLR. Many believe these dynamic measures (DH, KGR) are the best in vivo markers of the functional capacity of the liver. Therefore, in conjunction with sFLR >20 %, DH > 5 % and a KGR of >2 %/week following PVE are considered minimal acceptable parameters for safe liver resection.

Portal vein ligation (PVL) is another technique in which hypertrophy of the FLR may be achieved. Results with this technique appear to be equivalent to those obtained with PVE [55]. However, PVL, is significantly more invasive requiring either mini-laparotomy or laparoscopy to complete and at present, outside of its use in two-stage resections, it is rarely used. Most recently, in attempts to induce more rapid and greater hypertrophy of the FLR a surgical procedure has been described in which partitioning of the liver is combined with portal vein ligation (Associating liver partition and portal vein ligation for staged hepatectomy-ALPPS) [56–58]. The concept behind this procedure is that combination of PVL with in situ splitting of the liver prevents the development of collateral circulation between segments and leads to more complete vascular isolation of the FLR, optimizing conditions for hypertrophy of the FLR. Although initial studies show significant and rapid increases in FLR (median increase 74 %, median time 9 days) the overall complication rate exceeds 60 %, with major complications occurring in over 40 % of patients, and in hospital death reported in 12 % [58]. Furthermore, the procedure requires two laparotomies within 7–10 days of each other which can be exceedingly arduous and taxing for patients. It appears that although novel in concept, the risks associated with ALPPS are significant and the benefits have yet to be seen, as such general application is not recommended.

Assessment of Prognosis

Over the past 20 years multiple different scoring systems and predictive models have been developed to help prognosticate patients with resectable CRLM (Table 2) [59–70]. Despite the heterogeneity in patient populations and era of study, the majority of these systems incorporate some variation of factors related to the pathology of the primary CRC, extent of disease (primary tumor and metastases), and timing of CRLM development relative to primary CRC. To date there is no uniformly accepted or "ideal" prognostic scoring system, however, the clinical risk score (CRS) as reported by Fong et al. in 1999 [60] is the most widely used [71, 72]. Based on multivariate analysis of preoperative clinicopathologic factors it is comprised of five criteria including, disease-free interval (DFI) < 12 months, size >5 cm,

Table 2 Comparison of prognostic scoring systems

Author (year, location)	Number of patients	Time frame	Prognostic factors	Risk groups (score)	Outcome (5-year)
Nordlinger et al., 1996; France [59]	1568	1968–1990	– Age ≥ 60	Low (0–2)	2 year—79 %
			– Serosal invasion of primary	Intermediate (3–4)	60 %
			– Node + primary	High (5–7)	43 %
			– DFI < 2 years		
			– Size ≥ 5 cm		
			– ≥ 4 tumors		
			– Margin ≤ 1 cm		
Fong et al., 1999; USA [60]	1001	1985–1998	– Margin +	0 (0)	60 %
			– EHD	1 (1)	44 %
			– Node + primary	2 (2)	40 %
			– DFI ≤ 12 month	3 (3)	20 %
			– Size ≥ 5 cm	4 (4)	25 %
			– > 1 tumor	5 (5)	14 %
			– CEA ≥ 200 ng/mL		
Iwatsuki et al., 1999; USA [61]	305	1981–1996	– ≥ 2 tumors	Grade 1 (0)	48 %
			– Size ≥ 8 cm	Grade 2 (1)	34 %
			– Bilobar distribution	Grade 3 (2)	18 %
			– DFI ≤ 30 months	Grade 4 (3)	6 %
			– Margin +	Grade 5 (4)	1 %
			– EHD	Grade 6 (R1 or EHD)	0 %
Ueno et al., 2000; Japan [62]	85	1985–1996	– Primary tumor with marked budding and/or node +	Stage A (0–1)	55 %
			– DFI < 1 year	Stage B (2)	14 %
			– ≥ 3 tumors	Stage C (3)	0 %
Lise et al., 2001; Italy [63]	132	1977–1997	– > 30 % liver invasion	Group A (0–2)	3 Year
			– Node + primary	Group B (3–5)	80 %
			– > 1 tumor	Group C (≥6)	55 %
			– GPT ≥ 55U/L		10 %
			– Non-anatomic resection		
Nagashima et al., 2004; Japan [64]	81	1981–1997	– Serosal invasion of primary	Grade A (0–1)	85 %
			– Node + primary	Grade B (2–3)	56 %
			– Resectable EHD	Grade C (>3)	0 %
			– >1 tumor		
			– Size > 5 cm		

(continued)

Table 2 (continued)

Author (year, location)	Number of patients	Time frame	Prognostic factors	Risk groups (score)	Outcome (5-year)
Schindl et al., 2005; UK [65]	270	1988– 2002	– Duke stage C	Good (0–10)	Median OS
			– CEA level	Moderate (11–25)	60 months
			– ALP	Poor (>25)	32 months
			– Albumin		22 months
			– >3 tumors		
Malik et al., 2007; UK [66]	687	1993– 2006	– Inflammatory response to tumor	0 (0)	49 %
			– ≥ 8 tumors	1 (1)	34 %
				2 (2)	0 %
Zakaria et al., 2007; USA [67]	662	1960– 1995	– DFI ≤ 30 months	Group 1 (0)	55 %
			– Size ≥ 8 cm	Group 2 (BT)	39 %
			– Blood Transfusion	Group 3 (HDN)	20 %
			– Hepatoduodenal lymph node +		
Lee et al., 2008; Korea [68]	135	1994– 2005	– Margin ≤5 mm	Low (0–1)	46 %
			– CEA > 5 ng/mL	Intermediate (2)	41 %
			– Node + primary	High (3–4)	11 %
			– > 1 tumor		
Rees et al., 2008; UK [69] Evaluated preoperative and postoperative risk[a]	929	1987– 2005	– > 1 tumor	0 (0)	Pre/Post
			– Node + primary	1–5 (1–5)	66 %/64 %
			– Poorly differentiate primary	6–10 (6–10)	51 %/49 %
			– EHD	11–15 (11–15)	35 %/34 %
			– Size ≥ 5 cm	>15 (>15)	21 %/21 %
			– CEA > 60 ng/mL		2 %/2 %
			– Margin +		
Konopke et al., 2009; Germany [70]	201	1993– 2006	– ≥ 4 tumors	Low (0)	Median OS
			– Synchronous metastases	Intermediate (1)	67 months
			– CEA ≥ 200 ng/mL	High (≥2)	47 months
					38 months

EHD = extrahepatic disease, CEA = carcinoembryonic antigen, GPT = glutamic pyruvic transaminase, ALP = alanine phosphatase, R1 = involved margin, BT = blood transfusion, HDN = hepatoduodenal lymph nodes tumor number >1, CEA >200 ng/mL, and node positive primary, each of which is given a single point and a sum total score is generated. In the initial study by Fong et al. the total score was highly predictive of OS ($p<0.0001$), with actuarial 5 year OS of 60 % and 14 %, for scores of 0 and 5, respectively. Since its inception the clinical utility of this scoring system has been evaluated extensively and has been validated in other study cohorts [67, 71, 73–75], however, its external validity has not been universally observed [67].

More recently, the value and relevance of these clinical scoring systems has been called into question [9, 72, 76, 77]. The primary issue surrounding these models is the fact that they were developed using retrospective analysis of historical cohorts, including patients from over 40 years ago. Within that time frame the management of CRLM has drastically changed and our ability to assess patient-specific tumor biology and evaluate molecular markers of prognosis has increased exponentially. To date multiple studies have attempted to identify potential radiologic, pathologic and molecular markers of prognosis. To this end, KRAS, a GTPase that when activated induces the mitogen-activated protein kinase (MAPK) cascade, has been the most extensively evaluated with respect to prognosis. CRLM with mutant KRAS have not only been associated with resistance to epidermal growth factor targeted antibodies, but in recent studies have been associated with significantly worse OS, DSS, and RFS [78, 79]. A variety of other molecular markers have also been assessed with respect to outcome in patients with CRLM and are outlined in Box 1.

Modern chemotherapeutics are increasingly being used in the neoadjuvant setting, and have generated significant interest in the evaluation of the relationship between response to therapy and prognosis. Degree of tumor response to chemotherapy can be assessed radiographically, most commonly using size-based measures such as

Box 1: Association of Molecular Markers and Survival in CRLM

Biomarker	Prevalence	Impact on survival
K-RAS mutation [78, 79]	40 %	Independent predictor of worse OS, DSS, and RFS
BRAF mutation [80]	5–10 %	Independent predictor of worse OS
Thymidylate synthase [81, 82]	20–80 % (overexpression)	Overexpression is associated with worse OS and RFS
hTERT [83, 84]	– N/A	Independent predictor of worse OS; correlation with survival better than CRS
Ki-67 [78, 84]	– N/A	Independent predictor of worse OS; correlation with survival better than CRS
Hypoxia inducible factor-1α [85]	30 % (overexpression)	Overexpression is an independent risk factor for disease recurrence

OS = overall survival, DSS = disease-specific survival, RFS = recurrence-free survival, CRS = clinical risk score response evaluation criteria in solid tumors (RECIST). Using these criteria multiple studies have revealed that patients with CRLM who demonstrate radiographic progression while on treatment have worse OS, DSS, and RFS [86–88]. More recent reports, however, suggest that even with disease progression on chemotherapy, patients who remain resectable may have OS similar to those in whom complete or partial responses are observed [89]. Response to treatment may also be evaluated pathologically. The extent of pathologic response, measured as a percentage of remaining viable tumor cells, has repeatedly been shown to positively correlate with survival and recurrence outcomes [90–92]. More recent investigations suggest that the type of pathologic response, assessed by pathologic tumor regression (fibrosis overgrowing on tumor cells, decreased necrosis, and tumor glands at the periphery), is a better indicator of tumor response to chemotherapy and is an independent predictor of DFS [93]. Molecular risk scores (MRS), generated from gene expression profiling have recently been reported [94]. The MRS appears to have prognostic value in terms of DSS as well as liver recurrence-free survival (LRFS) alone as well as in conjunction with the CRS. Parallel innovations in many different realms; radiology, pathology, molecular biology, and genetics, has led to an insurgence of data regarding CRLM biomarkers. At present, no comprehensive prognostic scoring system incorporating these new potential biomarkers with clinical criteria has been developed. However, it is certain that as cancer care becomes increasingly personalized, integration of clinical and biologic factors will be essential in determining optimal therapeutic interventions.

Resectable Colorectal Liver Metastases

General Approach

Historically, of the over 50 % of patients with CRC who develop CRLM, only 15–20 % will have disease that is amenable to surgical resection [6]. However, as advancements in all areas of treatment of CRLM continue and the boundaries of surgical resection expand, this number is certain to increase. In general, resection for CRLM may be undertaken only when patient operability has been established, resectability confirmed, and FLR adequacy verified. Once the decision to proceed with resection is made, an operative plan, with the aim of removing all tumor(s) with a clear margin while simultaneously preserving as much functional liver parenchyma as feasible, is formulated. The importance of an R0 resection on disease recurrence has been well established; however, what constitutes R0 or negative margins remains a point of some debate. Previously, surgical margins with evidence of microscopic tumor present within 1 cm of the transected parenchyma (R1) were associated with significantly worse clinical outcomes [95, 96]. In attempts to avoid margin positivity, large volume anatomic resections (hemi-hepatectomies and trisegmentectomy) were commonly employed. This approach was bolstered by early studies suggesting that non-anatomic wedge resections (WR) were associated with increased rates of margin positivity when compared to anatomic lobar and segmental resection (AR) and subsequent worse clinical outcome [97, 98]. More recently, multiple large studies call to question the need for a 1 cm negative resection margin and suggest that although a negative margin (R0 resection) is critical, the width of that margin in millimeters is not [99–102]. As the definition of adequate surgical margins changed, surgical practice shifted towards greater use of parenchymal preservation techniques (WR). With this paradigm shift away from large volume resections, concerns arose regarding oncologic outcomes. In recent studies, however, no differences in terms of margin positivity or clinical outcome have been observed between parenchymal preservation WR and AR [18, 103, 104].

Open liver resection is typically performed under low central venous pressure (LCVP) anesthesia (CVP<5 mmHg), through an upper midline or a subcostal hockey stick (right subcostal with midline vertical extension) incision. LCVP anesthesia consists of a prehepatic resection phase where crystalloid administration is limited. CVP is kept at or below 5 mmHg in an attempt to minimize bleeding from hepatic veins during parenchymal transection and facilitate control of venous injury should it occur. Following hepatic transection, a resuscitation phase begins, where patients are returned to euvolemic state. Use of this technique is associated with reduced intraoperative blood loss, decreased perioperative blood transfusion, and has contributed significantly to lower surgical morbidity in patients undergoing liver resection [105]. Upon entering the abdominal cavity a full laparotomy is performed and a search for evidence of EHD is completed and any concerning findings are biopsied and sent for frozen section analysis. The liver is then mobilized, examined by palpation and intraoperative ultrasound (IOUS) is performed to confirm the location of all known tumors, to identify any new lesions (or residual tumor in the setting of neoadjuvant chemotherapy), and to assess tumor location relative to critical structures. Currently some controversy exists as to the overall utility of routine IOUS in the setting of CRLM. Initial studies indicated that IOUS changed operative management plan in 44–67 % of cases [106, 107] and clearly supported its value. However, some argument exists, that in the current era of high-resolution preoperative imaging routine use of IOUS is low yield and should be reserved for use only in cases in which preoperative imaging elicits concerns regarding involvement of critical structures, or in the setting of disappearing CRLM following neoadjuvant chemotherapy [108]. Despite this, IOUS adds little time to the procedure and continues to be performed routinely in most centers.

After a thorough evaluation, if no unexpected findings are encountered, preparation for liver transection begins. In all liver resections control of hepatic inflow structures at the hilum should be obtain such that, if required, a Pringle maneuver may be applied. For tumors in precarious locations, isolation and encirclement of hepatic veins should be considered, as rapid control may be obtained should it be required. For major resections, typically inflow is taken followed by outflow. The line of transection is marked on the liver and parenchymal transection initiated. Many different techniques and instruments have been described for division of hepatic tissue including clamp-crush, ultrasound or harmonic vibration, water jet, and ablative devices none of which is superior to another and use is typically dictated by surgeon preference. Regardless of instrument the goal of parenchymal transection is to safely and efficiently come through the liver tissue with minimal damage to the parenchyma that will remain. Transection should be cautious and all visible vessels and bile ducts formally secured. Blind coagulation of these structures increases the risk of postoperative bleeding and bile leak. At the completion of transection the specimen is checked to ensure grossly negative margins. The raw edge of the liver is assessed for hemostasis and biliostasis, the patient is resuscitated, and the abdomen closed. The evolution of these operative techniques combined with meticulous LCVP anesthesia and fastidious perioperative care, have significantly decreased the morbidity and mortality of liver resection, such that even large volume resection may safely be performed in experienced centers.

Synchronous Colorectal Liver Metastases

CRLM present at the time of primary diagnosis and/or those diagnosed within the following 12 months, are arbitrarily defined as synchronous. Patients presenting in this fashion may have less favorable disease biology and worse clinical outcomes [59, 60]. Simultaneous diagnosis of primary CRC and CRLM represents a unique, often challenging, clinical scenario requiring special consideration and multidisciplinary management [109]. In the setting of resectable synchronous CRLM three different surgical approaches have been described. The "*classic*" approach is most commonly employed and includes upfront resection of the primary CRC followed by subsequent liver resection at a later date. However, as morbidity associated with hepatectomy continues to decrease, there is increased enthusiasm for the use of a "*combined*" resection strategy, in which both the primary tumor and CRLM are removed simultaneously. Most recently, a third approach, referred to as the "*reverse*" or, liver first, approach has been described, in which hepatectomy precedes resection of the primary lesion. With the addition of chemotherapy, many permutations of these general approaches exist [110]. Each approach is associated with specific surgical and oncologic risks and benefits (Table 3). To date, no good clinical evidence exists to suggest superiority of one approach over the other [111].

Staged Resection Strategies

The "classic" or primary first approach is the most commonly employed. Typically patients undergo resection of their primary disease followed by some duration of adjuvant chemotherapy followed by hepatectomy. Proponents of this strategy suggest that it offers significant advantages including: (1) delivery of chemotherapy prior to liver resection ensuring all patients receive some treatment, (2) disease progression on chemotherapy identifies aggressive tumor biology and prevents unnecessary and morbid hepatic resection, (3) assessment of tumor responsiveness

Table 3 Comparison of surgical approaches for management of synchronous colorectal liver metastases

Approach	Advantages	Pitfalls
Classic (primary first)	– delivery of chemotherapy prior to liver resection is more reliable	– chemotherapy induced liver injury
	– test of time to assess tumor biology	– disappearing CRLM
	– in vivo assessment of tumor responsiveness facilitating postoperative therapy	– progression of disease
	– removal of the "source" of subsequent metastases	
Reverse (liver first)	– progression of disease unlikely	– primary CRC related complication (rare)
	– removal of "lethal" disease first	– decreased ability to deliver chemotherapy postoperatively
Simultaneous (combined liver and primary)	– single surgery	– relatively contraindication with major hepatic resection or low rectal resection (LAR/APR)
	– +/– reduced morbidity	– prolonged recovery may delay adjuvant chemotherapy

CRC = colorectal cancer, LAR = low anterior resection, APR = abdominoperineal resection

to chemotherapy prior to resection allows better selection of postoperative chemotherapy, and (4) resection of the primary removes the "source" of subsequent metastases. However, these assumptions for the most part are theoretical in nature and have not been substantiated. For instance, no prospective trial of neoadjuvant or perioperative chemotherapy in the setting of resectable CRLM has shown benefit in terms of overall survival; therefore, whether or not a patient receives, or does not receive, therapy may in fact be a moot point. Furthermore, in randomized trials of modern short course perioperative chemotherapy for resectable CRLM, disease progression is rare (7–8 %) [88, 112], as such identification of biologically aggressive disease is unlikely. Additionally, administration of chemotherapeutic agents such as oxaliplatin and irinotecan prior to liver resection may cause injury to the non-tumoral liver, and potentially increase the risk of subsequently hepatic resection [24]. This staged approach has been extensively evaluated and compared to the alternatives, and in some studies is has been associated with increased combined morbidity [113] while in others it has not [114]. Most importantly, to date, no differences have been observed in terms of long-term clinical outcomes [111]. At present no consensus exists regarding when and in whom this approach for synchronous CRLM is indicated.

In the past it was thought that resection of the primary tumor was essential to prevent complication (bleeding, perforation, obstruction), however, in the era of current combination chemotherapy regimens, these events are rare [115] and leaving the primary tumor in situ is acceptable and safe. Consequently, an alternative staged approach to synchronous CRLM has recently been described. This "reverse" or liver first approach entails resection of the CRLM followed by interval resection of the primary. The initial rationale of liver resection prior to primary resection stems from the belief that it is the burden of disease within the liver that dictates the development of subsequent metastases. Although commonly stated by proponents of a liver first approach, this popular theory lacks scientific evidence. With this strategy chemotherapy is typically given prior to liver resection. Consequently, it has been suggested as an approach well suited to rectal primaries, where evidence exists to support the use of preoperative chemoradiotherapy [116], and in the setting of more advanced CRLM [117] where reducing hepatic tumor burden may improve resectability of the CRLM. Recent systematic reviews evaluating the reverse approach in synchronous CRLM suggests that it is feasible and safe [118] and not inferior to other suggested management strategies [111].

Simultaneous Resection Strategies

Recent advances in perioperative care and surgical technique have reduced morbidity and mortality of both colorectal and liver surgeries, leading many to consider combined surgery in the setting of patients with resectable synchronous CRLM. Numerous retrospective studies published over the last two decades, support this shift in paradigm, and suggest that simultaneous colon and liver resection is not associated with increase morbidity when compared to either resection performed alone [114, 119]. In fact, given the need for a single operation, some suggest a reduction in cumulative morbidity when compared to staged interventions [113]. Simultaneous resection offers the benefits of a single operation without increased morbidity and is a viable option in the majority of patients with synchronous CRLM. There is however debate as to whether simultaneous resection should be undertaken in cases where major hepatectomy would be required to extirpate all disease. Investigations to date are all retrospective and the patients undergoing simultaneous procedures are highly selected with characteristically low volume, unilobar, CRLM [120]. Given this heavy selection bias towards minimal disease and minor resections the safety of simultaneous resection should not arbitrarily be extrapolated to all liver resections, but rather reviewed on a case by case basis. This approach is not appropriate for patients requiring emergency colorectal surgery for complications related to the primary, or in those with underlying liver dysfunction, poor functional status, or where concern regarding surgical margin exist. With the exception of performing major hepatectomy in combination with major pelvic surgery for low rectal cancer (i.e., abdominal perineal resection), in high volume centers, combined resection of synchronous CRLM is increasingly being employed and outcomes appear to be acceptable. Currently, outcomes in highly selected patients, undergoing simultaneous resection are similar to those observed with staged resections and in this setting appear safe and oncologically sound [111]. In general, we favor the combined approach for the great majority of cases. Cases requiring an extensive hepatectomy, especially when combined with complex pelvic resection, require special consideration and appropriateness is determined on a case by case basis after multidisciplinary review.

Multiple and/or Bilobar Colorectal Liver Metastases

The landscape of surgery for CRLM is rapidly changing and advancements in all areas of patient care and disease management continue to allow liberalization of the definition of surgically "resectable" CRLM. In the past, presence of four or more metastases, and/or bilobar disease distribution, were contraindications to resection. However, newer techniques and surgical adjuncts have resulted in a proportion of patients with multiple and/or bilobar disease distribution to undergo successful resection with 5 year disease-free survival (DFS) of up to 20 % and OS rates ranging from 33 to 50 % [18, 121]. Two basic approaches for surgical management in this group have been described, staged and parenchymal sparing. Staged resection typically consists of three phases; (1) clearing of the FLR of all disease, (2) PVE/PVL to induce hypertrophy of the FLR, and (3) interval hemi or extended major hepatectomy to remove all remaining disease. Depending on the center, chemotherapy may be given before, between, and/or after resections. The major limitation of this strategy is the need for multiple surgeries to achieve complete resection. It has been shown that between 20 and 50 % of patients fail to complete the second stage of resection and survival outcomes of this cohort are no different from those patients receiving palliative chemotherapy alone [122, 123]. These findings raise concern as to the regular use of this strategy as many patients are exposed to the potential harms of surgical intervention with no obvious benefit. However, failure to complete the second stage of two staged resection is reportedly lower (12–30 %) in modern series from specialized centers [124–126] and without this attempt there is no chance of complete resection. Conversely, parenchymal sparing surgery entails a single curative intent operation with treatment of all sites of disease using multiple segmental or sub-segmental resections WR with or without ablative techniques. Some studies suggest increase risk of liver recurrence with this approach as compared to more extensive resections. This may be due, in part, to the increased use of ablative therapies to achieve an RO resection, which has been associated with increased local recurrence when compared to resection [121]. However, this increase recurrence appears to be size dependent. A recent review of over 300 CRLM treated with ablation suggest that tumor size <1 cm is associated with 92 % local control rate at 2 years and is highly effective treatment for these lesions [127] Furthermore, it is of note that patients treated with parenchymal sparing techniques are inherently different, and clinical outcomes are not directly comparable to those in whom extensive resection achieves complete tumor removal. In general, if complete extirpation of disease can be achieved 5 year OS of 40–50 % have been observed [18, 121]. Regardless of approach, morbidity associated with both of these strategies is high but acceptable, and similar to other liver surgeries, morbidity remains low.

Despite some limitations, in this cohort of patients with advanced CRLM, surgery is feasible however controversy exists as to the routine implementation and multi-disciplinary planning is essential to optimize patient outcomes.

Chemotherapy for Resectable Colorectal Liver Metastases

Adjuvant Systemic Chemotherapy

Depending on selection criteria, approximately 70 % of patients undergoing complete resection of CRLM will experience recurrence. Half of these patients will have the liver as the only site of disease recurrence [128]. As such there is a strong rationale behind the desire to provide adjuvant systemic therapy in this setting with the goal of improving long-term outcomes. To date, several retrospective studies have suggested benefit of adjuvant systemic therapy. In a review of 792 patients by Parks et al. [129] adjuvant chemotherapy was associated with significant improvement in OS ($p=0.007$) and was an independent predictor of outcomes for all categories of clinical risk. This finding was mirrored in a retrospective review by Figueras et al. [130], where patients receiving adjuvant chemotherapy had an associated longer OS (RR 0.3, $p<0.001$). Despite impressive retrospective findings, similar outcomes have not been observed in randomized trials. To date, four trials of adjuvant systemic therapy alone in patients with resectable CRLM have been completed [131–134], all of which failed to show a significant benefit in terms of OS. In 2008, Mitry et al. published a pooled analysis of 278 patients with resectable CRLM from two randomized trials of 5FU based adjuvant systemic chemotherapy versus surgery alone and found no differences in terms of PFS or OS between the groups [135] Furthermore, recent randomized evidence published by Ychou et al., revealed no difference in DFS between patients randomized to receive adjuvant FOLFIRI versus those receiving 5FU/LV [134]. Direct evidence to support the use of adjuvant systemic chemotherapy for resectable CRLM is lacking and its usefulness in this setting is debated. Proponents of adjuvant therapy note several limitations to the interpretation of the aforementioned trial findings including, variability in the actual delivery of chemotherapy leading some trials to be underpowered, heterogeneity of baseline disease characteristics, and use of chemotherapy considered inadequate by current standards [128]. These limitations call to question the clinical applicability of these trial results in the modern era and use of adjuvant systemic therapy in patients with resectable CRLM is commonly employed.

Neoadjuvant Systemic Chemotherapy

Chemotherapy delivered prior to liver resection in patients with upfront resectable CRLM is controversial. Proponents of this approach suggest that neoadjuvant chemotherapy with modern drug combinations (5FU + Oxaliplatin/Irinotecan with or without targeted antibodies) has significant advantages, including; (1) facilitation of hepatic resection by reducing tumor size, (2) eradication of micrometastatic occult disease, (3) avoidance of unnecessary surgery for those who progress, (4) identification of tumor chemosensitivity prior to resection [128]. However, opponents suggest that administration of toxic chemotherapy in the setting of CRLM that are already resectable introduces the unnecessary risk of chemotherapy induced liver injury and increased perioperative morbidity [136]. Additionally, neoadjuvant therapy may result in "disappearance" of some tumors. This poses a significant challenge for surgeons, because although these tumors are not evident clinically, viable cancer cells are likely still present, and failure to resect these sites is associated with high rates of recurrence [137]. Furthermore, the argument that neoadjuvant treatment allows assessment of tumor biology is likely overstated. In a recent systematic review evaluating 23 different studies of neoadjuvant therapy in the setting of resectable CRLM median rate of disease progression while on treatment was 15 % (range 0–37 %) [138] whilst randomized trials of modern chemotherapy regimens found rates to be even lower (7–8 %) [88, 112] suggesting that the ability to select out "bad biology" with preoperative chemotherapy is uncommon. Neoadjuvant chemotherapy may also result in liver parenchymal injury that appears to portend higher postoperative morbidity [136, 139] Moreover, although tumor progression while on chemotherapy is associated with increased recurrence; there are conflicting data on the impact on OS and many series show no differences in long term outcome if completely resected [89, 140].

To date no randomized trial addressing neoadjuvant systemic chemotherapy alone for resectable CRLM has been completed. Its use has primarily been extrapolated from the initial findings of a single randomized trial of perioperative systemic chemotherapy (chemotherapy before and after resection). In this trial [112], Nordlinger et al. randomized 364 patients with resectable CRLM to surgery alone versus surgery + perioperative chemotherapy (six cycles preoperative 5FU-LV/oxaliplatin FOLFOX and six cycles FOLFOX postoperatively) with a primary end point of progression-free survival (PFS). Intent to treat analysis revealed a borderline absolute improvement in PFS of 7.3 % at 3 years in the treatment arm. Given these findings, use of chemotherapy perioperatively for resectable CRLM was considered standard practice. More recently, however, the long-term results of this trial were published [139]. No difference in median OS was observed between study arms at 8.5 years of follow-up (61.3 months (95 % CI 51.0–83.4) perioperative chemotherapy group versus 54.3 months (41.9–79.4) in the surgery-only group, $p = 0.34$). The authors suggest that despite the lack of OS benefit, the improvement in PFS with perioperative FOLFOX is evidence enough to warrant perioperative treatment in patients with CRLM.

Current practice guidelines typically recommend 6 months of perioperative systemic therapy in the setting of clinically resectable CRLM, however there is no indication or recommendation as to when this should be given, reflecting the lack of direct evidence for a single treatment regimen. It does appear that regardless of timing (neoadjuvant, adjuvant, or perioperative), arguments for and against the use of systemic chemotherapy in patients with resectable CRLM (Table 4) exist. At present, no study of chemotherapy in the setting of resectable

Table 4 Comparison of potential advantages and disadvantages of systemic chemotherapy for resectable colorectal liver metastases

Strategy	Advantages	Disadvantages
Neoadjuvant	– more reliable delivery of chemotherapy before liver resection	– chemotherapy induced liver injury
	– eradication of micro-metastases	– disappearing CRLM
	– in vivo assessment of tumor responsiveness to chemotherapy	– disease progression
	– assess tumor biology (avoidance of unnecessary surgery)	– may delay surgical recovery
	– facilitate/minimize hepatic resection	
Adjuvant	– treatment of potential micro-metastatic disease in the remnant liver	– chemotherapy more difficult to tolerate postoperatively
	– avoids risk of preoperative chemotherapy induced liver injury	– extensive surgery and/or complications may delay initiation
		– inability to assess in vivo tumor responsiveness to chemotherapy
Perioperative	– as per above (adjuvant + neoadjuvant)	– as per above (adjuvant + neoadjuvant)

CRLM has shown a benefit in terms of OS. Despite this, the large majority of patients with CRLM will receive chemotherapy at some time point in the course of their disease.

Disappearing Colorectal Liver Metastases

Modern combination chemotherapy regimens for metastatic CRC are associated with tumor response rates (RR) of over 50 %. Enthusiasm for the preoperative administration of these agents in patients with CRLM is increasing. This has led to the relatively new clinical problem of "disappearing" colorectal liver metastases (DCRLM). DCRLM may broadly be defined as CRLM that undergo complete radiologic response to chemotherapy such that they are no longer visible on cross-sectional imaging (Fig. 3). Risk of developing DCRLM is dependent on tumor size prior to treatment (<2 cm increase risk) and duration of preoperative chemotherapy [142]. With current preoperative treatment approximately 5–25 % of patients will develop DCRLM [137]. The wide variation in reported rates reflects the fact that diagnosis is dependent on the type of cross sectional imaging utilized to evaluate the liver. MRI has been shown to have greater ability to detect and differentiate lesions <1 cm, and with fat suppression techniques is more sensitive than other imaging modalities following the delivery of preoperative chemotherapy [33]. Not surprisingly, DCRLM diagnosed with preoperative MRI are associated with a decreased risk of finding residual tumor in the resected specimen or recurrence if the lesion is

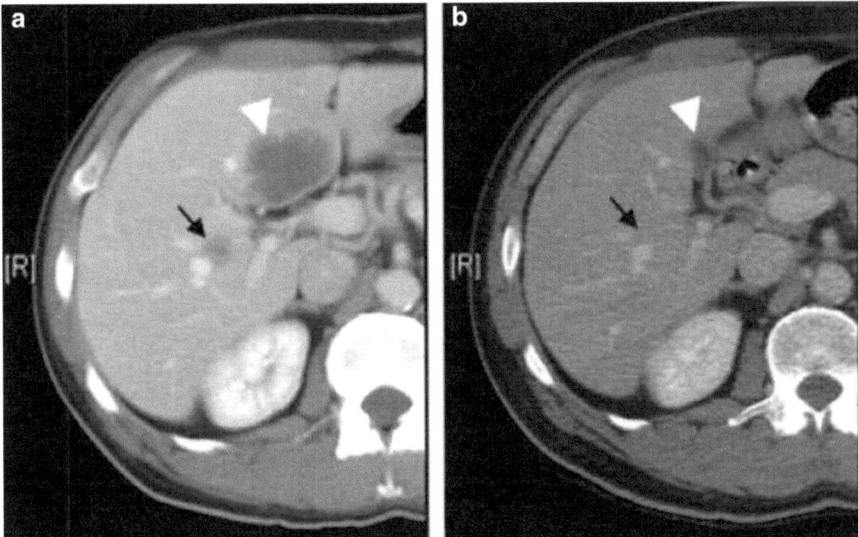

Fig. 3 CT images of colorectal cancer liver metastases at the time of diagnosis (**a**) and after 4 months of neoadjuvant chemotherapy with 5FU/LV + Irinotecan (**b**) *White arrowhead* denotes largest metastases with dramatic response on post therapy CT, *black arrowhead* denotes smaller metastases and subsequent "disappearance" on post therapy CT. *Reprinted with permission from Auer* et al. *Cancer 2010;116:1502–9* [141]

not resected [141]. Other predictors of a true complete response include normalization of CEA, and use of hepatic arterial infusion chemotherapy [141]. The clinical conundrum these lesions present is related to the fact that at present, regardless of imaging modality, complete radiologic response (CR) is poorly correlated with complete pathologic response and in fact, 25–45 % of lesions described as having a CR preoperatively are found to have residual macroscopic disease at the time of operation. Furthermore, disease recurrence, in cases where sites of DCRLM are left in situ, is significantly higher compared to cases where all site of DCRLM are resected ($p=0.04$) [142]. Currently, no standard of care for the management of DCRLM exists. Some suggest an interval period of surveillance to delineate the durability of response at site of DCRLM, with treatment reserved for those sites where lesions reveal themselves. More commonly, given the absence of a reliable predictor of durable response at the site of DCRLM, poor correlation between clinical and pathological response, and high rates of recurrence when left in situ, all sites of visible disease on pre-chemotherapy imaging are resected [143]. At present, a simple algorithm to manage DCRLM may include the following; CRLM that achieve CR on follow-up CT scan should be further evaluated with MRI (higher sensitivity), if lesions are not visualized on MRI the morbidity and extent of resection required to remove all sites must be considered. If resection is feasible with minimal morbidity this should be carried out; however, in those patients in whom resection of all sites would entail major complex resection a period of observation may be reasonable. Rapid advances in imaging technology and novel approaches to assessing tumor response to preoperative chemotherapy are likely to alter our management of DCRLM in the future.

Unresectable CRLM

General Approach

The majority of patients with CRLM will have disease that is not amenable to resection at the time of presentation (70–80 %) [144]. Despite significant advances in medical therapy, long-term survival in patients treated with systemic therapy alone is poor (<5 %). Alternatively, 10-year survival of patients undergoing complete surgical resection may be as high as 20 % [23]. Given that resection is associated with significantly improved long-term outcomes the primary goal of treatment, in appropriately selected patients, is down staging of disease and conversion to resection. In general this requires upfront use of the best available systemic therapy and fastidious surveillance of disease with surgical intervention as soon as feasible. The addition of specific liver directed therapies such as, hepatic arterial infusion chemotherapy (HAI), ablation, embolization, and stereotactic body radiation therapy (SBRT) to the treatment armamentarium may be useful in some patients with unresectable liver dominant disease.

Chemotherapy is the standard first-line therapy in the management of patients with unresectable CRLM. First-line therapy in the metastatic setting typically includes infusional 5FU/LV with oxaliplatin and/or irinotecan (FOLFOX, FOLFIRI, FOLFIRINOX). Overall clinical response rates (RR) with modern therapy range from 45 to 70 % [145]. Some patients that have an objective clinical response may become candidates for curative intent surgery. In a pooled analysis of 196 patients from three different prospective trials of FOLFOXIRI (5FU/LV + Oxaliplatin + Irinotecan) 37 (19 %) were able to undergo curative intent resection [23]. The median number of pre hepatectomy chemotherapy cycles was 11 and duration of treatment was 5.5 months. Despite this aggressive chemotherapy regimen, morbidity rate was acceptable at 27 % and 90 day mortality 0 %. The authors conclude that, in patients who are down-staged with chemotherapy, surgical resection is acceptable and safe. Multiple other series have been published regarding rates of conversion to resection with systemic therapy and depending on the type/duration of chemotherapy, the extent of disease, and the definition of resectability, rates of conversion vary from 6 to 38 % [145].

Strategies for complete tumor extirpation in this group are complex and often require staged resections or major hepatectomies, as well as the use of surgical adjuncts such as ablation. Given the need for more extensive surgery and use of non-resectional techniques concerns exists as to the impact of this on long-term outcomes. However, in a study by Masi et al. [23] the 5- and 8-year survival rates of those patients converted to resection were 42 % and 33 %, respectively, and median

OS was 40 months. This was significantly greater than OS observed in the group who had an objective response to chemotherapy but remained unresectable (23 months, $p<0.001$), as well as those who did not have a response (14 months, $p<0.001$). Furthermore, a recent review of over 10,000 patients undergoing resection of CRLM from the LiverMetSurvey registry, suggests that regardless of whether CRLM were resectable at presentation or down-staged to resectable with conversion therapy, survival is similar, so long as all disease is removed [143].

These results are encouraging; however, the majority of patients treated with standard first-line chemotherapy will not be candidates for resection and will inevitably develop disease progression. Second-line systemic therapy is associated with notoriously poor RR. Patients failing first-line irinotecan therapy treated with oxaliplatin-based regimens have RR ranging from 4 to 10 %. Similarly, failure of first-line oxaliplatin treated with second-line irinotecan is associated with RR of 12–15 % [146]. Addition of anti-VEGF (bevacizumab) therapy to modern chemotherapy regimens is associated with only modest improvements in RR (12–15 % vs. 4–10 %) over chemotherapy alone in the second-line setting [145]. On the other hand, in a retrospective review of 151 patients with unresectable CRLM who progressed on first-line therapy, subsequent treatment with anti-EGFR (cetuximab) and chemotherapy was associated with conversion to resection in 18 % of patients [147]. Although less likely to observe an objective response to therapy in the second-line setting there does appear to be a small fraction of patients in whom response occurs and subsequent resection may be achieved. This is not the case for most and those who remain unresectable following second-line chemotherapy should be offered novel treatment on clinical trials.

Colorectal Liver Metastases with Extrahepatic Spread

The presence of EHD in the setting of CRLM is a poor prognosticator and in the past was an absolute contraindication to resection [148]. However, innovation in the surgical and medical treatment of metastatic CRC has resulted in an expansion of criteria for resection with the goal of improving long-term outcomes. Although debate exists as to the role of surgical resection for patient with CRLM and EHD, multiple single institution series have been reported suggesting that in appropriately selected patients, with minimal EHD in which complete resection/ablation can be achieved, survival outcomes are better than those observed in patients treated with chemotherapy alone [149, 150]. It is of note however, that patients amenable to complete resection of both liver and EHD are not directly comparable to their unresectable counterparts. In a recent systematic review of 1142 patients with CRLM and concomitant EHD in whom resection was completed median DFS was 12 months, OS 30 months and 5 year OS 19 % [138].

Not only the presence of EHD but its location has been shown to impact outcomes (Table 5). CRLM with lung metastases appear to have prolonged OS compared to all other EHD sites (5 year OS 27 %). Furthermore, in terms of abdominal

Table 5 Outcomes of resection for colorectal liver metastases with concomitant extrahepatic disease stratified by site

EHD site	Incidence (as % of all EHD)	Median overall survival (months)	3-year survival (%)	5-year survival (%)
Lung	33 (3–51)	41 (32–46)	60 (40–80)	27 (0–33)
Lymph Node[a]	23 (15–68)	25 (19–48)	33 (20–56)	17 (0–27)
Peritoneal	15 (12–35)	25 (18–32)	28 (19–41)	8 (0–30)
>1 EHD Site	11	17 (13–25)	25 (10–28)	7 (0–28)

[a]Lymph nodes included: portocaval, celiac, retroperitoneal/aortocaval
EHD = extrahepatic disease
Data obtained from: Carpizo et al. Ann Surg Oncol. 2009;16(8):2138–46 and Pulitano et al. Ann Surg Oncol. 2011;18(5):1380–8

lymph node involvement, not all nodes are created equal. Pulitano et al. [151] found that survival outcomes were significantly worse in patients undergoing resection of aortocaval lymph nodes as compared to hepatic pedicular nodes (5 year OS 7 % vs. 27 %, respectively, $p < 0.0001$). Similarly, more than a single site of EHD has consistently been associated with very poor long-term outcomes. Disease recurrence in patients undergoing resection of CRLM and EHD sites is common and occurs in almost all patients; however, salvage medical and/or surgical intervention is often feasible. Overall, patients with CRLM and concomitant EHD have a worse prognosis than their counterparts with no EHD. However, surgical resection in patients with limited EHD, amenable to complete resection/ablation, is associated with improved long-term outcomes and may be considered in highly selected patients.

Recurrent Colorectal Liver Metastases

Over the past two decades, advances in surgical and medical treatment of CRLM have undoubtedly improved survival outcomes; however, recurrence of disease remains a considerable problem occurring in 70–85 % of patients [152]. Salvage therapies in this setting include; repeat surgery, locoregional interventions, and chemotherapy. A recent systematic review of the literature suggests that 10–15 % of patients with recurrent CRLM are candidates for repeat hepatectomy [153], however, concerns regarding the safety and overall efficacy of repeat hepatectomy exist. A second operative intervention requiring repeat exposure of a friable regenerated, often chemotherapy treated, liver with distorted vasculobiliary anatomy at the porta hepatis is obviously challenging. However, in high volume centers repeat intervention has been associated with morbidity and mortality rates comparable to those observed with initial hepatectomy. Additionally, the ability to achieve a negative margin does not appear to be compromised, with R0 resection being achieved in 77–96 % of cases [154]. Oncologic and technical criteria used to select patients for initial hepatectomy should be employed in identifying appropriate candidates for repeat operation. Short time interval between initial hepatectomy and recurrence and/or recurrence while on systemic therapy are poor prognosticators, and although not absolute contraindications to repeat resection should be approached with caution. In terms of survival, repeat hepatectomy for recurrent CRLM is associated with median OS of 35 months (19–56), 3 year OS 55 % (11–82), and 5 year OS 42 % (31–73) [155]. Nevertheless, recurrence following repeat hepatectomy is common (65–70 %). There is general agreement that systemic therapy should also be employed in the setting of recurrent CRLM, regardless of resectability, and most patients (>80 %) will receive chemotherapy [153]. At present no consensus exists as to the timing of administration relative to surgical intervention (neoadjuvant, adjuvant, perioperative). Recurrent CRLM are common and in those patients deemed appropriate, repeat hepatectomy is safe and is associated with acceptable survival outcomes.

Other Locoregional Therapies for Colorectal Liver Metastases

Ablation

Radiofrequency ablation (RFA) is the most well studied and most commonly used form of ablation in the treatment of CRLM. It may be performed via open, laparoscopic, or percutaneous approaches; furthermore, it may be performed alone, or in combination with open hepatic resection. Regardless of approach the premise is the same; under image guidance probes are strategically inserted into the lesion and alternating current radiofrequency energy is delivered to the tumor. This results in the development of increasing temperatures in the tumor tissue, leading to protein denaturation, tissue coagulation, and tissue desiccation which limits current flow and stops further ablation [156]. Technical limitations to the application of RFA include, potential injury to adjacent tissues, ineffectiveness in tumors >3 cm, and ineffectiveness in tumors adjacent to large blood vessels which act as heat sinks and limit thermal damage to surrounding cells [157]. Local recurrence following RFA ranges from 10 to 50 % and is higher than after resection. In a recent meta-analysis tumor size >3 cm and percutaneous approach were independently associated with higher rates of recurrence [158]. This latter finding is likely related to better tumor visualization and subsequent probe placement with IOUS and surgical mobilization of the liver. Survival data pertaining to RFA is difficult to compare to resection given the inherent heterogeneity of patients and tumor biology secondary to selection bias. At present, there is general consensus that, given the increased rates of local recurrence, RFA should not be used as an alternative to definitive surgical resection. It is, however, considered reasonable as a salvage treatment for recurrence following resection, as an adjunct to facilitated staged resections, and in patients with liver only disease who are unable to tolerate resection [159].

More recently the use of microwave ablation (MWA) has been described for treatment of CRLM. This form of ablation is administered in a similar fashion to RFA. MWA, however, is dependent on high frequency electromagnetic radiation to create thermal tissue damage and subsequent coagulation necrosis. The advantages and disadvantages of MWA relate to the fact that it employs a more powerful energy source than RFA. This form of ablation is associated with less tissue charring, reduced heat sink effect, and larger ablation zones created more rapidly. However, the use of a greater energy source may lead to higher rates of injury to adjacent tissues [157]. Complication rates reported in series of MWA for liver tumors range from 6 to 30 % [127, 160] and local recurrence rates range from 3 to 50 %; likely reflecting the heterogeneity of tumor types included in most series. Similarly, interpretation of reported survival rates is inappropriate given the variety of different tumor types treated. It does, however, appear that MWA is associated with similar rates of complication as RFA, and recurrence rates are at least equivalent, as such indication for MWA in CRLM is similar to those discussed for RFA.

External Beam Radiation

Historically, external beam radiation was not used to treat liver tumors as the risk of radiation induced liver injury was prohibitive. More recently, improvement in the planning and delivery of radiation allows for more focused delivery of large doses of radiation with high precision and accuracy to targeted organs. This is referred to as stereotactic body radiation (SBRT) [161]. More specifically, in the setting of CRLM, SBRT may be used to deliver ablative radiation doses directly to metastases, in few fractions, with precise radiation dose gradients, minimizing injury to surrounding liver [159]. To date the use of SBRT in the treatment of CRLM has not been well studied, however, an obvious advantage is its noninvasive nature compared to other local therapies. A retrospective review of 65 patients with CRLM treated with SBRT, suggested factors associated with improved local control included increase dose per fraction and total radiation dose [162]. The majority of investigations with SBRT have included multiple tumor types and focused primarily on the safety and feasibility of delivering adequate doses of therapy to tumors while limiting toxicity to surrounding tissues. However, results from a recent well-designed dose escalation study of SBRT for malignant liver tumors are encouraging, revealing a RR of 90 % and a 2-year local control rate of 100 % [163]. Use of SBRT for CRLM is in its infancy, and at present may be offered in specialized centers after other standard treatment options have been exhausted.

Hepatic Artery Infusion Chemotherapy

The rationale for delivery of therapy via the hepatic artery (HA) for treatment of CRLM is based on two primary concepts; (1) in many patients the liver is the only site of metastatic disease, and (2) the primary blood supply of CRLM >1 mm in size is the HA whereas normal liver parenchyma is supplied predominantly by the portal vein [164]. Direct administration of chemotherapy to the liver via the HA allows the delivery of higher concentration of cytotoxic drugs to cancer cells while at the same time exposure to normal hepatocytes and systemic circulation is limited.

Hepatic artery infusion chemotherapy (HAI) is typically administered via an arterial catheter inserted into the gastroduodenal artery (GDA) with the tip at the HA/GDA junction. Infusion systems consist of either a surgically placed subcutaneous port or continuous infusion pump, placed via laparotomy. Floxuridine (FUDR) is the most commonly used agent for HAI because it has over 90 % first pass extraction in the liver which leads to a 400-fold increase in concentration as compared to systemic circulation, it limits systemic exposure and toxicity allowing for concomitant administration of systemic chemotherapy [165]. However, FUDR is not approved for use in many countries; consequently, other agents with less favorable regional pharmacokinetic profiles have been utilized including, 5-FU, mitomycin-c, and oxaliplatin. Although systemic toxicity is reduced with HAI chemotherapy overall complication rates are concerning. Technical complications related to catheter, or pump, occur in up to 20 % of patients. Surgeon inexperience, as well as catheter insertion into a vessel other than the GDA, have been found to be independent risk factors for technical complication [166]. These complications are typically salvageable (80 %) and therapy can still be delivered. Hepatotoxicity in the form of liver enzyme elevation with therapy is a common complication that is most often rectified with dose modification. It is essential that patients treated with HAI be followed fastidiously for clinical and/or laboratory signs of complication so that immediate modification can be made. Biliary sclerosis is the most feared complication of HAI chemotherapy, and reported rates range from 1 to 26 % depending on the study. However, in modern series from experienced centers where rigorous follow-up is employed the observed risk is less than 5 % [167]. Furthermore, addition of dexamethasone has been shown to reduce this risk and is routinely combined with FUDR for this purpose [168].

Use of HAI chemotherapy in the setting of unresectable CRLM has been studied extensively. Multiple trials have been published comparing the use of HAI chemotherapy alone to systemic therapies. The results of these trials consistently report improved tumor RR in the HAI arm compared to the systemic therapy arms. However, despite the improvements in RR, only the CALGB trial found an improvement in OS with HAI chemotherapy. This trial design was optimal when compared to others in that no cross over was allowed between groups and unlike many other trials HAI FUDR was employed as oppose to HAI 5FU. In this trial 135 patients were randomized to HAI FUDR or systemic therapy with 5FU/LV. Median OS was significantly different between the two arms (median OS 24.4 months HAI FUDR vs. 20 months 5FU/LV, $p=0.003$) [169]. Pooled meta-analysis of these trials found RR for HAI chemotherapy to be 43 % in comparison to 18 % in the systemic chemotherapy arms; however, no overall survival benefit was obtained, mean weighted median OS were 15.9 months for the HAI group compared to 12.4 months in the systemic therapy group ($p=0.24$) [168]. The implications of these trial findings are difficult to employ clinically as the systemic therapy arms of these trials consisted of outdated chemotherapy regimens that would be considered inadequate by today's standards.

More recently phase I and II trials of HAI chemotherapy in combination with modern system chemotherapy have been completed in patients with advanced unresectable CRLM who have failed first-line systemic therapies. Combination of HAI FUDR with systemic irinotecan was associated with RR or 74 %, median time to progression (TTP) of 8.1 months, and median OS of 17.2 months [168]. A second trial of HAI FUDR in combination with oxaliplatin based systemic therapy was similarly impressive with RR of 87 % in the HAI FUDR + FOLFOX group and 90 % in the HAI FUDR + oxaliplatin/irinotecan group, median OS was 22 months and 36 months, respectively [170]. Considering RR observed with second-line systemic therapy are at best 12–15 %, the results of these trials, although small and non-randomized suggest that HAI FUDR in combination with modern systemic chemotherapy regimens is safe and is associated with improved RR over systemic therapy alone in the second-line setting. Perhaps of more clinical significance than RR, the use of HAI chemotherapy in combination with irinotecan/oxaliplatin in 49 patients with technically unresectable CRLM was associated with conversion to resection in 23 (47 %) and DFS following resection was 7.6 months [145]. These findings were further confirmed by a prospective phase II trial of 49 previously treated patients with unresectable CRLM treated with HAI with systemic therapy. The primary end point of conversion to resection was achieved in 23 (47 %) of patients at a median of 6 months of therapy and on multivariate analysis conversion was the only factor associated with improved OS and PFS [171] Furthermore, a retrospective review of 373 patients treated with HAI chemotherapy and modern systemic therapy over two decades at MSKCC found that 25 % of patients were converted to resectable disease which was associated with median OS of 59 months. This was significantly higher than that observed in those patients in whom resection was not feasible [172].

Multiple randomized trials have been conducted evaluating adjuvant HAI chemotherapy following liver resection. In general, the findings have been consistent with HAI + systemic therapy providing significant improvements in DFS without concomitant improvements in OS [128]. To date, the only trial in which an improvement in OS was observed was published in 1999 by Kemeny et al. [173] in which 156 patients with resected CRLM were randomized to receive six cycles of adjuvant systemic 5FU +/− LV with or without HAI FUDR. In this trial OS at 2 years was 86 % in the HAI group and was significantly greater than the systemic therapy alone group (72 % OS ($p = 0.03$)). PFS was not different between groups (57 % HAI vs. 42 % systemic ($p = 0.07$)), respectively. These survival benefits, did not persist at a median of 10.3 years FUP, however, the trial was not powered to assess this. All of these adjuvant trials were completed in an era where best systemic chemotherapy was 5FU/LV and there is question as to the applicability in the current clinical setting. More recent single arm Phase I/II trials of HAI combined with modern systemic chemotherapy (oxaliplatin/irinotecan) have shown 5-year OS rates of 59 % [168]. Furthermore, a trial of adjuvant HAI + modern systemic chemotherapy with or without bevacizumab revealed 4 year OS of 85 % and RFS of 46 % [168]. Retrospective review of over 1000 patients undergoing hepatectomy for CRLM at a single institution found use of HAI chemotherapy to be an independent predictor of improved OS (HR 0.64; 95 % CI, 0.51–0.81; $p<0.001$) [174]. Furthermore, House et al. reported on 250 patients who underwent hepatectomy and received postoperative FOLFOX or FOLFIRI alone or FOLFOX or FOLFIRI + HAI FUDR, 5 year OS was 72 % in the HAI arm vs. 52 % in the systemic arm ($p<0.004$) [175]. Despite consistent findings of improved DFS, and suggestion of OS benefits from retrospective series, use of HAI in the adjuvant setting is highly controversial and its application is relegated to a few select centers.

Embolization

A second means by which the HA can be exploited for the treatment of CRLM is in the form of embolization. The most common type of embolization therapy in the setting of CRLM is chemoembolization [176]. Traditional chemoembolization consists of infusion of chemotherapeutic agent directly into the segmental artery supplying the CRLM followed by injection of an embolic agent to induce stasis and prevent washout (TACE). For CRLM a variety of drugs have been used for infusion, including cisplatin, 5FU, mitomycin, and doxorubicin all of which have historically been associated with minimal success. More recently, drug-eluting beads have been introduced for use in chemoembolization (DEB TACE) [177]. These beads can be loaded with chemotherapeutic agents, such as irinotecan (DEBIRI), and because they cause permanent embolization can provide prolonged local drug delivery. Although the role of TACE is well defined in the setting of hepatocellular carcinoma little data regarding its use in CRLM exists and its role in this setting is poorly defined. Over the past 20 years multiple small single center phase I trials have been completed with TACE for unresectable CRLM, typically as a salvage treatment in patients failing standard first or second-line therapy. Median OS observed with standard TACE in this setting ranges from 7 to 14 months and is associated with acceptable complications and minimal toxicities [176]. To date a single randomized trial of DEBIRI alone versus systemic FOLFIRI as first-line treatment in patients with unresectable CRLM has been conducted [178]. 74 patients were randomized to receive DEBIRI alone or systemic FOLFIRI. The primary end point of the trial was survival. At a total follow-up of 50 months, median OS in the DEBIRI arm was significantly longer (22 months) compared to the FOLFIRI group (15 months) ($p=0.031$). PFS was also longer in the DEBIRI group compared to the FOLFIRI group (7 months vs. 4 months, $p=0.006$). These findings suggest an advantage of local DEBIRI therapy over systemic FOLFIRI in the setting of unresectable CRLM. However, these results should be interpreted with caution as this was a highly select group with liver only disease effecting <50 % of the liver in the setting of a very small trial subject to significant risk of statistical error. At present chemoembolization therapy in CRLM is typically reserved as a salvage treatment following failure of standard therapies. Future trials of DEBIRI combined with systemic therapy in the unresectable setting are warranted.

Even with significant improvements in RR with new chemotherapeutics and targeted agents for metastatic CRC, there are a proportion of patients who have disease that is resistant to all current forms of chemotherapy. Treatment options in this group are limited. Recently, the use of liver directed radioembolization with yttrium-90 (Y-90) has been considered as a possible treatment for unresectable chemo resistant CRLM. In a recent systematic review of 979 patients with CRLM treated with Y-90 the median number of treatment lines prior to Y-90 was 4, highlighting the last resort nature of this intervention [179]. In terms of RR, objective response was seen in up to 71.5 % of patients with 17.5 % having disease progression. On average 70 % of patients also received systemic therapy following Y-90. The pooled median PFS was 4.9 months (3.4–9.3) and OS was 12 month (8.3–16). Acute toxicity was common, but all were low grade with no need for intervention. Amongst the studies included there are no randomized trials; furthermore, there is significant heterogeneity of patients and techniques, such that definitive conclusions are impossible. However, it does appear that radioembolization with Y-90 as a salvage treatment in a sub select group of patients with chemo resistant disease is safe and may provide some benefit in this notoriously difficult to treat population.

Minimally Invasive Surgery for Colorectal Liver Metastases

Traditionally, surgery for CRLM has been completed in an open fashion, where access to the abdomen is achieved through an upper midline or hockey stick incision. Morbidity associated with this incision can be significant and lead to increased length of hospitalization. Laparoscopic surgery offers the benefit of smaller incisions, which may be beneficial in terms of reducing morbidity associated with liver resection. Innovation in laparoscopic equipment over the last decade has facilitated the performance of liver resection laparoscopically.

Prior to engaging in laparoscopic resections, it is essential for all liver surgeons to first become facile and comfortable in performing open liver surgery. Furthermore, a high level of laparoscopic skill is required [180]. The steps of resection do not differ from the open approach; however, they can be more challenging given the limited degree of motion related to laparoscopic instruments and port placement. Despite the increased technical difficulty of laparoscopic hepatectomy (LH) morbidity and mortality appear to be similar to open approaches. However, to date, cases amenable to laparoscopic resection are typically limited to minimal resections in which tumors are in accessible locations (i.e., left lateral segment). Major hepatic resection or resection for bilobar disease laparoscopically remains uncommon. The only consistently reported benefit to LH has been a decrease in hospital length of stay [181]. Given the minimal benefit of LH it is imperative that LH results in equivalent oncologic outcomes when compared to the accepted standard open procedure. In a retrospective matched cohort study of LH versus open hepatectomy for the treatment of CRLM OS at 1-, 3-, and 5-year was 97, 82, 64 % in the LH group and 97, 70, 56 %, in the open group and was not different between groups ($p=0.32$).

Evaluation of DFS similarly revealed no differences between LH and open hepatectomy ($p = 0.12$) [182], suggesting that oncologic results of LH for CRLM are equivalent to the open approach. As suggested above, one of the major limitations in LH is technical in nature. With long straight instruments, and an inability to reproduce wrist movements at the tips, some maneuvers are impossible. Robotic surgery may combat this issue with the ability to recapitulate normal hand and wrist movements. To date little has been published on the use of robotic surgery in the management of CRLM. Currently, open hepatectomy is the gold standard for resection of CRLM; however, LH is a reasonable alternative in high volume experienced centers.

Summary

Significant evolution in the management of CRLM has occurred over the last two decades. Improvement in disease detection, refinement of surgical techniques, development of more effective chemotherapy, and greater use of local adjuncts, have resulted in more patients, with greater disease burden, surviving longer. Surgery remains the only treatment option with the potential to cure CRLM. In the past, this was an option in only a minority of cases. Ongoing refinement and optimization of newer therapies in the future will likely increase the number of patient with CRLM in whom resection is possible and ultimately improve outcomes. At present many controversies exist regarding optimal treatment of CRLM, and as the number of treatment options/regimens continue to expand, so do will the controversy surrounding implementation. Overall, management of CRLM is becoming increasingly complex and the landscape is rapidly changing, as such ongoing evaluation of short and long term outcomes is essential.

Financial Disclosures/Conflicts of Interest None

References

1. GLOBOCAN 2012 v1.0, Cancer Incidence and Mortality Worldwide: IARC CancerBase. [Internet]. International Agency for Research on Cancer. 2013. Accessed on July 14, 2014. Available from: http://globocan.iarc.fr
2. U.S. Cancer Statistics Working Group. United States cancer statistics: 1999–2010 incidence and mortality web-based report. Atlanta, GA: U.S. Department of Health and Human Services, Centers for Disease Control and Prevention, and National Cancer Institute; 2013.
3. van der Pool AE, Damhuis RA, Ijzermans JN, de Wilt JH, Eggermont AM, Kranse R, et al. Trends in incidence, treatment and survival of patients with stage IV colorectal cancer: a population-based series. Colorectal Dis. 2012;14(1):56–61.
4. Siegel RL, Ward EM, Jemal A. Trends in colorectal cancer incidence rates in the United States by tumor location and stage, 1992-2008. Cancer Epidemiol Biomarkers Prev. 2012;21(3): 411–6.
5. Frankel TL, D'Angelica MI. Hepatic resection for colorectal metastases. J Surg Oncol. 2014;109(1):2–7.

6. Abdalla EK, Adam R, Bilchik AJ, Jaeck D, Vauthey JN, Mahvi D. Improving resectability of hepatic colorectal metastases: expert consensus statement. Ann Surg Oncol. 2006;13(10):1271–80.

7. Tomlinson J, Jarnagin W, DeMatteo R, Fong Y, Kornprat P, Gonen M, et al. Actual 10-year Survival after resection of colorectal liver metastases. J Clin Oncol. 2007;25:4575–82.

8. House MG, Ito H, Gonen M, Fong Y, Allen PJ, DeMatteo RP, et al. Survival after hepatic resection for metastatic colorectal cancer: trends in outcomes for 1,600 patients during two decades at a single institution. J Am Coll Surg. 2010;210(5):744–52. 52–5.

9. Spolverato G, Ejaz A, Azad N, Pawlik TM. Surgery for colorectal liver metastases: the evolution of determining prognosis. World J Gastrointest Oncol. 2013;5(12):207–21.

10. Choti MA, Sitzmann JV, Tiburi MF, Sumetchotimetha W, Rangsin R, Schulick RD, et al. Trends in long-term survival following liver resection for hepatic colorectal metastases. Ann Surg. 2002;235(6):759–66.

11. Wood CB, Gillis CR, Blumgart LH. A retrospective study of the natural history of patients with liver metastases from colorectal cancer. Clin Oncol. 1976;2(3):285–8.

12. Wagner JS, Adson MA, Van Heerden JA, Adson MH, Ilstrup DM. The natural history of hepatic metastases from colorectal cancer. A comparison with resective treatment. Ann Surg. 1984;199(5):502–8.

13. Schwarz RE, Berlin JD, Lenz HJ, Nordlinger B, Rubbia-Brandt L, Choti MA. Systemic cytotoxic and biological therapies of colorectal liver metastases: expert consensus statement. HPB (Oxford). 2013;15(2):106–15.

14. Kornprat P, Jarnagin WR, Gonen M, DeMatteo RP, Fong Y, Blumgart LH, et al. Outcome after hepatectomy for multiple (four or more) colorectal metastases in the era of effective chemotherapy. Ann Surg Oncol. 2007;14(3):1151–60.

15. Bittoni A, Scartozzi M, Giampieri R, Faloppi L, Maccaroni E, Del Prete M, et al. The Tower of Babel of liver metastases from colorectal cancer: are we ready for one language. Crit Rev Oncol Hematol. 2013;85:332–41.

16. Pawlik TM, Schulick RD, Choti MA. Expanding criteria for resectability of colorectal liver metastases. Oncologist. 2008;13(1):51–64.

17. Charnsangavej C, Clary B, Fong Y, Grothey A, Pawlik TM, Choti MA. Selection of patients for resection of hepatic colorectal metastases: expert consensus statement. Ann Surg Oncol. 2006;13(10):1261–8.

18. Gold JS, Are C, Kornprat P, Jarnagin WR, Gonen M, Fong Y, et al. Increased use of parenchymal-sparing surgery for bilateral liver metastases from colorectal cancer is associated with improved mortality without change in oncologic outcome: trends in treatment over time in 440 patients. Ann Surg. 2008;247(1):109–17.

19. Adams RB, Aloia TA, Loyer E, Pawlik TM, Taouli B, Vauthey JN. Selection for hepatic resection of colorectal liver metastases: expert consensus statement. HPB (Oxford). 2013;15(2):91–103.

20. de Gramont A, Figer A, Seymour M, Homerin M, Hmissi A, Cassidy J, et al. Leucovorin and fluorouracil with or without oxaliplatin as first-line treatment in advanced colorectal cancer. J Clin Oncol. 2000;18(16):2938–47.

21. Pozzo C, Basso M, Cassano A, Quirino M, Schinzari G, Trigila N, et al. Neoadjuvant treatment of unresectable liver disease with irinotecan and 5-fluorouracil plus folinic acid in colorectal cancer patients. Ann Oncol. 2004;15(6):933–9.

22. Nuzzo G, Giuliante F, Ardito F, Vellone M, Pozzo C, Cassano A, et al. Liver resection for primarily unresectable colorectal metastases downsized by chemotherapy. J Gastrointest Surg. 2007;11(3):318–24.

23. Masi G, Loupakis F, Pollina L, Vasile E, Cupini S, Ricci S, et al. Long-term outcome of initially unresectable metastatic colorectal cancer patients treated with 5-fluorouracil/leucovorin, oxaliplatin, and irinotecan (FOLFOXIRI) followed by radical surgery of metastases. Ann Surg. 2009;249(3):420–5.

24. Reddy SK, Barbas AS, Clary BM. Synchronous colorectal liver metastases: is it time to reconsider traditional paradigms of management? Ann Surg Oncol. 2009;16(9):2395–410.

25. Sheth KR, Clary BM. Management of hepatic metastases from colorectal cancer. Clin Colon Rectal Surg. 2005;18(3):215–23.
26. Charlson ME, Pompei P, Ales KL, MacKenzie CR. A new method of classifying prognostic comorbidity in longitudinal studies: development and validation. J Chronic Dis. 1987;40(5):373–83.
27. Kinkel K, Lu Y, Both M, Warren RS, Thoeni RF. Detection of hepatic metastases from cancers of the gastrointestinal tract by using noninvasive imaging methods (US, CT, MR imaging, PET): a meta-analysis. Radiology. 2002;224(3):748–56.
28. Wilson SR, Burns PN. Microbubble-enhanced US in body imaging: what role? Radiology. 2010;257(1):24–39.
29. Leen E, Ceccotti P, Moug SJ, Glen P, MacQuarrie J, Angerson WJ, et al. Potential value of contrast-enhanced intraoperative ultrasonography during partial hepatectomy for metastases: an essential investigation before resection? Ann Surg. 2006;243(2):236–40.
30. Sahani DV, Bajwa MA, Andrabi Y, Bajpai S, Cusack JC. Current status of imaging and emerging techniques to evaluate liver metastases from colorectal carcinoma. Ann Surg. 2014;259(5):861–72.
31. Wiering B, Ruers TJ, Krabbe PF, Dekker HM, Oyen WJ. Comparison of multiphase CT, FDG-PET and intra-operative ultrasound in patients with colorectal liver metastases selected for surgery. Ann Surg Oncol. 2007;14(2):818–26.
32. Benoist S, Brouquet A, Penna C, Julie C, El Hajjam M, Chagnon S, et al. Complete response of colorectal liver metastases after chemotherapy: does it mean cure? J Clin Oncol. 2006;24(24):3939–45.
33. van Kessel CS, Buckens CF, van den Bosch MA, van Leeuwen MS, van Hillegersberg R, Verkooijen HM. Preoperative imaging of colorectal liver metastases after neoadjuvant chemotherapy: a meta-analysis. Ann Surg Oncol. 2012;19(9):2805–13.
34. Ward J, Robinson PJ, Guthrie JA, Downing S, Wilson D, Lodge JP, et al. Liver metastases in candidates for hepatic resection: comparison of helical CT and gadolinium- and SPIO-enhanced MR imaging. Radiology. 2005;237(1):170–80.
35. Holalkere NS, Sahani DV, Blake MA, Halpern EF, Hahn PF, Mueller PR. Characterization of small liver lesions: added role of MR after MDCT. J Comput Assist Tomogr. 2006;30(4):591–6.
36. Van Beers BE, Pastor CM, Hussain HK. Primovist, Eovist: what to expect? J Hepatol. 2012;57(2):421–9.
37. Eiber M, Fingerle AA, Brugel M, Gaa J, Rummeny EJ, Holzapfel K. Detection and classification of focal liver lesions in patients with colorectal cancer: retrospective comparison of diffusion-weighted MR imaging and multi-slice CT. Eur J Radiol. 2012;81(4):683–91.
38. Bipat S, van Leeuwen MS, Comans EF, Pijl ME, Bossuyt PM, Zwinderman AH, et al. Colorectal liver metastases: CT, MR imaging, and PET for diagnosis--meta-analysis. Radiology. 2005;237(1):123–31.
39. Wiering B, Krabbe PF, Jager GJ, Oyen WJ, Ruers TJ. The impact of fluor-18-deoxyglucose-positron emission tomography in the management of colorectal liver metastases. Cancer. 2005;104(12):2658–70.
40. Floriani I, Torri V, Rulli E, Garavaglia D, Compagnoni A, Salvolini L, et al. Performance of imaging modalities in diagnosis of liver metastases from colorectal cancer: a systematic review and meta-analysis. J Magn Reson Imaging. 2010;31(1):19–31.
41. Niekel MC, Bipat S, Stoker J. Diagnostic imaging of colorectal liver metastases with CT, MR imaging, FDG PET, and/or FDG PET/CT: a meta-analysis of prospective studies including patients who have not previously undergone treatment. Radiology. 2010;257(3):674–84.
42. Ruers TJ, Wiering B, van der Sijp JR, Roumen RM, de Jong KP, Comans EF, et al. Improved selection of patients for hepatic surgery of colorectal liver metastases with (18)F-FDG PET: a randomized study. J Nucl Med. 2009;50(7):1036–41.
43. Moulton CA, Gu CS, Law CH, Tandan VR, Hart R, Quan D, et al. Effect of PET before liver resection on surgical management for colorectal adenocarcinoma metastases: a randomized clinical trial. JAMA. 2014;311(18):1863–9.

44. Chun YS, Ribero D, Abdalla EK, Madoff DC, Mortenson MM, Wei SH, et al. Comparison of two methods of future liver remnant volume measurement. J Gastrointest Surg. 2008;12(1):123–8.
45. Schroeder RA, Marroquin CE, Bute BP, Khuri S, Henderson WG, Kuo PC. Predictive indices of morbidity and mortality after liver resection. Ann Surg. 2006;243(3):373–9.
46. Imamura H, Sano K, Sugawara Y, Kokudo N, Makuuchi M. Assessment of hepatic reserve for indication of hepatic resection: decision tree incorporating indocyanine green test. J Hepatobiliary Pancreat Surg. 2005;12(1):16–22.
47. Abdalla EK, Denys A, Chevalier P, Nemr RA, Vauthey JN. Total and segmental liver volume variations: implications for liver surgery. Surgery. 2004;135(4):404–10.
48. Rous P, Larimore LD. Relation of the portal blood to liver maintenance: a demonstration of liver atrophy conditional on compensation. J Exp Med. 1920;31(5):609–32.
49. Kinoshita H, Sakai K, Hirohashi K, Igawa S, Yamasaki O, Kubo S. Preoperative portal vein embolization for hepatocellular carcinoma. World J Surg. 1986;10(5):803–8.
50. Makuuchi M, Thai BL, Takayasu K, Takayama T, Kosuge T, Gunven P, et al. Preoperative portal embolization to increase safety of major hepatectomy for hilar bile duct carcinoma: a preliminary report. Surgery. 1990;107(5):521–7.
51. Farges O, Belghiti J, Kianmanesh R, Regimbeau JM, Santoro R, Vilgrain V, et al. Portal vein embolization before right hepatectomy: prospective clinical trial. Ann Surg. 2003;237(2):208–17.
52. Abulkhir A, Limongelli P, Healey AJ, Damrah O, Tait P, Jackson J, et al. Preoperative portal vein embolization for major liver resection: a meta-analysis. Ann Surg. 2008;247(1):49–57.
53. Ribero D, Abdalla EK, Madoff DC, Donadon M, Loyer EM, Vauthey JN. Portal vein embolization before major hepatectomy and its effects on regeneration, resectability and outcome. Br J Surg. 2007;94(11):1386–94.
54. Shindoh J, Truty MJ, Aloia TA, Curley SA, Zimmitti G, Huang SY, et al. Kinetic growth rate after portal vein embolization predicts posthepatectomy outcomes: toward zero liver-related mortality in patients with colorectal liver metastases and small future liver remnant. J Am Coll Surg. 2013;216(2):201–9.
55. Capussotti L, Muratore A, Baracchi F, Lelong B, Ferrero A, Regge D, et al. Portal vein ligation as an efficient method of increasing the future liver remnant volume in the surgical treatment of colorectal metastases. Arch Surg. 2008;143(10):978–82. discussion 82.
56. de Santibanes E, Clavien PA. Playing Play-Doh to prevent postoperative liver failure: the "ALPPS" approach. Ann Surg. 2012;255(3):415–7.
57. de Santibanes E, Alvarez FA, Ardiles V. How to avoid postoperative liver failure: a novel method. World J Surg. 2012;36(1):125–8.
58. Schnitzbauer AA, Lang SA, Goessmann H, Nadalin S, Baumgart J, Farkas SA, et al. Right portal vein ligation combined with in situ splitting induces rapid left lateral liver lobe hypertrophy enabling 2-staged extended right hepatic resection in small-for-size settings. Ann Surg. 2012;255(3):405–14.
59. Nordlinger B, Guiguet M, Vaillant JC, Balladur P, Boudjema K, Bachellier P, et al. Surgical resection of colorectal carcinoma metastases to the liver. A prognostic scoring system to improve case selection, based on 1568 patients. Association Francaise de Chirurgie. Cancer. 1996;77(7):1254–62.
60. Fong Y, Fortner J, Sun R, Brennan M, Blumgart L. Clinical score for predicting recurrence after hepatic resection for metastatic colorectal cancer. Ann Surg. 1999;230:309–21.
61. Iwatsuki S, Dvorchik I, Madariaga JR, Marsh JW, Dodson F, Bonham AC, et al. Hepatic resection for metastatic colorectal adenocarcinoma: a proposal of a prognostic scoring system. J Am Coll Surg. 1999;189(3):291–9.
62. Ueno H, Mochizuki H, Hatsuse K, Hase K, Yamamoto T. Indicators for treatment strategies of colorectal liver metastases. Ann Surg. 2000;231(1):59–66.
63. Lise M, Bacchetti S, Da Pian P, Nitti D, Pilati P. Patterns of recurrence after resection of colorectal liver metastases: prediction by models of outcome analysis. World J Surg. 2001;25(5):638–44.

64. Nagashima I, Takada T, Matsuda K, Adachi M, Nagawa H, Muto T, et al. A new scoring system to classify patients with colorectal liver metastases: proposal of criteria to select candidates for hepatic resection. J Hepatobiliary Pancreat Surg. 2004;11(2):79–83.
65. Schindl M, Wigmore SJ, Currie EJ, Laengle F, Garden OJ. Prognostic scoring in colorectal cancer liver metastases: development and validation. Arch Surg. 2005;140(2):183–9.
66. Malik H, Hamandy Z, Adair R, Finch R, Al-Mukhtar A, Toogood G, et al. Prognostic influence of multiple hepatic metastases from colorectal cancer. Eur J Surg Oncol. 2007;33: 468–73.
67. Zakaria S, Donohue JH, Que FG, Farnell MB, Schleck CD, Ilstrup DM, et al. Hepatic resection for colorectal metastases: value for risk scoring systems? Ann Surg. 2007;246(2): 183–91.
68. Lee WS, Kim MJ, Yun SH, Chun HK, Lee WY, Kim SJ, et al. Risk factor stratification after simultaneous liver and colorectal resection for synchronous colorectal metastasis. Langenbecks Arch Surg. 2008;393(1):13–9.
69. Rees M, Tekkis PP, Welsh FK, O'Rourke T, John TG. Evaluation of long-term survival after hepatic resection for metastatic colorectal cancer: a multifactorial model of 929 patients. Ann Surg. 2008;247(1):125–35.
70. Konopke R, Kersting S, Distler M, Dietrich J, Gastmeier J, Heller A, et al. Prognostic factors and evaluation of a clinical score for predicting survival after resection of colorectal liver metastases. Liver Int. 2009;29(1):89–102.
71. Merkel S, Bialecki D, Meyer T, Muller V, Papadopoulos T, Hohenberger W. Comparison of clinical risk scores predicting prognosis after resection of colorectal liver metastases. J Surg Oncol. 2009;100(5):349–57.
72. Gomez D, Cameron IC. Prognostic scores for colorectal liver metastasis: clinically important or an academic exercise? HPB (Oxford). 2010;12(4):227–38.
73. Mala T, Bohler G, Mathisen O, Bergan A, Soreide O. Hepatic resection for colorectal metastases: can preoperative scoring predict patient outcome? World J Surg. 2002;26(11): 1348–53.
74. Mann CD, Metcalfe MS, Leopardi LN, Maddern GJ. The clinical risk score: emerging as a reliable preoperative prognostic index in hepatectomy for colorectal metastases. Arch Surg. 2004;139(11):1168–72.
75. Arru M, Aldrighetti L, Castoldi R, Di Palo S, Orsenigo E, Stella M, et al. Analysis of prognostic factors influencing long-term survival after hepatic resection for metastatic colorectal cancer. World J Surg. 2008;32(1):93–103.
76. Ayez N, Lalmahomed ZS, van der Pool AE, Vergouwe Y, van Montfort K, de Jonge J, et al. Is the clinical risk score for patients with colorectal liver metastases still useable in the era of effective neoadjuvant chemotherapy? Ann Surg Oncol. 2011;18(10):2757–63.
77. Nathan H, de Jong MC, Pulitano C, Ribero D, Strub J, Mentha G, et al. Conditional survival after surgical resection of colorectal liver metastasis: an international multi-institutional analysis of 949 patients. J Am Coll Surg. 2010;210(5):755–64. 64–6.
78. Nash GM, Gimbel M, Shia J, Nathanson DR, Ndubuisi MI, Zeng ZS, et al. KRAS mutation correlates with accelerated metastatic progression in patients with colorectal liver metastases. Ann Surg Oncol. 2010;17(2):572–8.
79. Karagkounis G, Torbenson MS, Daniel HD, Azad NS, Diaz Jr LA, Donehower RC, et al. Incidence and prognostic impact of KRAS and BRAF mutation in patients undergoing liver surgery for colorectal metastases. Cancer. 2013;119(23):4137–44.
80. Teng HW, Huang YC, Lin JK, Chen WS, Lin TC, Jiang JK, et al. BRAF mutation is a prognostic biomarker for colorectal liver metastasectomy. J Surg Oncol. 2012;106(2):123–9.
81. Bathe OF, Franceschi D, Livingstone AS, Moffat FL, Tian E, Ardalan B. Increased thymidylate synthase gene expression in liver metastases from colorectal carcinoma: implications for chemotherapeutic options and survival. Cancer J Sci Am. 1999;5(1):34–40.
82. Gonen M, Hummer A, Zervoudakis A, Sullivan D, Fong Y, Banerjee D, et al. Thymidylate synthase expression in hepatic tumors is a predictor of survival and progression in patients with resectable metastatic colorectal cancer. J Clin Oncol. 2003;21(3):406–12.

83. Domont J, Pawlik TM, Boige V, Rose M, Weber JC, Hoff PM, et al. Catalytic subunit of human telomerase reverse transcriptase is an independent predictor of survival in patients undergoing curative resection of hepatic colorectal metastases: a multicenter analysis. J Clin Oncol. 2005;23(13):3086–93.

84. Smith DL, Soria JC, Morat L, Yang Q, Sabatier L, Liu DD, et al. Human telomerase reverse transcriptase (hTERT) and Ki-67 are better predictors of survival than established clinical indicators in patients undergoing curative hepatic resection for colorectal metastases. Ann Surg Oncol. 2004;11(1):45–51.

85. Shimomura M, Hinoi T, Kuroda S, Adachi T, Kawaguchi Y, Sasada T, et al. Overexpression of hypoxia inducible factor-1 alpha is an independent risk factor for recurrence after curative resection of colorectal liver metastases. Ann Surg Oncol. 2013;20 Suppl 3:S527–36.

86. Adam R, Pascal G, Castaing D, Azoulay D, Delvart V, Paule B, et al. Tumor progression while on chemotherapy: a contraindication to liver resection for multiple colorectal metasta-ses? Ann Surg. 2004;240(6):1052–61. discussion 61–4.

87. Allen PJ, Kemeny N, Jarnagin W, DeMatteo R, Blumgart L, Fong Y. Importance of response to neoadjuvant chemotherapy in patients undergoing resection of synchronous colorectal liver metastases. J Gastrointest Surg. 2003;7(1):109–15. discussion 16–7.

88. Gruenberger B, Scheithauer W, Punzengruber R, Zielinski C, Tamandl D, Gruenberger T. Importance of response to neoadjuvant chemotherapy in potentially curable colorectal cancer liver metastases. BMC Cancer. 2008;8:120.

89. Gallagher DJ, Zheng J, Capanu M, Haviland D, Paty P, Dematteo RP, et al. Response to neo-adjuvant chemotherapy does not predict overall survival for patients with synchronous colorectal hepatic metastases. Ann Surg Oncol. 2009;16(7):1844–51.

90. Adam R, Wicherts DA, de Haas RJ, Aloia T, Levi F, Paule B, et al. Complete pathologic response after preoperative chemotherapy for colorectal liver metastases: myth or reality? J Clin Oncol. 2008;26(10):1635–41.

91. Blazer 3rd DG, Kishi Y, Maru DM, Kopetz S, Chun YS, Overman MJ, et al. Pathologic response to preoperative chemotherapy: a new outcome end point after resection of hepatic colorectal metastases. J Clin Oncol. 2008;26(33):5344–51.

92. Tanaka K, Takakura H, Takeda K, Matsuo K, Nagano Y, Endo I. Importance of complete pathologic response to prehepatectomy chemotherapy in treating colorectal cancer metasta-ses. Ann Surg. 2009;250(6):935–42.

93. Rubbia-Brandt L, Giostra E, Brezault C, Roth AD, Andres A, Audard V, et al. Importance of histological tumor response assessment in predicting the outcome in patients with colorectal liver metastases treated with neo-adjuvant chemotherapy followed by liver surgery. Ann Oncol. 2007;18(2):299–304.

94. Ito H, Mo Q, Qin L-X, Viale A, Maithel SK, Maker AV, et al. Gene expression profiles accurately predict outcome following liver resection in patients with metastatic colorectal cancer. PLoS One. 2013;8(12):e81680.

95. Ekberg H, Tranberg KG, Andersson R, Lundstedt C, Hagerstrand I, Ranstam J, et al. Determinants of survival in liver resection for colorectal secondaries. Br J Surg. 1986; 73(9):727–31.

96. Cady B, Jenkins RL, Steele Jr GD, Lewis WD, Stone MD, McDermott WV, et al. Surgical margin in hepatic resection for colorectal metastasis: a critical and improvable determinant of outcome. Ann Surg. 1998;227(4):566–71.

97. DeMatteo RP, Palese C, Jarnagin WR, Sun RL, Blumgart LH, Fong Y. Anatomic segmental hepatic resection is superior to wedge resection as an oncologic operation for colorectal liver metastases. J Gastrointest Surg. 2000;4(2):178–84.

98. Welsh FK, Tekkis PP, O'Rourke T, John TG, Rees M. Quantification of risk of a positive (R1) resection margin following hepatic resection for metastatic colorectal cancer: an aid to clinical decision-making. Surg Oncol. 2008;17(1):3–13.

99. Elias D, Cavalcanti A, Sabourin JC, Lassau N, Pignon JP, Ducreux M, et al. Resection of liver metastases from colorectal cancer: the real impact of the surgical margin. Eur J Surg Oncol. 1998;24(3):174–9.

100. Pawlik TM, Scoggins CR, Zorzi D, Abdalla EK, Andres A, Eng C, et al. Effect of surgical margin status on survival and site of recurrence after hepatic resection for colorectal metastases. Ann Surg. 2005;241(5):715–22. discussion 22–4.
101. Are C, Gonen M, Zazzali K, Dematteo RP, Jarnagin WR, Fong Y, et al. The impact of margins on outcome after hepatic resection for colorectal metastasis. Ann Surg. 2007;246(2): 295–300.
102. Pawlik TM, Vauthey JN. Surgical margins during hepatic surgery for colorectal liver metastases: complete resection not millimeters defines outcome. Ann Surg Oncol. 2008;15(3):677–9.
103. Guzzetti E, Pulitano C, Catena M, Arru M, Ratti F, Finazzi R, et al. Impact of type of liver resection on the outcome of colorectal liver metastases: a case-matched analysis. J Surg Oncol. 2008;97(6):503–7.
104. Lalmahomed ZS, Ayez N, van der Pool AE, Verheij J, IJzermans JN, Verhoef C. Anatomical versus nonanatomical resection of colorectal liver metastases: is there a difference in surgical and oncological outcome? World J Surg. 2011;35(3):656–61.
105. Melendez JA, Arslan V, Fischer ME, Wuest D, Jarnagin WR, Fong Y, et al. Perioperative outcomes of major hepatic resections under low central venous pressure anesthesia: blood loss, blood transfusion, and the risk of postoperative renal dysfunction. J Am Coll Surg. 1998;187(6):620–5.
106. Solomon MJ, Stephen MS, Gallinger S, White GH. Does intraoperative hepatic ultrasonography change surgical decision making during liver resection? Am J Surg. 1994;168(4):307–10.
107. Cervone A, Sardi A, Conaway GL. Intraoperative ultrasound (IOUS) is essential in the management of metastatic colorectal liver lesions. Am Surg. 2000;66(7):611–5.
108. Lordan JT, Stenson KM, Karanjia ND. The value of intraoperative ultrasound and preoperative imaging, individually and in combination, in liver resection for metastatic colorectal cancer. Ann R Coll Surg Engl. 2011;93(3):246–9.
109. Fahy B, D'Angelica M, DeMatteo R, Blumgart L, Weiser M, Ostrovnaya I, et al. Synchronous hepatic metastases from colon cancer: changing treatment strategies and results of surgical intervention. Ann Surg Oncol. 2009;16(2):361–70.
110. Aloia TA, Fahy BN. A decision analysis model predicts the optimal treatment pathway for patients with colorectal cancer and resectable synchronous liver metastases. Clin Colorectal Cancer. 2008;7(3):197–201.
111. Lykoudis PM, O'Reilly D, Nastos K, Fusai G. Systematic review of surgical management of synchronous colorectal liver metastases. Br J Surg. 2014;101(6):605–12.
112. Nordlinger B, Sorbye H, Glimelius B, Poston G, Schlag P, Rougier P, et al. Perioperative chemo with FOLFOX4 and surgery versus surgery alone for resectable liver metastases from colorectal cancer; a RCT. Lancet. 2008;371:1007–16.
113. de Haas RJ, Adam R, Wicherts DA, Azoulay D, Bismuth H, Vibert E, et al. Comparison of simultaneous or delayed liver surgery for limited synchronous colorectal metastases. Br J Surg. 2010;97(8):1279–89.
114. Brouquet A, Mortenson MM, Vauthey J-N, Rodriguez-Bigas MA, Overman MJ, Chang GJ, Kopetz S, Garrett C, Curley SA, Abdalla EK. Surgical strategies for synchronous colorectal liver metastases in 156 consecutive patients: classic, combined, or reverse strategy? J Am Coll Surg. 2010;210:934–41.
115. Poultsides GA, Servais EL, Saltz LB, Patil S, Kemeny NE, Guillem JG, et al. Outcome of primary tumor in patients with synchronous stage IV colorectal cancer receiving combination chemotherapy without surgery as initial treatment. J Clin Oncol. 2009;27(20):3379–84.
116. Rodel C. Radiotherapy: preoperative chemoradiotherapy for rectal cancer. Nat Rev Clin Oncol. 2010;7(3):129–30.
117. Mentha G, Majno PE, Andres A, Rubbia-Brandt L, Morel P, Roth AD. Neoadjuvant chemotherapy and resection of advanced synchronous liver metastases before treatment of the colorectal primary. Br J Surg. 2006;93(7):872–8.
118. Jegatheeswaran S, Mason JM, Hancock HC, Siriwardena AK. The liver-first approach to the management of colorectal cancer with synchronous hepatic metastases: a systematic review. JAMA Surg. 2013;148(4):385–91.

119. Reddy SK, Pawlik TM, Zorzi D, Gleisner AL, Ribero D, Assumpcao L, et al. Simultaneous resections of colorectal cancer and synchronous liver metastases: a multi-institutional analysis. Ann Surg Oncol. 2007;14(12):3481–91.

120. Mentha G, Majno P, Terraz S, Rubbia-Brandt L, Gervaz P, Andres A, et al. Treatment strategies for the management of advanced colorectal liver metastases detected synchronously with the primary tumour. Eur J Surg Oncol. 2007;33 Suppl 2:S76–83.

121. Pawlik TM, Abdalla EK, Ellis LM, Vauthey JN, Curley SA. Debunking dogma: surgery for four or more colorectal liver metastases is justified. J Gastrointest Surg. 2006;10(2): 240–8.

122. Jamal MH, Hassanain M, Chaudhury P, Tran TT, Wong S, Yousef Y, et al. Staged hepatectomy for bilobar colorectal hepatic metastases. HPB (Oxford). 2012;14(11):782–9.

123. Tsai S, Marques HP, de Jong MC, Mira P, Ribeiro V, Choti MA, et al. Two-stage strategy for patients with extensive bilateral colorectal liver metastases. HPB (Oxford). 2010;12(4):262–9.

124. Cardona K, Donataccio D, Kingham TP, Allen PJ, DeMatteo RP, Fong Y, et al. Treatment of extensive metastatic colorectal cancer to the liver with systemic and hepatic arterial infusion chemotherapy and two-stage hepatic resection: the role of salvage therapy for recurrent disease. Ann Surg Oncol. 2014;21(3):815–21.

125. Chun YS, Vauthey JN, Ribero D, Donadon M, Mullen JT, Eng C, et al. Systemic chemotherapy and two-stage hepatectomy for extensive bilateral colorectal liver metastases: perioperative safety and survival. J Gastrointest Surg. 2007;11(11):1498–504. discussion 504–5.

126. Wicherts DA, Miller R, de Haas RJ, Bitsakou G, Vibert E, Veilhan LA, et al. Long-term results of two-stage hepatectomy for irresectable colorectal cancer liver metastases. Ann Surg. 2008;248(6):994–1005.

127. Kingham TP, Tanoue M, Eaton A, Rocha FG, Do R, Allen P, et al. Patterns of recurrence after ablation of colorectal cancer liver metastases. Ann Surg Oncol. 2012;19(3):834–41.

128. Power DG, Kemeny NE. Role of adjuvant therapy after resection of colorectal cancer liver metastases. J Clin Oncol. 2010;28(13):2300–9.

129. Parks R, Gonen M, Kemeny N, Jarnagin W, D'Angelica M, DeMatteo R, et al. Adjuvant chemotherapy improves survival after resection of hepatic colorectal metastases: analysis of data from two continents. J Am Coll Surg. 2007;204(5):753–61. discussion 61–3.

130. Figueras J, Torras J, Valls C, Llado L, Ramos E, Marti-Rague J, et al. Surgical resection of colorectal liver metastases in patients with expanded indications: a single-center experience with 501 patients. Dis Colon Rectum. 2007;50(4):478–88.

131. Langer B, Bleiberg H, Labianca R, et al. Fluorouracil (FU) plus I-Leucovorin (i-LV) versus observation after potentially curative resection of liver or lung metastases from colorectal cancer (CRC); Results of the ENG (EORTC/NCIC CTG/GIVIO) randomized trial. Proc Am Soc Clin Oncol. 2002;21(S1):149a.

132. Lopez-Ladron A, Salvador AJ, Bernabe R. Observation versus postoperative chemotherapy after resection of liver metastases in patients with advanced colorectal cancer. Proc Am Soc Clin Oncol 2003;22(373):abstr 1497.

133. Portier G, Elias D, Bouche O, Rougier P, Bosset JF, Saric J, et al. Multicenter randomized trial of adjuvant fluorouracil and folinic acid compared with surgery alone after resection of colorectal liver metastases: FFCD ACHBTH AURC 9002 trial. J Clin Oncol. 2006; 24(31):4976–82.

134. Ychou M, Hohenberger W, Thezenas S, Navarro M, Maurel J, Bokemeyer C, et al. A randomized phase III study comparing adjuvant 5-fluorouracil/folinic acid with FOLFIRI in patients following complete resection of liver metastases from colorectal cancer. Ann Oncol. 2009;20(12):1964–70.

135. Mitry E, Fields AL, Bleiberg H, Labianca R, Portier G, Tu D, et al. Adjuvant chemotherapy after potentially curative resection of metastases from colorectal cancer: a pooled analysis of two randomized trials. J Clin Oncol. 2008;26(30):4906–11.

136. Vauthey JN, Pawlik TM, Ribero D, Wu TT, Zorzi D, Hoff PM, et al. Chemotherapy regimen predicts steatohepatitis and an increase in 90-day mortality after surgery for hepatic colorectal metastases. J Clin Oncol. 2006;24(13):2065–72.

137. Bischof DA, Clary BM, Maithel SK, Pawlik TM. Surgical management of disappearing colorectal liver metastases. Br J Surg. 2013;100(11):1414–20.

138. Chua TC, Saxena A, Liauw W, Kokandi A, Morris DL. Systematic review of randomized and nonrandomized trials of the clinical response and outcomes of neoadjuvant systemic chemotherapy for resectable colorectal liver metastases. Ann Surg Oncol. 2010; 17(2):492–501.

139. Nordlinger B, Sorbye H, Glimelius B, Poston GJ, Schlag PM, Rougier P, et al. Perioperative FOLFOX4 chemotherapy and surgery versus surgery alone for resectable liver metastases from colorectal cancer (EORTC 40983): long-term results of a randomised, controlled, phase 3 trial. Lancet Oncol. 2013;14(12):1208–15.

140. Neumann UP, Thelen A, Rocken C, Seehofer D, Bahra M, Riess H, et al. Nonresponse to pre-operative chemotherapy does not preclude long-term survival after liver resection in patients with colorectal liver metastases. Surgery. 2009;146(1):52–9.

141. Auer RC, White RR, Kemeny NE, Schwartz LH, Shia J, Blumgart LH, et al. Predictors of a true complete response among disappearing liver metastases from colorectal cancer after chemotherapy. Cancer. 2010;116(6):1502–9.

142. van Vledder MG, de Jong MC, Pawlik TM, Schulick RD, Diaz LA, Choti MA. Disappearing colorectal liver metastases after chemotherapy: should we be concerned? J Gastrointest Surg. 2010;14(11):1691–700.

143. Adam R, De Gramont A, Figueras J, Guthrie A, Kokudo N, Kunstlinger F, et al. The oncosurgery approach to managing liver metastases from colorectal cancer: a multidisciplinary international consensus. Oncologist. 2012;17(10):1225–39.

144. Adam R, Wicherts DA, de Haas RJ, Ciacio O, Levi F, Paule B, et al. Patients with initially unresectable colorectal liver metastases: is there a possibility of cure? J Clin Oncol. 2009;27(11):1829–35.

145. Kemeny N. The management of resectable and unresectable liver metastases from colorectal cancer. Curr Opin Oncol. 2010;22(4):364–73.

146. Tournigand C, Andre T, Achille E, Lledo G, Flesh M, Mery-Mignard D, et al. FOLFIRI followed by FOLFOX6 or the reverse sequence in advanced colorectal cancer: a randomized GERCOR study. J Clin Oncol. 2004;22(2):229–37.

147. Adam R, Aloia T, Levi F, Wicherts DA, de Haas RJ, Paule B, et al. Hepatic resection after rescue cetuximab treatment for colorectal liver metastases previously refractory to conventional systemic therapy. J Clin Oncol. 2007;25(29):4593–602.

148. Chua TC, Saxena A, Liauw W, Chu F, Morris DL. Hepatectomy and resection of concomitant extrahepatic disease for colorectal liver metastases--a systematic review. Eur J Cancer. 2012;48(12):1757–65.

149. Elias D, Liberale G, Vernerey D, Pocard M, Ducreux M, Boige V, et al. Hepatic and extrahepatic colorectal metastases: when resectable, their localization does not matter, but their total number has a prognostic effect. Ann Surg Oncol. 2005;12(11):900–9.

150. Carpizo DR, Are C, Jarnagin W, Dematteo R, Fong Y, Gonen M, et al. Liver resection for metastatic colorectal cancer in patients with concurrent extrahepatic disease: results in 127 patients treated at a single center. Ann Surg Oncol. 2009;16(8):2138–46.

151. Pulitano C, Bodingbauer M, Aldrighetti L, de Jong MC, Castillo F, Schulick RD, et al. Liver resection for colorectal metastases in presence of extrahepatic disease: results from an international multi-institutional analysis. Ann Surg Oncol. 2011;18(5):1380–8.

152. Jones RP, Jackson R, Dunne DF, Malik HZ, Fenwick SW, Poston GJ, et al. Systematic review and meta-analysis of follow-up after hepatectomy for colorectal liver metastases. Br J Surg. 2012;99(4):477–86.

153. Lam VW, Pang T, Laurence JM, Johnston E, Hollands MJ, Pleass HC, et al. A systematic review of repeat hepatectomy for recurrent colorectal liver metastases. J Gastrointest Surg. 2013;17(7):1312–21.

154. Antoniou A, Lovegrove RE, Tilney HS, Heriot AG, John TG, Rees M, et al. Meta-analysis of clinical outcome after first and second liver resection for colorectal metastases. Surgery. 2007;141(1):9–18.

155. Lam VW, Laurence JM, Johnston E, Hollands MJ, Pleass HC, Richardson AJ. A systematic review of two-stage hepatectomy in patients with initially unresectable colorectal liver metastases. HPB (Oxford). 2013;15(7):483–91.
156. Mayo SC, Pawlik TM. Thermal ablative therapies for secondary hepatic malignancies. Cancer J. 2010;16(2):111–7.
157. Abdalla EK, Bauer TW, Chun YS, D'Angelica M, Kooby DA, Jarnagin WR. Locoregional surgical and interventional therapies for advanced colorectal cancer liver metastases: expert consensus statements. HPB (Oxford). 2013;15(2):119–30.
158. Mulier S, Ni Y, Jamart J, Ruers T, Marchal G, Michel L. Local recurrence after hepatic radiofrequency coagulation: multivariate meta-analysis and review of contributing factors. Ann Surg. 2005;242(2):158–71.
159. Johnston FM, Mavros MN, Herman JM, Pawlik TM. Local therapies for hepatic metastases. J Natl Compr Canc Netw. 2013;11(2):153–60.
160. Rocha FG, D'Angelica M. Treatment of liver colorectal metastases: role of laparoscopy, radiofrequency ablation, and microwave coagulation. J Surg Oncol. 2010;102(8):968–74.
161. Swaminath A, Dawson LA. Emerging role of radiotherapy in the management of liver metastases. Cancer J. 2010;16(2):150–5.
162. Chang DT, Swaminath A, Kozak M, Weintraub J, Koong AC, Kim J, et al. Stereotactic body radiotherapy for colorectal liver metastases: a pooled analysis. Cancer. 2011;117(17):4060–9.
163. Rule W, Timmerman R, Tong L, Abdulrahman R, Meyer J, Boike T, et al. Phase I dose-escalation study of stereotactic body radiotherapy in patients with hepatic metastases. Ann Surg Oncol. 2011;18(4):1081–7.
164. Kingham TP, D'Angelica M, Kemeny NE. Role of intra-arterial hepatic chemotherapy in the treatment of colorectal cancer metastases. J Surg Oncol. 2010;102(8):988–95.
165. Ensminger WD, Gyves JW. Clinical pharmacology of hepatic arterial chemotherapy. Semin Oncol. 1983;10(2):176–82.
166. Allen PJ, Nissan A, Picon AI, Kemeny N, Dudrick P, Ben-Porat L, et al. Technical complications and durability of hepatic artery infusion pumps for unresectable colorectal liver metastases: an institutional experience of 544 consecutive cases. J Am Coll Surg. 2005; 201(1):57–65.
167. Ito K, Ito H, Kemeny NE, Gonen M, Allen PJ, Paty PB, et al. Biliary sclerosis after hepatic arterial infusion pump chemotherapy for patients with colorectal cancer liver metastasis: incidence, clinical features, and risk factors. Ann Surg Oncol. 2012;19(5):1609–17.
168. Mocellin S, Pilati P, Lise M, Nitti D. Meta-analysis of hepatic arterial infusion for unresectable liver metastases from colorectal cancer: the end of an era? J Clin Oncol. 2007; 25(35):5649–54.
169. Kemeny NE, Niedzwiecki D, Hollis DR, Lenz HJ, Warren RS, Naughton MJ, et al. Hepatic arterial infusion versus systemic therapy for hepatic metastases from colorectal cancer: a randomized trial of efficacy, quality of life, and molecular markers (CALGB 9481). J Clin Oncol. 2006;24(9):1395–403.
170. Kemeny N, Jarnagin W, Paty P, Gonen M, Schwartz L, Morse M, et al. Phase I trial of systemic oxaliplatin combination chemotherapy with hepatic arterial infusion in patients with unresectable liver metastases from colorectal cancer. J Clin Oncol. 2005;23(22):4888–96.
171. D'Angelica MI, Correa-Gallego C, Paty PB, Cercek A, Gewirtz AN, Chou JF, et al. Phase II trial of hepatic artery infusional and systemic chemotherapy for patients with unresectable hepatic metastases from colorectal cancer: conversion to resection and long-term outcomes. Ann Surg. 2014;261:353.
172. Ammori JB, Kemeny NE, Fong Y, Cercek A, Dematteo RP, Allen PJ, et al. Conversion to complete resection and/or ablation using hepatic artery infusional chemotherapy in patients with unresectable liver metastases from colorectal cancer: a decade of experience at a single institution. Ann Surg Oncol. 2013;20(9):2901–7.
173. Kemeny N, Huang Y, Cohen AM, Shi W, Conti JA, Brennan MF, et al. Hepatic arterial infusion of chemotherapy after resection of hepatic metastases from colorectal cancer. N Engl J Med. 1999;341(27):2039–48.

174. Ito H, Are C, Gonen M, D'Angelica M, Dematteo RP, Kemeny NE, et al. Effect of postoperative morbidity on long-term survival after hepatic resection for metastatic colorectal cancer. Ann Surg. 2008;247(6):994–1002.

175. House MG, Kemeny NE, Gonen M, Fong Y, Allen PJ, Paty PB, et al. Comparison of adjuvant systemic chemotherapy with or without hepatic arterial infusional chemotherapy after hepatic resection for metastatic colorectal cancer. Ann Surg. 2011;254(6):851–6.

176. Fiorentini G, Aliberti C, Mulazzani L, Coschiera P, Catalano V, Rossi D, et al. Chemoembolization in colorectal liver metastases: the rebirth. Anticancer Res. 2014; 34(2):575–84.

177. Taylor RR, Tang Y, Gonzalez MV, Stratford PW, Lewis AL. Irinotecan drug eluting beads for use in chemoembolization: in vitro and in vivo evaluation of drug release properties. Eur J Pharm Sci. 2007;30(1):7–14.

178. Fiorentini G, Aliberti C, Tilli M, Mulazzani L, Graziano F, Giordani P, et al. Intra-arterial infusion of irinotecan-loaded drug-eluting beads (DEBIRI) versus intravenous therapy (FOLFIRI) for hepatic metastases from colorectal cancer: final results of a phase III study. Anticancer Res. 2012;32(4):1387–95.

179. Saxena A, Bester L, Shan L, Perera M, Gibbs P, Meteling B, et al. A systematic review on the safety and efficacy of yttrium-90 radioembolization for unresectable, chemorefractory colorectal cancer liver metastases. J Cancer Res Clin Oncol. 2014;140(4):537–47.

180. Primrose JN. Surgery for colorectal liver metastases. Br J Cancer. 2010;102(9):1313–8.

181. Nguyen KT, Gamblin TC, Geller DA. World review of laparoscopic liver resection-2,804 patients. Ann Surg. 2009;250(5):831–41.

182. Castaing D, Vibert E, Ricca L, Azoulay D, Adam R, Gayet B. Oncologic results of laparoscopic versus open hepatectomy for colorectal liver metastases in two specialized centers. Ann Surg. 2009;250(5):849–55.

Incidentalomas of the Pancreas

John C. McAuliffe and John D. Christein

Introduction: The Scope of the Problem

Pancreatic ductal adenocarcinoma (PDAC)is the fourth leading cause of cancer-related mortality in the United States. Approximately 43,000 will be diagnosed with PDAC within the United States this year and up to 230,000 people worldwide will die of the cancer this year [1–3]. The estimated overall 1-year survival is only 22 % with less than 5 % survival at 5 years. The only potentially curative modality is surgical resection. Unfortunately, only 15–20 % of patients will have disease amenable to extirpation at presentation [1]. Even with intended curative resection, survival is limited.

Clearly, with such a poor prognosis, early detection or ideally diagnosis of a malignant precursor would be beneficial. And yet, no validated means of screening for PDAC exist.

Over the last 20 years, utilization of cross-sectional imaging has increased dramatically. At the same time, improved technological capabilities and spatial resolution have increased the number of incidental findings [4]. As a result, a veritable epidemic of newly discovered asymptomatic pancreatic lesions has occurred. The term "pancreatic incidentaloma" or an asymptomatic pancreatic lesion was coined in 2001 [4]. The frequency of pancreatic incidentalomas seen by CT and MRI is 1.2–20 % [5, 6]. An list of potential diagnoses can be found in Table 1.

J.C. McAuliffe, M.D., Ph.D.
Department of Surgery, Memorial Sloan Kettering Cancer Center,
1275 York Ave, C-1272, New York, NY 10065, USA
e-mail: jmcauliffe78@gmail.com

J.D. Christein, M.D. (✉)
Division of Gastrointestinal Surgery, Department of Surgery,
University of Atlanta at Birmingham, 1720 2nd Avenue South,
Kracke Building (KB) Room 428, Birmingham, AL 35294-0016, USA
e-mail: jchristein@uabmc.edu

© Springer International Publishing Switzerland 2016
K.A. Morgan (ed.), *Current Controversies in Cancer Care
for the Surgeon*, DOI 10.1007/978-3-319-16205-8_6

Table 1 Etiology of pancreatic lesions

Neoplastic	Non-neoplastic
Ductal adenocarcinoma	Lymphoepithelial cyst
Mucinous cystadenocarcinoma	Congential cyst
Pancreatoblastoma	Mucinous non-neoplastic cyst
Neuroendocrine tumor	Enterogeneous cyst
Solid pseudopapillary tumor	Retention cyst
Serous cystadenoma	Duodenal cyst
Mucinous cystadenoma	Endometrial cyst
Intraductal papillary mucinous neoplasm	Pseudocyst
Sarcoma	Parasitic cyst
Lymphoma	Autoimmune pancreatitis
Metastatic lesion	Splenule
Dermoid cyst	Fat necrosis
Hamartoma	
Acinar cell cystadenoma	
von Hippel-Lindau cystic neoplasm	
Cholangiocarcinoma	
Gastrointestinal stromal tumor	

The diagnosis of incidentaloma may be a great opportunity for eradication of a malignancy or precursor even at high volume centers, mortality and morbidity following pancreatic surgery is 3 and 50 %, respectively [3]. In addition, surgical intervention and management of these patients carries a financial burden [7].

In the context of an incidentaloma, the benefit of early detention with subsequent aggressive surgical resection versus the morbidity and mortality is a delicate balance for both patient and the health care institution. The following review will discuss the risk of malignancy, etiology of, and the current recommendations for management of pancreatic incidentalomas, particularly cystic lesions. Excluded from this review are lesions of the pancreas that are symptomatic including sequelae of acute, autoimmune, or chronic pancreatitis (i.e. pancreatic pseudocyst) and advanced carcinoma (primary or metastatic).

The Threat: Risk of Malignancy

The concern of any lesion in the pancreas is malignancy. Reports indicate that up to 60 % of lesions of the pancreas harbor malignant or pre-malignant diagnoses [8]. Early detection and resection leads to favorable survival for those with malignancy [9]. In one report, 5-year survival was 64 % for incidental lesions as compared to 47 % for non-incidental lesions with a median survival of 145 versus 46 months. Disease-specific survival for adenocarcinoma was improved by 3 months for incidental lesions compared to non-incidental lesions [10].

Multiple high volume pancreatic groups have presented their experience with pancreatic incidentalomas. Vollmer et al. presented a 5-year experience showing 17 % of incidentalomas were invasive cancer [11]. Lahat et al. showed that 34 % of patients with pancreatic incidentalomas harbored malignancy [10]. Importantly, this rate was half of those with symptomatic lesions. But, 23 % of the incidental group had the diagnosis of intraductal papillary mucinous neoplasm (IPMN), a pre-malignant lesion.

In these reports, invasive lesions were adenocarcinoma of the pancreas. However, neuroendocrine tumors, cholangiocarcinoma, and metastatic lesions can also be seen in a minority of cases [10, 12]. The operations required to extirpate these lesions include pancreaticoduodenectomy (approx. 30 % of the time), central (8 %) and distal pancreatectomy (30 %), total pancreatectomy (4 %), and enucleation (2–22 %) [12]. Features of the each common incidentaloma are summarized in Table 2. Important to note, lesions of the pancreas that are symptomatic have an indication for surgery in surgically fit patients. Extensive laboratory and invasive workup is not necessary for these patients. However, in those without symptoms better definition of the disease is required to tailor intervention or surveillance.

Cystic Incidentalomas

Most of pancreatic incidental lesions (52 %) are cystic rather than solid [11]. Cystic lesions can be classified into congenital (serous and multicystic syndromes), inflammatory (pseudocysts), and neoplastic (serous cystadenoma/SCN and mucinous cystic neoplasms/MCN, and intraductal papillary mucinous neoplasms (IPMN, main-duct and branched-duct)). Typically inflammatory and main-duct IPMN lesions are symptomatic. The cystic neoplasms represent 90 % of incidental cystic lesions of the pancreas [13]. Patients present with CT of the chest, abdomen, or pelvis that lacks the resolution to adequately define the pancreatic lesion and its resectability. Following a comprehensive history and physical, repeat CT or MRI with a pancreatic protocol is optimal to better define the lesion and predict its natural history.

SCNs have a well-demarcated wall with multiple septated cysts within its mass described as a honey-comb lesion. Most SCNs are found in the pancreatic head. Symptoms relate to mass effect: gastric outlet obstruction, early satiety, and jaundice. Each cyst is <2 cm filled with clear fluid void of mucin (carcinoembryonic antigen/CEA). SCNs are typically single and located in the pancreatic parenchyma but can become quite large (up to 25 cm). Importantly, these lesions are considered benign but as they enlarge can cause symptoms. Once symptomatic, surgically fit patients should undergo an appropriate resection. If these lesions have mural nodularity, however, the diagnosis of SCN should be questioned. Further workup or early resection is warranted as nodularity is a worrisome finding for malignancy. Only 25 cases of a malignancy have been reported [14]. The long-term survival for these lesions appears to be very favorable following resection.

Table 2 Summary of clinical feature of common incidentalomas

Entity	Serum	Cystic contents	Ultrasound	ERCP	CT/MRI
IPMN	Normal	High CEA	Mural nodules, ductal dilation	Communicates with duct, ductal dilation	Mural nodules, ductal dilation
MCN	Normal	High CEA, CA 19-9, low amylase	Round, smooth, large cyst	No ductal involvement	Round, well circumscribed, septations, macrocystic
SCN	Normal	Low CEA, CA 19-9, amylase	Septations, calcifications	No ductal involvement	Septations, honeycomb, central scar, hypervascular
Pseudocyst	Normal	High amylase, low CEA, CA 19-9	Anechoic, smooth, round	Ductal communication possible	Round, fluid filled, smooth, unilocular
Lymphoepithelial Cyst	Normal	High CEA, CA 19-9	Hypoechoic, internal debris	No ductal involvement	Low attenuation, internal keratin
PNET	High chromogranin, GI hormone if functioning	Low or normal CEA, CA 19-9	Smooth, round, loculations variable	Normal duct	Hyperattenuation
SPT	Normal	NA	Hypoechoic	Ductal involvement variable	Cystic degeneration, solid and cystic

MCNs are the most common cystic lesion of the pancreas [15]. They do have malignant potential. Ten to 50 % of MCNs harbor malignancy. These lesions, as their name implies, produce mucin from their mucin-producing epithelial wall. MCNs do not communicate with the pancreatic duct. Histologically, the cyst wall is mucin-rich with ovarian-like stoma with estrogen and progesterone receptors in most cases. Most lesions are found in the body and tail but can, though less commonly, be in the pancreatic head and uncinate. Usually these present as a single cyst with fine septations with a rim of calcification and considered macrocytic in contrast to SCNs, which are microcytic. Following appropriate abdominal imaging, endoscopic ultrasound (EUS) is recommended for biopsy and cyst fluid analysis. A cyst fluid level of CEA>192 ng/mL (which implies a mucinous lesion) with a low amylase has an 80 % diagnostic accuracy for MCN. In contrast, a pseudocyst has a high amylase and low CEA level [16]. Once the diagnosis is made, resection is recommended for all surgically fit patients [17]. Prognosis is dependent on pathology: benign, borderline, or malignant. In the setting of malignancy, 5-year survival following resection is 57 % [18]. Survival is better than those with pancreatic adenocarcinoma.

Much like MCNs, IPMN can present anywhere in the spectrum of tumor progression from a benign adenoma, to borderline or dysplastic, carcinoma in situ (PanIN), and invasive carcinoma. IPMNs are described based on the pancreatic duct morphology in relation to the cyst. Branch-duct IPMN do not involve the main duct of Wirsung. Lesions affecting the main duct are labeled main-duct IPMN. Side-branch IPMNs that extend to the main duct are called mixed-type IPMN. These lesions are characterized by dilation of the pancreatic duct. All these subtypes are pre-malignant and invasive cancer is found in 20–50 % of resected pancreatic specimens [19]. Features that are worrisome for malignant degeneration are cysts >3 cm, main duct diameter of 1 cm, mural nodules, size, main-duct disease, cyst wall thickening, and elevated CA 19-9. Likewise, symptoms such as jaundice are associated with an increased likelihood of a malignancy.

International, contemporary management of mucinous neoplasms of the pancreas is summarized by Tanaka et al. in 2012 [17]. These guidelines are a revision of the 2006 consensus statement, or Sendai Criteria, and highlight advances in endoscopy, CT, MRI, as well as elucidation of the natural history of these diseases at high volume centers. We strongly recommend the reader to this consensus statement. The working group clearly defines high-risk stigmata of malignancy and "worrisome" features aiding in the management and follow up for these lesions. The algorithmic approach given by this group is displayed in Fig. 1.

Another type of incidentaloma are lymphoepithelial cysts. They are rare compared to other etiologies of incidentalomas of the pancreas. They are cysts composed of a mature keratinizing squamous epithelial surrounded by lymphoid tissue. They are born from ectopic pancreatic tissue arising in a lymph node that undergoes metaplasia. In contrast to other cystic lesions of the pancreas, most are found in men. They can have a high CA 19-9 and mucin level confusing their diagnosis with IPMN. They are well demarcated with low attenuation by CT and are hypoechoic with internal debris by sonography. The use of MRI differentiates the internal

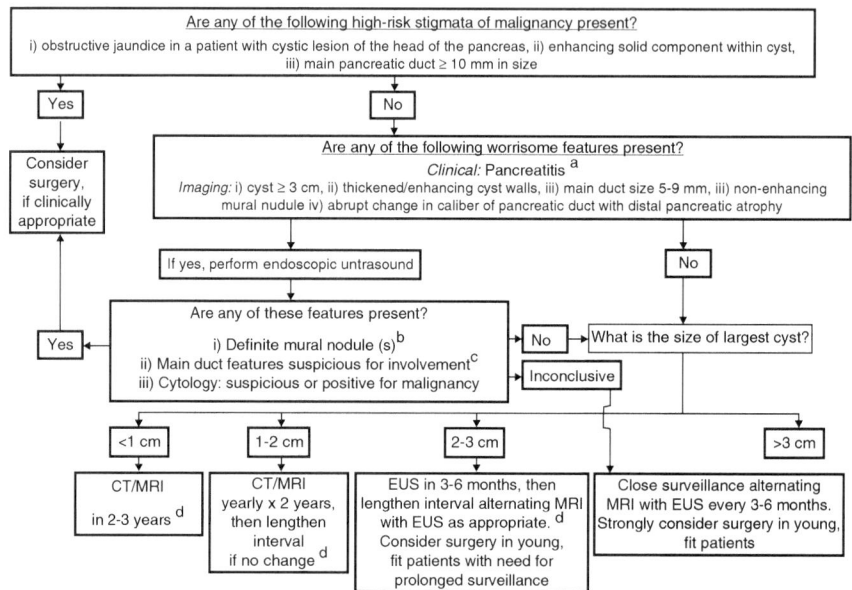

a. Pancreatitis may be an indication for surgery for relief of symptoms.

b. Differential diagnosis includes mucin. Mucin can move with change in patient position, may be dislodged on cyst lavage and does not have Doppler flow. Features of true tumor nodule include lack of mobility, presence of Doppler flow and FNA of nodule showing tumor tissue

c. Presence of any one of thickened walls, intraductal mucin or mural nodules is suggestive of main duct involvement. In their absence main duct involvement is incolclusive.

d. Studies from Japan suggest that on follow-up of subjects with suspected BD-IPMN there is increased incidence of pancreatic ductal adenocarcinoma unrelated to malignant transformation of the BD-IPMN(s) being followed. However, it is unclear if imaging surveillance can detect early ductal adenocarcinoma, and, if so, at what interval surveillance imaging should be performed.

Fig. 1 Algorithim for evaluating and managing cystic neoplams of the pancreas as defined by the International consensus guidelines 2012 [17]

keratin debris of the cyst with high T1 and low T2 signals. Characteristic MRI findings, no ductal dilatation, and biopsy help differentiate this benign lesion from more ominous entities. Resection is not warranted unless severe symptoms occur.

Solid Lesions

As stated previously, a minority of incidentalomas of the pancreas are solid. To the exhaustive clinician, the majority of solid lesions manifest albeit at times subtle. The discovery of a solid lesion should provoke anxiety. As reported, only 13 % of solid lesions are benign. Up to 38 % were overtly malignant with another 49 % having malignant potential [11]. Solid incidentalomas have a myriad of diagnoses but adenocarcinoma and pancreatic neuroendocrine tumors principally. Other diagnosis can be solid pseudopapillary tumors, metastatic implants or lymphomas. Rarely do solid lesions present as incidental findings. We will discuss neuroendocrine tumor (PNET) and solid pseudopapillary tumors (SPPS).

Pancreatic Neuroendocrine Tumor

PNET represent only 1–2 % of neoplasms of the pancreas and have unique clinical characteristics. While histologically similar to other neuroendocrine tumors throughout the gut, PNETs differ in their biology. PNETs are classified as functional and non-functional. Functional tumors secrete products of the islet cells (either insulin, glucagon, somatostatin, VIP, or gastrin) and manifest in fascinating ways [20]. Most PNETs are sporadic neoplasms. However, rarely PNETs arise in the constellation of hereditary syndromes; namely, multiple endocrine neoplasia type 1, neurofibromatosis type 1, von Hippel-Lindau, and tuberous sclerosis [21]. Outside of the hereditary syndrome, non-functional typically present with a vague or non-specific symptoms. They can also be incidentalomas.

Up to 50 % of patients with PNET present with locally advanced or metastatic disease. While not secreting a functional gastrointestinal hormone, non-functioning PNETs typically secrete chromogranin A, a neuron-specific enolase, and pancreatic polypeptide. Serum chromogranin A is a good biomarker for PNETs, a surrogate for disease burden, and response to therapy [22]. Serum levels should be measured prior to and after interventions for PNETs.

If adequate imaging is not available at diagnosis, a pancreas protocol CT or MRI will evaluate all lesions greater than 1 cm, metastatic implants, and orientation to pertinent anatomy for a planned resection. These lesions are hypervascular providing easy visualization during arterial phase contrasted studies. An alternative to radiographic imaging is endoscopic ultrasound which may also provide biopsy capability [23]. To improve the staging workup, somatostatic receptor scintigraphy should be considered prior to intervention on PNETs [24, 25].

The main stay of therapy for PNETs is surgical resection for locoregional disease. Extipation provides the only means of cure and symptom relief if functional. Save for insulinomas, PNETs are malignant and resection should include formal pancreatectomy and en-bloc lymphadenectomy [26]. Currently, enucleation is not a recommended modality but is being explored for tumor <2 cm [27]. Following resection, metastasis is common in usually an indolent course with 48 % of patients having liver metastasis at 3 years following resection [28]. Thus oncologic surveillance annually is required. For unresectable, recurrent, or metastatic disease combination cytotoxic chemotherapy has shown efficacy for PNET with response rates as high as 70 % using capecitabine and temozolomide [29]. Multiple other regiments utilizing streptozotocin, 5-flourouracil, and doxorubicin can be used as well. In addition, targeted therapies such as mTOR and receptor tyrosine kinase inhibitors have shown promise alone or in combination with cytotoxic therapies [30–32]. As one would expect, survival and response to therapy depends on the tumor stage and the tumor biology in each individual patient.

Solid Pseudopapillary Tumor

Solid pseudopapillary tumors (SPTs)) are solid lesions of the pancreas that undergo cystic degeneration due to hemorrhage or necrosis. These account for a mere 3 % of all pancreatic resections. Diagnosis in the female predominates and typically in the mid-20s. A minority of patients present without symptoms will most present with pain or mass effect [33].

Cross-sectional imaging reveals a well-circumscribed lesion with calcified deposits in the wall with irregular hypodensities signifying necrosis and hemorrhage. The key to differentiating this tumor from pseudocysts is the combination of solid and cystic components with degenerative components (pseudopapillae) [34]. Importantly, these tumors do not cause pancreatic ductal dilation.

SPTs do have malignant potential and should be resected if able. They are indolent and cured with partial pancreatectomy. Up to 15 % however are metastatic at presentation. Resection is not precluded by metastasis however, and durable survival is possible [35].

Conclusion

With the increased resolution and use of abdominal imaging for a variety of complaints, lesions of the pancreas are more prevalent. The discovery of a small, asymptomatic pancreatic lesion requires a rational workup to determine malignant potential and surgical resection. The natural history of incidentalomas is being better defined at high volume centers of excellence in pancreatic diseases. We have reviewed the workup and indications for treatment for each of the common incidentalomas of the pancreas.

References

1. Sharma C, Eltawil KM, Renfrew PD, Walsh MJ, Molinari M. Advances in diagnosis, treatment and palliation of pancreatic carcinoma: 1990-2010. World J Gastroenterol. 2011;17(7):867–97.
2. Vincent A, Herman J, Schulick R, Hruban RH, Goggins M. Pancreatic cancer. Lancet. 2011;378(9791):607–20.
3. Vollmer CM, Sanchez N, Gondek S, McAuliffe J, Kent TS, Christein JD, et al. A root-cause analysis of mortality following major pancreatectomy. J Gastrointest Surg. 2012;16(1):89–102. discussion 3.
4. Berland LL, Silverman SG, Gore RM, Mayo-Smith WW, Megibow AJ, Yee J, et al. Managing incidental findings on abdominal CT: white paper of the ACR incidental findings committee. J Am Coll Radiol. 2010;7(10):754–73.
5. Spinelli KS, Fromwiller TE, Daniel RA, Kiely JM, Nakeeb A, Komorowski RA, et al. Cystic pancreatic neoplasms: observe or operate. Ann Surg. 2004;239(5):651–7. discussion 7–9.
6. Laffan TA, Horton KM, Klein AP, Berlanstein B, Siegelman SS, Kawamoto S, et al. Prevalence of unsuspected pancreatic cysts on MDCT. AJR Am J Roentgenol. 2008;191(3):802–7.

7. Vollmer CM. The economics of pancreas surgery. Surg Clin North Am. 2013;93(3):711–28.

8. Fernández-del Castillo C, Targarona J, Thayer SP, Rattner DW, Brugge WR, Warshaw AL. Incidental pancreatic cysts: clinicopathologic characteristics and comparison with symptomatic patients. Arch Surg. 2003;138(4):427–34. discussion 33-4.

9. Winter JM, Cameron JL, Lillemoe KD, Campbell KA, Chang D, Riall TS, et al. Periampullary and pancreatic incidentaloma: a single institution's experience with an increasingly common diagnosis. Ann Surg. 2006;243(5):673–80. discussion 80-3.

10. Lahat G, Ben Haim M, Nachmany I, Sever R, Blachar A, Nakache R, et al. Pancreatic incidentalomas: high rate of potentially malignant tumors. J Am Coll Surg. 2009;209(3):313–9.

11. Sachs T, Pratt WB, Callery MP, Vollmer CM. The incidental asymptomatic pancreatic lesion: nuisance or threat? J Gastrointest Surg. 2009;13(3):405–15.

12. Kent TS, Vollmer CM, Callery MP. Intraductal papillary mucinous neoplasm and the pancreatic incidentaloma. World J Gastrointest Surg. 2010;2(10):319–23.

13. Allen PJ, Jaques DP, D'Angelica M, Bowne WB, Conlon KC, Brennan MF. Cystic lesions of the pancreas: selection criteria for operative and nonoperative management in 209 patients. J Gastrointest Surg. 2003;7(8):970–7.

14. King JC, Ng TT, White SC, Cortina G, Reber HA, Hines OJ. Pancreatic serous cystadenocarcinoma: a case report and review of the literature. J Gastrointest Surg. 2009;13(10):1864–8.

15. Compagno J, Oertel JE. Mucinous cystic neoplasms of the pancreas with overt and latent malignancy (cystadenocarcinoma and cystadenoma). A clinicopathologic study of 41 cases. Am J Clin Pathol. 1978;69(6):573–80.

16. Brugge WR, Lewandrowski K, Lee-Lewandrowski E, Centeno BA, Szydlo T, Regan S, et al. Diagnosis of pancreatic cystic neoplasms: a report of the cooperative pancreatic cyst study. Gastroenterology. 2004;126(5):1330–6.

17. Tanaka M, Fernández-del Castillo C, Adsay V, Chari S, Falconi M, Jang JY, et al. International consensus guidelines 2012 for the management of IPMN and MCN of the pancreas. Pancreatology. 2012;12(3):183–97.

18. Goh BK, Ooi LL, Kumarasinghe MP, Tan YM, Cheow PC, Chow PK, et al. Clinicopathological features of patients with concomitant intraductal papillary mucinous neoplasm of the pancreas and pancreatic endocrine neoplasm. Pancreatology. 2006;6(6):520–6.

19. D'Angelica M, Brennan MF, Suriawinata AA, Klimstra D, Conlon KC. Intraductal papillary mucinous neoplasms of the pancreas: an analysis of clinicopathologic features and outcome. Ann Surg. 2004;239(3):400–8.

20. Metz DC, Jensen RT. Gastrointestinal neuroendocrine tumors: pancreatic endocrine tumors. Gastroenterology. 2008;135(5):1469–92.

21. Jensen RT, Berna MJ, Bingham DB, Norton JA. Inherited pancreatic endocrine tumor syndromes: advances in molecular pathogenesis, diagnosis, management, and controversies. Cancer. 2008;113 Suppl 7:1807–43.

22. Campana D, Nori F, Piscitelli L, Morselli-Labate AM, Pezzilli R, Corinaldesi R, et al. Chromogranin A: is it a useful marker of neuroendocrine tumors? J Clin Oncol. 2007;25(15):1967–73.

23. Anderson MA, Carpenter S, Thompson NW, Nostrant TT, Elta GH, Scheiman JM. Endoscopic ultrasound is highly accurate and directs management in patients with neuroendocrine tumors of the pancreas. Am J Gastroenterol. 2000;95(9):2271–7.

24. Kulke MH, Anthony LB, Bushnell DL, de Herder WW, Goldsmith SJ, Klimstra DS, et al. NANETS treatment guidelines: well-differentiated neuroendocrine tumors of the stomach and pancreas. Pancreas. 2010;39(6):735–52.

25. Kunz PL, Reidy-Lagunes D, Anthony LB, Bertino EM, Brendtro K, Chan JA, et al. Consensus guidelines for the management and treatment of neuroendocrine tumors. Pancreas. 2013;42(4):557–77.

26. Kouvaraki MA, Solorzano CC, Shapiro SE, Yao JC, Perrier ND, Lee JE, et al. Surgical treatment of non-functioning pancreatic islet cell tumors. J Surg Oncol. 2005;89(3):170–85.

27. Fernández-Cruz L, Molina V, Vallejos R, Jiménez Chavarria E, López-Boado MA, Ferrer J. Outcome after laparoscopic enucleation for non-functional neuroendocrine pancreatic tumours. HPB (Oxford). 2012;14(3):171–6.

28. Solorzano CC, Lee JE, Pisters PW, Vauthey JN, Ayers GD, Jean ME, et al. Nonfunctioning islet cell carcinoma of the pancreas: survival results in a contemporary series of 163 patients. Surgery. 2001;130(6):1078–85.

29. Strosberg JR, Fine RL, Choi J, Nasir A, Coppola D, Chen DT, et al. First-line chemotherapy with capecitabine and temozolomide in patients with metastatic pancreatic endocrine carcinomas. Cancer. 2011;117(2):268–75.

30. Yao JC, Shah MH, Ito T, Bohas CL, Wolin EM, Van Cutsem E, et al. Everolimus for advanced pancreatic neuroendocrine tumors. N Engl J Med. 2011;364(6):514–23.

31. Yao JC, Phan AT, Jehl V, Shah G, Meric-Bernstam F. Everolimus in advanced pancreatic neuroendocrine tumors: the clinical experience. Cancer Res. 2013;73(5):1449–53.

32. Raymond E, Dahan L, Raoul JL, Bang YJ, Borbath I, Lombard-Bohas C, et al. Sunitinib malate for the treatment of pancreatic neuroendocrine tumors. N Engl J Med. 2011;364(6):501–13.

33. Papavramidis T, Papavramidis S. Solid pseudopapillary tumors of the pancreas: review of 718 patients reported in English literature. J Am Coll Surg. 2005;200(6):965–72.

34. Tang LH, Aydin H, Brennan MF, Klimstra DS. Clinically aggressive solid pseudopapillary tumors of the pancreas: a report of two cases with components of undifferentiated carcinoma and a comparative clinicopathologic analysis of 34 conventional cases. Am J Surg Pathol. 2005;29(4):512–9.

35. Reddy S, Cameron JL, Scudiere J, Hruban RH, Fishman EK, Ahuja N, et al. Surgical management of solid-pseudopapillary neoplasms of the pancreas (Franz or Hamoudi tumors): a large single-institutional series. J Am Coll Surg. 2009;208(5):950–7. discussion 7–9.

Current Controversies in the Surgical Management of Pancreatic Cancer

Ammar Asrar Javed, Kanza Aziz, and Christopher Lee Wolfgang

Introduction

Pancreatic ductal adenocarcinoma (PDAC) is one of the deadliest of all solid malignancies and ranks as the fourth leading cause of cancer-related deaths in the United States [1]. It is estimated that in 2014, 46,420 people were diagnosed with pancreatic cancer and 39,590 people died from it [1]. The 5-year survival rate remains approximately 5 % despite advancements in surgery and oncologic therapies.

A.A. Javed, M.B.B.S.
The Center for Surgical Trials and Outcomes Research, Johns Hopkins
University School of Medicine, Baltimore, MD USA

Department of Surgery, Johns Hopkins University School of Medicine,
685 Blalock, 600N. Wolfe Street, Baltimore, MD 21287, USA
e-mail: ajaved1@jhmi.edu

K. Aziz, M.B.B.S.
Department of Surgery, Johns Hopkins University School of Medicine,
685 Blalock, 600N. Wolfe Street, Baltimore, MD 21287, USA
e-mail: kanza.aku@gmail.com

C.L. Wolfgang, M.D., Ph.D., F.A.C.S. (✉)
Department of Surgery, Johns Hopkins University School of Medicine,
685 Blalock, 600N. Wolfe Street, Baltimore, MD 21287, USA

Department of Pathology, Johns Hopkins University School of Medicine,
685 Blalock, 600N. Wolfe Street, Baltimore, MD 21287, USA

The Sidney Kimmel Comprehensive Cancer Center, Johns Hopkins
University School of Medicine, Baltimore, MD, USA

The Skip Viragh Center for Pancreatic Cancer, Johns Hopkins
University School of Medicine, Baltimore, MD, USA

The Sol Goldman Pancreatic Cancer Center, Johns Hopkins
University School of Medicine, Baltimore, MD, USA
e-mail: cwolfga2@jhmi.edu

© Springer International Publishing Switzerland 2016
K.A. Morgan (ed.), *Current Controversies in Cancer Care*
for the Surgeon, DOI 10.1007/978-3-319-16205-8_7

Early diagnosis is difficult due to the absence of specific symptoms and early systemic spread. Therefore, a majority of patients are diagnosed late in the course of the disease when the cancer has already spread to other organs [2]. Unfortunately, 80 % of patients at the time of diagnosis are not surgical candidates [3]. Surgical resection remains the only potential form of curative management.

The natural history of PDAC is characterized by early systemic spread and major vessel involvement, resistance to chemotherapy, and rapid progression which make the treatment challenging. The complexity of treatment of PDAC has led to several controversies over the optimal approach to managing certain aspects of this disease. This chapter aims to review the overall management of pancreatic adenocarcinoma with a focus on a few controversial issues regarding diagnosis and treatment as it relates to surgical practice. In particular four main controversies have specific importance to surgeons, including (1) the use of diagnostic laparoscopy, (2) surgery-first versus neoadjuvant approach, (3) definition of borderline resectable disease, and (4) ablative therapies for locally advanced unresectable pancreatic cancer.

Summary of Pancreatic Cancer

Patients with pancreatic cancer present with vague and nonspecific symptoms, thus most often leading to a late diagnosis. Two-thirds of these lesions occur in the head of the pancreas [4] and commonly present with symptoms related to the obstruction of the biliary tree [5]: jaundice, dark urine, acholic stools, and pruritus. Tumors of the tail, on the other hand, present later on and are more commonly associated with abdominal pain with or without back pain and nonspecific findings like unexplained weight loss, anorexia, early satiety, dyspepsia, nausea, and depression [6]. Pancreatic cancer can also present with new-onset diabetes mellitus or signs and symptoms of chronic pancreatitis. Sudden onset of a difficult to control, atypical type 2 diabetes mellitus in a thin patient, 50 years or older may suggest presence of a pancreatic neoplasm [7, 8]. Interestingly, depression is also a common finding and in some instances, a diagnosis of depression precedes the diagnosis of cancer [6].

Multiple risk factors contribute to the development of pancreatic adenocarcinoma including both environmental and inherited ones [9, 10]. Environmental agents include cigarette smoking [11–13], heavy alcohol consumption, increased body mass index (BMI) [14], long-standing type 2 diabetes [15, 16], and chronic pancreatitis. The best documented of these risk factors is cigarette smoking. Approximately one-quarter of all pancreatic cancers can be attributed to exposure to tobacco [7, 13]. Studies have reported a 2.2-fold increase in risk of pancreatic cancer in smokers as compared to non-smokers, and more importantly that it decreases to 1.64- and 1.12-fold in patients who quit smoking 1–10 and 15–20 years ago, respectively [12]. In addition to these modifiable risk factors, hereditary factors may play a role in a small proportion of pancreatic cancers. A 1.9- to 13-fold increased risk has been reported in patients with a positive family history of pancreatic cancer

[17–20]. Familial pancreatic cancer is defined as having at least a pair of first-degree relatives with pancreatic cancer in the family. Family registries such as the National Familial Pancreas Tumor Registry (NFPTR) at Johns Hopkins have revealed a 6.8-fold increased risk of developing pancreatic cancer in first-degree relatives of familial cancer patients, as opposed to the general population of United States [21].

The treatment of pancreatic cancer is difficult and requires a multidisciplinary approach. Decision for treatment is usually made after a thorough discussion that involves the oncological surgeons, pathologists, radiologists, medical oncologists, radiation oncologists, and pain management specialists. The multidisciplinary approach leads to an improvement in categorization of the disease prior to initiation of treatment and also at times leads to a change in diagnosis and/or management decisions [22].

Accurate staging of PDAC is essential, as management decisions directly depend on the stage of the disease. The most commonly used staging system is the one proposed by the American Joint Committee on Cancer (AJCC) which includes the TNM classification [23–25]. This staging system divides the disease into stage I and stage II which are resectable and a subgroup of stage II which is borderline resectable. Stage III is locally advanced disease which is unresectable and stage IV which takes into account presence of metastatic disease [26] (Table 1). The treatment of pancreatic cancer is dependent on the stage and resectability of the disease and different institutions have proposed staging systems which determine whether the disease is resectable, borderline resectable, unresectable, or metastatic [27].

Surgical resection followed by adjuvant therapy is the main stay of treatment for patients with Stage I/II disease. The use of neoadjuvant therapy for these patients is controversial. Patients with Stage II borderline resectable disease should receive neoadjuvant therapy preoperatively [28]. Patients with stage III locally advanced

Table 1 AJCC TNM staging of pancreatic adenocarcinoma

Stage	Description	Tumor extent	Surgical category
IA	Tumor is <2 cm and limited to the pancreas	Localized	Resectable
IB	Tumor is >2 cm and limited to the pancreas		
IIA	Tumor extends directly beyond the pancreas No arterial involvement. LN−	Locally advanced	Resectable or borderline resectable
IIB	Tumor may or may not extend beyond the pancreas No arterial involvement. LN+		
III	Tumor involves major local arteries (SMA, celiac). LN− or LN+	Locally advanced	Unresectable
IV	Primary tumor may be any size. Metastatic disease is present	Metastatic	Unresectable

disease should be treated with chemotherapy and/or chemoradiotherapy. A great number of these patients tend to develop metastatic disease later on; however, a few select cases can still be considered suitable for surgical resection. Systemic therapy is administered to patients with Stage IV disease with a good performance status while those with poor overall health are given supportive and palliative therapy [2, 27].

Controversies

The Role of Diagnostic Laparoscopy

Radiological diagnosis of pancreatic cancer has improved greatly due to advancement in imaging technology leading to increased sensitivity of available modalities. The first step in the diagnosis of suspected pancreatic adenocarcinoma is a pancreas protocol CT and a chest CT [27]. The pancreas protocol CT is a detailed examination of the pancreas. It includes both a non-contrast scan and contrast enhancement of arterial, pancreatic parenchymal, and portovenous phases. The difference between the tumor and the pancreatic parenchyma is most prominent during the late arterial phase during contrast enhancement. Post processing three-dimensional reconstructions of images assist in determining the relationship of the tumor to its surrounding vasculature, thus helping to determine tumor resectability. MRI scans are helpful in finding small metastatic deposits especially in the liver and peritoneum. It can also be used in patients who cannot tolerate contrast for CT. CT scans and MRIs have comparable sensitivities [27]. Endoscopic ultrasound can be used to visualize the tumor and also to obtain tissue for diagnosis. PET scanning has a role in select cases [29] and retrospective studies have shown that it has increased sensitivity to identifying metastatic disease compared to CT scan alone [30]. It can also be used to determine the extent of soft tissue invasion before planning radiotherapy [31]. Evidence of extrapancreatic spread, involvement of celiac axis and the SMA, and the patency of the SMV-PV confluence are all factors that can be identified on imaging and help determine tumor resectability [32].

Although CT remains the main tool for staging, the major variability in false negatives, is small peritoneal disease. One older study reported that 20–30 % of patients who appear to have resectable disease on CT were found to have undetected local spread or hepatic and peritoneal implants [33]. For this reason, some centers advocate the routine use of diagnostic laparoscopy. Laparoscopy has the potential to better establish tumor resectability by allowing direct visualization of the tumor and detecting hepatic and peritoneal metastases, particularly when coupled with laparoscopic ultrasound. Doppler techniques can also be used to assess vascular involvement [34, 35]. Moreover, in-depth laparoscopic staging in which celiac, periportal, and peripancreatic lymph nodes are examined has been reported [36]. Thus, laparoscopy potentially prevents the morbidity associated with a non-therapeutic laparotomy in patients with unresectable tumors. These patients can then receive chemotherapy without delay [37]. In patients who are found to have resectable disease using frozen section evaluation of specimens during laparoscopy, the surgeon can proceed with a laparotomy during the same operation [34, 38].

However, diagnostic laparoscopy is time consuming and costly. In addition, data demonstrating benefit to diagnostic laparoscopy are dated. In the contemporary period with high-quality cross-sectional imaging, the finding of unexpected metastatic disease is low. More recent reports demonstrate radiographic failure to detect metastatic disease in only approximately 15 % of all cases [39, 40]. Fisher et al. have recommended the use of laparoscopy in cases where there is a large primary tumor, substantial weight loss, a tumor located in the body or tail of the pancreas, hypoalbuminemia or considerable elevated CA 19-9 levels [41]. The use of diagnostic laparoscopy, at large well-established centers for pancreatic surgery, given the availability of powerful diagnostic modalities and the expertise of the treating physicians, is probably best applied in select cases [37].

Surgery-First Versus Neoadjuvant Approach

Approximately 15–20 % of patients with PDAC have resectable disease at the time of diagnosis. The goal of a potentially curative operation in this cohort is to achieve a margin free of cancer (R0) leaving the patient in a condition that allows systemic treatment for micrometastatic disease [42–44]. There is still no definite consensus on whether patients who initially have resectable tumors should undergo a neoadjuvant approach or a surgery-first approach. Advocates of the surgery-first approach believe that the single most important treatment for a chance of cure is resection of the tumor and this should be accomplished prior to systemic therapy. On the other hand, potential advantages of the neoadjuvant approach include earlier control of micrometastatic disease with systemic therapy and an opportunity for better selecting patients for pancreatectomy by excluding those with more aggressive disease that progresses on therapy. Based on current studies, it is still unclear whether a neoadjuvant approach improves survival as a better treatment modality or whether tumors with favorable tumor biology are simply selected. Designing a randomized clinical trial to make this differentiation is challenging.

Several well-done trials have evaluated the outcomes of the neoadjuvant approach (Table 2). In summary, when taking into account intention to treat, it appears that that both initial surgery and neoadjuvant therapy have comparable survival rates and that the major advantage of neoadjuvant approach is with patient selection. In this regard, several studies reported that patients who receive neoadjuvant therapy have a better median survival than what has traditionally been reported for the surgery-first approach, but 10.71–36.58 % do not make it to surgery [28, 45–48]. The reasons for not making it to surgery included rapid progression in 20 % ($n=17$) of the patients of which 9.4 % ($n=8$) were deemed unresectable at the time of restaging while 10.6 % ($n=9$) were found to have metastatic disease [28].

A retrospective study identified 199 patients out of a total of 1562 patients who received neoadjuvant therapy. The percentage of patients who underwent preoperative

Table 2 Neoadjuvant therapy for resectable pancreatic cancer

Study	Treatment	Patients	Median survival (months)	Median survival mo. (resected)	Median survival mo.(unresected)
Desai [69]	Gem/Ox + XRT> Gem/Ox	12(44)[a]	12.5 (44 pts.)	NR	NR
Varadhachary [45]	Gem + Cis > Gem + XRT	79	17.4	31 (52 pts.)	10.5 (27 pts.)
Evans [28]	Gem + XRT	86	23	34 (64 pts.)	7.1 (22 pts.)
Heinrich [70]	Gem + Cis	28	26.5	19.1 (25 pts.)	NR (3 pts.)
Le Scodan [46]	5FU/Cis + XRT	41	9.4	9.5 (26 pts.)	5.6 (15 pts.)
Golcher [47]	Gem + Cis	33	17.4	25 (19 pts.)	NR

Gem gemcitabine, *Cis* cisplatin, *Ox* oxaliplatin, *RT* radiation, *pts* patients

[a]Twelve out of a total of 44 patients were enrolled as resectable

biliary stenting (57.9 vs. 44.7 %, $p=0.0005$), vascular resection (41.5 vs. 17.3 %, $p<0.0001$), and open resections (94.0 vs. 91.4 %, $p=0.008$) was higher in the neoadjuvant group. However, there was no significant difference between the 30 days mortality (2.0 vs. 1.5 %, $p=0.56$) and postoperative morbidity (56.3 vs. 52.8 %, $p=0.35$) between the two groups [49].

Another recent retrospective study evaluated patients with resectable disease who received neoadjuvant therapy and provided a classification by dividing them into three groups: those who had clinically resectable cancer with no extrapancreatic disease, those for whom there was a suspicion of extra pancreatic disease, and those who had poor performance status or significant co-morbidities. Resection rates in the three groups were 75, 46, and 37 % respectively ($p<0.001$). Old age, poor performance status, pain, and treatment complications ($p<0.05$) were factors which were identified for selection against surgery. The overall median survival was 21 months for all patients. Moreover, survival rates in resected and unresected patients who had suspicion of extra pancreatic disease and those who had poor performance status or co-morbidities were similar to those resected and unresected patients who did not have these adverse factors, respectively ($p>0.22$) [50].

The standard paradigm in PDAC treatment has involved bias toward a surgery-first approach in resectable tumors, driven by the relatively low efficacy of standard systemic therapies such as gemcitabine. With the advent of more potent chemotherapy regimens, such as FOLFIRINOX and gemcitabine/abraxane, the bias is shifting toward the increased use of neoadjuvant therapy. PDAC is a highly systemic disease and thus aggressive systemic therapy must be the goal in all patients [51].

In contrast to patients with resectable disease and no major vessel involvement, neoadjuvant chemotherapy with chemoradiation is given to all patients with borderline resectable disease as there is a general consensus that such patients will benefit from this therapy. There is a greater probability of positive margin resection if these patients are not given neoadjuvant therapy [52]. Patients who receive neoadjuvant therapy have an 80–90 % rate of margin-negative resection with comparable or sometimes even better survival outcomes than patients who have tumors that are initially classified as resectable [52].

Definition of Borderline Resectable Disease

The treatment of pancreatic cancer is dependent on the stage and resectability of the disease, therefore different institutions have proposed staging systems that determine whether the disease is resectable, borderline resectable, unresectable, or metastatic [27]. These institutions include the M.D. Anderson Cancer Center (MDACC) and the National Comprehensive Cancer Network (NCCN). Moreover a recent consensus guideline which modified the M.D. Anderson staging criteria was recommended by a joint committee of American Hepato-Pancreato-Biliary Association (AHPBA), Society of Surgical Oncology (SSO), and the Society for the Surgery of the Alimentary Tract (SSAT) [53].

Based on these guidelines, resectability is determined by the presence or absence of metastatic disease and involvement of major blood vessels. Both portovenous and arterial vessels are evaluated separately. A tumor involving the portovenous vessels is considered resectable as long as the vessels can be reconstructed after resection. On the other hand, assessing the involvement of arterial vasculature, most importantly the superior mesenteric, hepatic and celiac arteries, is crucial as the degree of involvement determines resectability of the tumor. The degree of involvement is assessed on axial planes of high-quality cross-sectional imaging [54–57]. Encasement (>180° involvement) by the tumor of any arterial vessel is considered unresectable. Abutment (<180° involvement) of the celiac arteries or the superior mesenteric artery is considered to be borderline resectable but is associated with margin-positive resections, high rates of recurrence, and a lower survival [27].

Although these guidelines have proven to be useful in the classifying resectability in the majority of patients, several controversies exist on what should be considered borderline resectable versus locally advanced. With regards to venous involvement, the term "technically reconstructable" varies depending on the experience of the surgeon and variations of anatomy in each patient. For example, involvement of the inferior superior mesenteric vein at the level of the confluence of ileal and jejunal branches is often considered to be locally advanced. However, examples exist in which one or more of these branches can be sacrificed or reconstructed based on the size of remaining branches and location to the tumor. Another example is encasement of the hepatic artery and celiac axis which is strictly considered to be locally advanced. However, in some cases of local involvement of these vessels resection is possible. This may include focal involvement of the hepatic artery that is amenable to reconstruction or in some cases a patient with an accessory right or left hepatic artery may make resection of the hepatic artery possible. In addition, focal encasement of the celiac artery and proximal common hepatic artery with preservation of the gastroduodenal artery may be resected through an Appleby's procedure [26]. Therefore, the definition of what is borderline resectable versus locally advanced unresectable may not be the same at all institutions. Ultimately, we believe that it is up to the surgeon's judgment to determine whether successful resection of the tumor is feasible

Ablative Therapy for Locally Advanced Disease

Management of locally advanced disease is difficult and is best managed through a multidisciplinary approach. The literature available to us is limited and as new data become available to us our approach to this stage of the disease will improve. A great deal of emphasis is given to the role of systemic chemotherapy in these patients given that there is a high probability of presence of microscopic systemic disease at the time of diagnosis and/or the risk of development of metastases during the course of radiation. It has been reported that in rare cases that the use of currently available regimens may result in a significant downstaging of the disease.

Moertel et al., in the largest randomized study in this field, demonstrated that concurrent use of radiation with 5-fluorouracil (5-FU) significantly prolonged the median overall survival of these patients, which now is the standard of care for this subset of our patient population [58]. Subsequent research studies support the use of systemic chemotherapy followed by chemoradiation. The team at Johns Hopkins in a retrospective analysis of data from these patients demonstrated better survival outcomes in patients who had a longer course of induction chemotherapy prior to the chemoradiation [59]. Unfortunately, a large-scale study comparing the multiple chemotherapeutic agents available is not available.

A new emerging frontier in the therapy of pancreatic cancer is irreversible electroporation (IRE) [60]. The use of IRE in pancreatic surgery is controversial given that it is a new technique, with only few centers having trained professionals who can use this modality. The current focus lies on the use of IRE to treat locally advanced pancreatic cancer. Careful selection of patients is vital. Experts usually treat only stage III disease using this method. It is a method that employees the use of short pulses of high voltage low energy electric current, to create nanoscale micropores in the lipid bilayer of cell membranes. This leads to an increased permeability to ions and macromolecules and subsequently, leads to cell swelling and subsequent apoptosis. Amplitude of the pulse, its duration, frequency, and number of pulses applied all determine the extent of cell damage and death [61, 62].

Since IRE causes cell death via apoptosis, structures formed by proteins such as vascular elastin and collagenous structures are not affected and, hence, surrounding vessels are preserved making it safe to use for tumors near vital structures. Literature available on IRE is limited to case series and case reports and a large-scale study is required to evaluate the safety and efficacy of IRE. The research available shows an improvement in survival and pain control in patients with unresectable LAPC.

Other ablative techniques include radiofrequency ablation, cryoablation, and microwave ablation. Radiofrequency ablation (RFA) uses alternating current to treat solid tumors by increasing local temperatures and causing coagulative necrosis. Though the use of RFA results in decreased tumor volume and improved pain symptoms, it is associated with high complication rates due to the damage of local tissue given the high temperatures [63, 64]. Cryoablation on the other hand uses the other extreme of temperature to damage tumor tissue. The tumor is frozen to temperatures as low as −160 °C, allowed to thaw and then frozen again [65]. Apart from damage to surrounding tissue, cryoablation can also lead to bleeding, bile leak and delayed gastric emptying, thus care must be taken when using this modality [66, 67]. A newer technique is microwave ablation, which has better outcomes as compared to the earlier two. Less heat-sink effect takes place thus the surrounding tissue is at a lesser risk of damage. Also, longer survival and a transient improvement in quality of life have been observed in patient who underwent microwave ablation [68].

Literature available to us related to the use of these modalities is limited and further research is necessary before any of these ablative methods become part of our common practices.

Conclusion

Pancreatic adenocarcinoma is one of the most fatal forms of malignancies. Given the low survival rates of these patients despite our current knowledge and the improvements that have been made in surgical techniques, chemotherapy and radiation therapy, there is still a lot more that needs to be known. Early detection of both premalignant lesions, such as cysts of the pancreas, and the malignant ones can lead to an improvement in the overall outcome and is ideal. PDAC management has to be multidisciplinary, involving surgery, pathology, medical oncology, and radiation oncology teams. The treatment that a patient receives is best individually tailored including disease response to the available treatment modalities. Exciting new and controversial therapies such as IRE are emerging to treat these patients.

Disclosure No relevant conflicts of interest to be disclosed.

References

1. Siegel R, et al. Cancer treatment and survivorship statistics, 2012. CA Cancer J Clin. 2012;62(4):220–41.
2. Wolfgang CL, Herman JM, Laheru DA, Klein AP, Erdek MA, Fishman EK, et al. Recent progress in pancreatic cancer. CA Cancer J Clin. 2013;63(5):318–48. doi:10.3322/caac.21190. Epub 2013 Jul 15. Review; PubMed PMID: 23856911; PubMed Central PMCID: PMC3769458.
3. Siegel R, et al. Cancer statistics, 2014. CA Cancer J Clin. 2014;64(1):9–29.
4. Kalser MH, Barkin J, Macintyre JM. Pancreatic cancer. Assessment of prognosis by clinical presentation. Cancer. 1985;56(2):397–402.
5. American gastroenterological association medical position statement: epidemiology, diagnosis, and treatment of pancreatic ductal adenocarcinoma. Gastroenterology. 1999;117(6):1463–84.
6. Mayr M, Schmid RM. Pancreatic cancer and depression: myth and truth. BMC Cancer. 2010;10:569.
7. De La Cruz MS, Young AP, Ruffin MT. Diagnosis and management of pancreatic cancer. Am Fam Physician. 2014;89(8):626–32.
8. Girelli CM, et al. Pancreatic carcinoma: differences between patients with or without diabetes mellitus. Recenti Prog Med. 1995;86(4):143–6.

9. Lochan R, et al. Genetic susceptibility in pancreatic ductal adenocarcinoma. Br J Surg. 2008;95(1):22–32.

10. Ojajarvi IA, et al. Occupational exposures and pancreatic cancer: a meta-analysis. Occup Environ Med. 2000;57(5):316–24.

11. Blackford A, et al. Genetic mutations associated with cigarette smoking in pancreatic cancer. Cancer Res. 2009;69(8):3681–8.

12. Bosetti C, et al. Cigarette smoking and pancreatic cancer: an analysis from the International Pancreatic Cancer Case-Control Consortium (Panc4). Ann Oncol. 2012;23(7):1880–8.

13. Maisonneuve P, Lowenfels AB. Epidemiology of pancreatic cancer: an update. Dig Dis. 2010;28(4–5):645–56.

14. Arslan AA, et al. Anthropometric measures, body mass index, and pancreatic cancer: a pooled analysis from the Pancreatic Cancer Cohort Consortium (PanScan). Arch Intern Med. 2010;170(9):791–802.

15. Huxley R, et al. Type-II diabetes and pancreatic cancer: a meta-analysis of 36 studies. Br J Cancer. 2005;92(11):2076–83.

16. Chari ST, et al. Probability of pancreatic cancer following diabetes: a population-based study. Gastroenterology. 2005;129(2):504–11.

17. Jacobs EJ, et al. Family history of cancer and risk of pancreatic cancer: a pooled analysis from the Pancreatic Cancer Cohort Consortium (PanScan). Int J Cancer. 2010;127(6):1421–8.

18. Ghadirian P, et al. Reported family aggregation of pancreatic cancer within a population-based case-control study in the Francophone community in Montreal, Canada. Int J Pancreatol. 1991;10(3–4):183–96.

19. Falk RT, et al. Life-style risk factors for pancreatic cancer in Louisiana: a case-control study. Am J Epidemiol. 1988;128(2):324–36.

20. Price TF, Payne RL, Oberleitner MG. Familial pancreatic cancer in south Louisiana. Cancer Nurs. 1996;19(4):275–82.

21. Brune KA, et al. Importance of age of onset in pancreatic cancer kindreds. J Natl Cancer Inst. 2010;102(2):119–26.

22. Pawlik TM, et al. Evaluating the impact of a single-day multidisciplinary clinic on the management of pancreatic cancer. Ann Surg Oncol. 2008;15(8):2081–8.

23. Tamm EP, et al. Imaging of pancreatic adenocarcinoma: update on staging/resectability. Radiol Clin North Am. 2012;50(3):407–28.

24. McIntyre CA, Winter JM. Diagnostic evaluation and staging of pancreatic ductal adenocarcinoma. Semin Oncol. 2015;42(1):19–27. doi:10.1053/j.seminoncol.2014.12.003. Epub 2014 Dec 9. Review; PubMed PMID: 25726049.

25. Edge S, American Joint Committee on Cancer. AJCC cancer staging manual. 7th ed. New York: Springer; 2010.

26. Siegel R, Naishadham D, Jemal A. Cancer statistics, 2013. CA Cancer J Clin. 2013;63:11–30.

27. Tempero MA, Arnoletti JP, Behrman SW, et al. Pancreatic adenocarcinoma, version 2.2012: featured updates to the NCCN guidelines. J Natl Comp Cancer Netw. 2012;10:703–13.

28. Evans DB, et al. Preoperative gemcitabine-based chemoradiation for patients with resectable adenocarcinoma of the pancreatic head. J Clin Oncol. 2008;26(21):3496–502.

29. Schellenberg D, et al. 18Fluorodeoxyglucose PET is prognostic of progression-free and overall survival in locally advanced pancreas cancer treated with stereotactic radiotherapy. Int J Radiat Oncol Biol Phys. 2010;77(5):1420–5.

30. Farma JM, et al. PET/CT fusion scan enhances CT staging in patients with pancreatic neoplasms. Ann Surg Oncol. 2008;15(9):2465–71.

31. Wahl RL, Herman JM, Ford E. The promise and pitfalls of positron emission tomography and single-photon emission computed tomography molecular imaging-guided radiation therapy. Semin Radiat Oncol. 2011;21(2):88–100.

32. Wray CJ, et al. Surgery for pancreatic cancer: recent controversies and current practice. Gastroenterology. 2005;128(6):1626–41.

33. Drebin JA, Metz JM, Furth EE. Carcinoma of the pancreas. In: Abeloff MD, Armitage JO, Niederhuber JE, Kastan MB, Gillies McKenna M, editors. Abeloff's clinical oncology. 4th ed. Philadelphia, PA: Churchill Livingstone Elsevier; 2008. p. 1595–608.

34. Callery MP, et al. Staging laparoscopy with laparoscopic ultrasonography: optimizing resectability in hepatobiliary and pancreatic malignancy. J Am Coll Surg. 1997;185(1):33–9.

35. John TG, et al. Carcinoma of the pancreatic head and periampullary region. Tumor staging with laparoscopy and laparoscopic ultrasonography. Ann Surg. 1995;221(2):156–64.

36. Conlon KC, et al. The value of minimal access surgery in the staging of patients with potentially resectable peripancreatic malignancy. Ann Surg. 1996;223(2):134–40.

37. Muniraj T, Barve P. Laparoscopic staging and surgical treatment of pancreatic cancer. N Am J Med Sci. 2013;5(1):1–9.

38. Vollmer CM, et al. Utility of staging laparoscopy in subsets of peripancreatic and biliary malignancies. Ann Surg. 2002;235(1):1–7.

39. Barreiro CJ, et al. Diagnostic laparoscopy for periampullary and pancreatic cancer: what is the true benefit? J Gastrointest Surg. 2002;6(1):75–81.

40. White R, et al. Current utility of staging laparoscopy for pancreatic and peripancreatic neoplasms. J Am Coll Surg. 2008;206(3):445–50.

41. Camacho D, et al. Value of laparoscopy in the staging of pancreatic cancer. JOP. 2005;6(6): 552–61.

42. Neoptolemos JP, et al. Adjuvant chemotherapy with fluorouracil plus folinic acid vs gemcitabine following pancreatic cancer resection: a randomized controlled trial. JAMA. 2010; 304(10):1073–81.

43. Richter A, et al. Long-term results of partial pancreaticoduodenectomy for ductal adenocarcinoma of the pancreatic head: 25-year experience. World J Surg. 2003;27(3):324–9.

44. Wagner M, et al. Curative resection is the single most important factor determining outcome in patients with pancreatic adenocarcinoma. Br J Surg. 2004;91(5):586–94.

45. Varadhachary GR, et al. Preoperative gemcitabine and cisplatin followed by gemcitabine-based chemoradiation for resectable adenocarcinoma of the pancreatic head. J Clin Oncol. 2008;26(21):3487–95.

46. Le Scodan R, et al. Histopathological response to preoperative chemoradiation for resectable pancreatic adenocarcinoma: the French Phase II FFCD 9704-SFRO Trial. Am J Clin Oncol. 2008;31(6):545–52.

47. Golcher H, Brunner TB, Witzigmann H, Marti L, Bechstein WO, Bruns C, et al. Neoadjuvant chemoradiation therapy with gemcitabine/cisplatin and surgery versus immediate surgery in resectable pancreatic cancer: results of the first prospective randomized phase II trial. Strahlenther Onkol. 2015;191(1):7–16. doi:10.1007/s00066-014-0737-7. Epub 2014 Sep 25. PubMed PMID: 25252602; PubMed Central PMCID: PMC4289008.

48. Heinrich S, et al. Neoadjuvant chemotherapy generates a significant tumor response in resectable pancreatic cancer without increasing morbidity: results of a prospective phase II trial. Ann Surg. 2008;248(6):1014–22.

49. Cooper AB, Parmar AD, Riall TS, Hall BL, Katz MH, Aloia TA, et al. Does the use of neoadjuvant therapy for pancreatic adenocarcinoma increase postoperative morbidity and mortality rates? J Gastrointest Surg. 2015;19(1):80–6. doi:10.1007/s11605-014-2620-3. Discussion 86–7; Epub 2014 Aug 5; PubMed PMID: 25091851; PubMed Central PMCID: PMC4289101.

50. Tzeng CW, et al. Defined clinical classifications are associated with outcome of patients with anatomically resectable pancreatic adenocarcinoma treated with neoadjuvant therapy. Ann Surg Oncol. 2012;19(6):2045–53.

51. Twombly R. Adjuvant chemoradiation for pancreatic cancer: few good data, much debate. J Natl Cancer Inst. 2008;100(23):1670–1.

52. Gillen S, et al. Preoperative/neoadjuvant therapy in pancreatic cancer: a systematic review and meta-analysis of response and resection percentages. PLoS Med. 2010;7(4):e1000267.

53. Callery MP, et al. Pretreatment assessment of resectable and borderline resectable pancreatic cancer: expert consensus statement. Ann Surg Oncol. 2009;16(7):1727–33.

54. Vincent A, et al. Pancreatic cancer. Lancet. 2011;378(9791):607–20.

55. Buchs NC, et al. Vascular invasion in pancreatic cancer: imaging modalities, preoperative diagnosis and surgical management. World J Gastroenterol. 2010;16(7):818–31.
56. Tseng JF, et al. Pancreaticoduodenectomy with vascular resection: margin status and survival duration. J Gastrointest Surg. 2004;8(8):935–49. discussion 949-50.
57. Leach SD, et al. Survival following pancreaticoduodenectomy with resection of the superior mesenteric-portal vein confluence for adenocarcinoma of the pancreatic head. Br J Surg. 1998;85(5):611–7.
58. Moertel CG, et al. Therapy of locally unresectable pancreatic carcinoma: a randomized comparison of high dose (6000 rads) radiation alone, moderate dose radiation (4000 rads + 5-fluorouracil), and high dose radiation + 5-fluorouracil: The Gastrointestinal Tumor Study Group. Cancer. 1981;48(8):1705–10.
59. Faisal F, Tsai HL, Blackford A, Olino K, Xia C, De Jesus-Acosta A, Le DT, Cosgrove D, Azad N, Rasheed Z, Diaz LA Jr, Donehower R, Laheru D, Hruban RH, Fishman EK, Edil BH, Schulick R, Wolfgang C, Herman J, Zheng L. Longer course of induction chemotherapy followed by chemoradiation favors better survival outcomes for patients with locally advanced pancreatic cancer. Am J Clin Oncol. 2013; Epub ahead of print. PubMed PMID: 24351782; PubMed Central PMCID:PMC4061284.
60. Chang DC, Reese TS. Changes in membrane structure induced by electroporation as revealed by rapid-freezing electron microscopy. Biophys J. 1990;58(1):1–12.
61. Breton M, Mir LM. Microsecond and nanosecond electric pulses in cancer treatments. Bioelectromagnetics. 2012;33(2):106–23. doi:10.1002/bem.20692. Epub 2011 Aug 3. PubMed PMID: 21812011.
62. Davalos RV, Mir IL, Rubinsky B. Tissue ablation with irreversible electroporation. Ann Biomed Eng. 2005;33(2):223–31.
63. Spiliotis JD, et al. Radiofrequency ablation combined with palliative surgery may prolong survival of patients with advanced cancer of the pancreas. Langenbecks Arch Surg. 2007; 392(1):55–60.
64. Girelli R, et al. Feasibility and safety of radiofrequency ablation for locally advanced pancreatic cancer. Br J Surg. 2010;97(2):220–5.
65. Xu KC, et al. Cryosurgery with combination of (125)iodine seed implantation for the treatment of locally advanced pancreatic cancer. J Dig Dis. 2008;9(1):32–40.
66. Li J, et al. Tumour cryoablation combined with palliative bypass surgery in the treatment of unresectable pancreatic cancer: a retrospective study of 142 patients. Postgrad Med J. 2011;87(1024):89–95.
67. Xu K, Niu L, Yang D. Cryosurgery for pancreatic cancer. Gland Surg. 2013;2(1):30–9.
68. Carrafiello G, et al. Microwave ablation of pancreatic head cancer: safety and efficacy. J Vasc Interv Radiol. 2013;24(10):1513–20.
69. Desai SP, et al. Phase I study of oxaliplatin, full-dose gemcitabine, and concurrent radiation therapy in pancreatic cancer. J Clin Oncol. 2007;25(29):4587–92.
70. Heinrich S, et al. Prospective phase II trial of neoadjuvant chemotherapy with gemcitabine and cisplatin for resectable adenocarcinoma of the pancreatic head. J Clin Oncol. 2008;26(15): 2526–31.

Current Controversies in Cancer Care: Breast Cancer

Megan K. Baker

Introduction

Breast cancer remains the most commonly diagnosed solid tumor malignancy amongst women in the United States with an estimated 232,000 cases to be diagnosed in the US in 2014. It is the second leading cause of cancer death in all American women accounting for more than 40,000 deaths in 2013. The incidence in breast cancer had continued to increase until 2003 when it leveled off. This stabilization of the curve has been commonly attributed to the nationwide decline in postmenopausal hormone therapy use seen following the publication of the Women's Health Initiative results in 2002. At the same time, breast cancer mortality has enjoyed a steady decline since 1989, likely due to increased screening efforts and new treatment paradigms [1].

Breast cancer screening, diagnosis, and management have undergone tremendous change in the past 20 years. In many cases the trend has been to scale back efforts with a few important exceptions where intensity of care has increased. No aspect of the breast cancer field has been spared by the swing in the care pendulum. Breast cancer screening continues to rely conventionally on mammography, although controversy exists regarding its frequency, age at initiation and cessation of screening, as well as its contribution to over-diagnosis. The actual diagnosis of breast cancer is best made with preoperative core biopsy. However, as our understanding of the biology of the disease becomes more sophisticated, what constitutes "diagnosis" is likely to be expanded to include subtype analysis and possible gene sequencing. Consequent to a more in-depth understanding of disease, the number of efficacious evidence-based treatment paradigms has grown largely allowing for a more personalized approach to breast cancer therapy.

M.K. Baker, M.D., F.A.C.S. (✉)
Department of Surgery, Roper St. Francis Health Care System,
316 Calhoun Street, Charleston, SC 29401, USA
e-mail: bakermk@musc.edu

© Springer International Publishing Switzerland 2016   133
K.A. Morgan (ed.), *Current Controversies in Cancer Care*
for the Surgeon, DOI 10.1007/978-3-319-16205-8_8

Imaging

Screening

Breast cancer screening classically involved both a clinical breast examination (CBE) and two-view bilateral mammograms to be performed every year or every other year starting at age 40. In 2009, the United States Preventative Services Task Force (USPSTF) released new and controversial guidelines that decreased the frequency of and narrowed the age window for screening mammography. Further, the USPSTF went so far as to recommend against the self-breast examination and clinical breast examinations at any age and screening mammography prior to age 50. These recommendations were revised within weeks to move clinical breast examination into the insufficient data to comment recommendation and softened the recommendation for mammography before age 50 to "discuss with your provider" [2, 3].

A more recent review by Bleyer and Welch using Surveillance, Epidemiology and End Results (SEER) database describe the 30-year impact of screening mammography on breast cancer incidence. They note a 30 % increase in the diagnosis of early stage (ductal carcinoma in situ or localized) breast cancer and an 8 % decrease in later stage (regional or distant) disease. This raises concerns for over-diagnosis. Critics of this study note that the inclusion of in situ disease incorrectly biased the sample and skewed the incidence rate. Even more recently, the Canadian National Breast Cancer Screening Study published its 25-year update showing no difference in survival between the observation (clinical breast examination alone) and the imaged group. Notably, this study has been fraught with controversy from its inception. It has been criticized for the absence of standardized mammography technique, its use of outdated equipment, and lack of study center credentialing. Interestingly however and in contrast to the claims made by the USPSTF 2009 guidelines, this study demonstrates that clinical breast examination is in fact effective at diagnosing breast cancer or at least as effective as substandard mammography [4].

High-Risk Surveillance

Significantly more concordance surrounds screening recommendations for those women noted to be at elevated risk for developing breast cancer. This group of patients is typically defined by either an estimated lifetime risk of breast cancer in excess of 20 % as calculated by risk models such as Tyer-Cusik or by identification as a carrier of a deleterious gene associated with increased breast cancer risk (i.e. BRCA1, BRCA2, pTEN, p53). For these women, the National Comprehensive Cancer Network guidelines recommend in addition to annual breast examination, starting annual MRI as early as age 20 (p53 mutations) and age 25 (BRCA mutations) and adding annual mammography at age 30 for both [5, 6]. Recommendations are slightly less clear for those women who have a personal history of lobular carcinoma in situ, atypical lobular hyperplasia, or atypical ductal hyperplasia as the only indication. It is recommended to use that information when calculating their lifetime risk with the various available validated risk models to determine screening MRI candidacy [6].

In addition to its screening application, great hope was held out that breast MRI when used preoperatively would impact surgical outcomes. Both retrospective studies as summarized in Houssami et al. review as well as a randomized controlled trial (COMICE) failed to demonstrate that the routine use of preoperative breast MRI could impact rates of breast conservation, need for margin re-excision or decrease local or disease-free survival [7, 8, 40]. As such, the routine use of preoperative MRI is discouraged.

New Technologies

New technologies and new applications of existing technologies are being proposed and in some cases legislated. The addition of an emerging technology, breast tomosynthesis to a standard digital screening mammogram, was found to increase breast cancer detection rates with decreased call back rates [9]. Concerns for radiation exposure although quite valid have largely been put to rest, as the radiation dose received with a tomosynthesis is equal to or less than standard 2D digital mammography [10]. While the technology for breast cancer screening has been evolving so too has our understanding of the observed density of the breast gland. Breast density, as defined for each individual using their mammogram, relationship to breast cancer risk is becoming better delineated. To that end, grass roots efforts have resulted in legislative mandates in more than one-third of the states in the US to report a woman's density as part of her mammogram results. Further, some of those states have mandated the availability of screening breast ultrasound as an adjunct for those women identified with dense breasts. Critics of this approach cite that the increased detection rate observed with the addition of breast ultrasound is accompanied by a significant increase in the false-positive rate [11].

Diagnosis

Breast cancer diagnosis remains critical for optimal operative care planning. The importance of a pretreatment core biopsy to best ascertain the nature and timing of multimodality treatment cannot be overstated. Routine preoperative image-guided core biopsy, ideally with clip placement, remains the gold standard for diagnosis [8]. Current national benchmark standards at both academic and community centers recommend fewer than 18 % of breast cancers to be diagnosed with excisional biopsy. The most common indications for excisional biopsy as a means of diagnosis included: symptomatic abnormalities, technical challenges that prohibit preoperative biopsy, and patient choice [12].

The concept of diagnosis has also expanded to include the molecular subtyping of breast cancer: luminal A, luminal B, or basal type. In fact, recent work has demonstrated that this sophisticated level of diagnosis may be instructive for the purposeful selection of neoadjuvant chemotherapy regimens so as to improve rates of complete pathologic response [13].

Surgery

Margin Adequacy

Historically no universally accepted standard for an adequate surgical margin in breast cancer care existed. The importance of this however cannot be overstated as local failure has been associated with decreased overall survival [14]. Improved local control in both the breast conserving setting and for patients undergoing mastectomy is associated with improved survival. As surgeons we directly impact rates of local control via margin status.

In the seminal trials that established the efficacy of breast conserving technique, only NSABP B-06 trial required a clear margin, using a standard of "no tumor on ink." The remaining trails required the gross removal of macroscopic tumor [14–18]. Most recently in careful review of fundamental trials as well as more contemporary data, the Society of Surgical Oncology and the American Society for Radiation Oncology issued a consensus recommendation for margin adequacy for those patients undergoing breast conserving surgery and whole-breast irradiation in the treatment of Stage I and II invasive breast cancer: no tumor on ink [19]. Such guidelines do not currently exist for mastectomy margins. A recent review noted detailed the contradictory data in this clinical setting. One meta-analysis which looked at women with non-inflammatory invasive breast cancer who had a close or positive margin experienced an increased relative risk of local failure of 2.6. Another meta-analysis however failed to show any increased risk for women who underwent skin sparing mastectomy with close or positive margins [20]. As such the management of a close or positive margin in the setting of mastectomy treatment remains a clinical interdisciplinary decision.

Nipple Sparing Mastectomy

The surgical techniques for mastectomy have experienced significant evolution over the past several decades: Halsted's radical mastectomy, modified radical mastectomy, total mastectomy, skin sparing mastectomy, and now nipple sparing mastectomy. With respect to the latter, concern existed for risk of nipple failure and as such the technique gained earlier traction in the prophylactic setting. Early work by authors such as Crowe and Stolier provided conservative inclusion criteria based on small personal series [21, 22]. More recent and larger single institution series have further established the technique's efficacy in the both the prophylactic and cancer setting. They have also detailed technical considerations for nipple preservation. In general, occult nipple involvement is present less than 3 % of cases but is more likely for those women with central tumors, N1, or N2 disease whereas the risk of nipple involvement in prophylactic cases is minimal. Further, a higher rate of nipple loss was associated with incisions that interrupt blood supply to the nipple areolar complex and should be avoided [23–25].

Axillary Management

No one aspect of breast cancer care has evolved more than axillary nodal surgery. Management of the axilla has dramatically changed in the past decade. The efficacy of sentinel node management was established with the results of NSABP B-32 which compared sentinel lymph node biopsy to axillary node dissection in patients with clinically negative nodes. Shortly thereafter, the American College of Surgeons Oncology Group (ACOSOG) sponsored the Z0011 trial which compared axillary observation to completion node dissection for women with clinical T1-T2, clinical node-negative disease undergoing breast conserving surgery, and whole breast radiation. Recent results demonstrate no difference in local, regional, or distant failure at 6.3 years between the two groups. The study group's recommendation for women that meet inclusion criteria and are found to have a 1–2 positive sentinel lymph nodes is for no further axillary surgery, but continue with adjuvant standard of care [26] (Table 1).

Published results from the AMAROS trial are eagerly awaited. Results were presented at the 2013 ASCO meeting and demonstrated that for women with tumors less than 3 cm and a positive sentinel lymph node that there was no difference in local recurrence or overall survival between the surgical arm (completion node dissection) and the radiation arm (regional nodal field). Notably, lymphedema rates were twice as high in the surgical arm [27]. The group therefore recommend against completion node dissection for this select group of patients.

The use of sentinel lymph node biopsy in the setting of neoadjuvant chemotherapy for the node-positive patient has also been studied. Researchers have attempted to clarify if sentinel lymph node biopsy is an appropriate surrogate to determine

Table 1 Patient selection criteria for avoidance of axillary lymph node dissection

Avoidance of Axillary Lymph Node Dissection Patient Selection Guidelines (ACOSOG Z0011)
Tumor size <5 cm (T1 or T2)
Fewer than 3 positive SLN
No evidence of extracapsular tumor extension in SLN
Planned whole breast radiation therapy
Planned standard of care adjuvant therapy

down-staging of the axilla following chemotherapy. The ACOSOG Z1071 (Alliance trial) reported a 12 % false-negative rate which exceeded their predetermined threshold of 10 %. Notably, for those patients whose sentinel lymph node was identified with dual tracer technique, a higher yield of nodes were identified and the false-negative rate was not exceeded. Nonetheless, as the primary aim null hypothesis was not negated, the study group does not recommend use of sentinel lymph node biopsy following the neoadjuvant treatment of patients with node-positive breast cancer [28].

Adjuvant Therapy

Breast cancer care has become more personalized and treatment more targeted. A more sophisticated understanding of the biology of the tumor is integral to making well-matched treatment selections. Disagreement exists however on the appropriateness of the tools that are currently available to aid in this effort. As a matter of gold standard, the OncotypeDx assay was quickly received and integrated into standard care. The RT-PCR test which assists in the risk–benefit analysis of adjuvant chemotherapy for women with ER+, node-negative tumors was validated on a prospectively collected data set. As such its application in treatment decision making, to add cytotoxic chemotherapy or not, has not met much disagreement. Its broader utility for patients who are node positive is currently being studied in the cooperative SWOG 0007 trial. Other contemporary assays, such as the Mammaprint microarray assay, have received FDA approval and are enjoying some practice uptake. The MINDACT trial (Micorarray in Node negative and 1–3 positive lymph node disease may avoid chemotherapy) results are eagerly awaited. This prospective, randomized Phase III trial exceeded its target enrollment with 6700 patients. Those patients were assessed concordantly by both microarray and traditional clinic-pathologic measures and placed into high risk or low risk categories. Those at high risk were treated with cytotoxic chemotherapy while those at low risk were given hormonal therapy. Those patients for whom discordance existed between the microarray analysis and traditional pathologic predictors were randomized to receive either chemotherapy or hormonal therapy based on clinic-pathologic risk assessment or Mammaprint. The results of this trial have significant potential to change how we determine adjuvant therapy for a large number of our patients.

Radiation

Radiation therapy has long enjoyed a pivotal role in the management of breast cancer. For well over 20 years now, whole breast radiation has been accepted as a critical and effective tool to reduce local recurrence following breast conserving therapy [14–18]. Similarly, the use of post-mastectomy radiation therapy (PMRT) in the setting of substantial node-positive disease burden (>3 nodes positive) has also been well established [29].

Partial Breast Irradiation

Recognition that the elsewhere in breast failure rate at 5 years equals that of the rate of occurrence in the unaffected breast spurred researches to consider treating what may be considered the area of the breast that can be impacted by radiation therapy. To this end, early researchers proposed and conducted small trials assessing the safety of partial breast irradiation. No significant difference thus far has been found to exist between the methods of accelerated partial breast irradiation: brachytherapy catheter, indwelling balloon, or 3-D conformal technique. Single institution studies have shown that in well selected patients (T < 3 cm, node-negative, absent lympho-vascular invasion, and age >50 years) that local failure rates are comparable to whole breast radiation treatment paradigms [30, 31]. In 2009, the American Society for Radiation Oncology (ASTRO) released a consensus guideline focused on the appropriate patient selection for accelerated partial breast radiation [32]. Other groups have subsequently challenged the lack of concordance between this proposed classification and actual patient outcome data stratified using the consensus criteria [33, 34]. NSABP B-39 was designed so that in a prospective randomized manner, a direct comparison may be made between accelerated partial breast and whole breast techniques for patients not only in low-risk categories, but also for women with stage 0, 1, and 2 breast cancer. Enrollment is complete and follow up data are pending.

Post-Mastectomy Radiation

The use of post-mastectomy radiation therapy has long been established as a means to improve both local control and improve survival for those patients with four or more positive lymph nodes. More recent meta-analyses have revisited its application for those patients with pN1a disease (3 or fewer positive lymph nodes). In summary, a benefit for both local recurrence and survival was attributable to the addition of chest wall and nodal radiation fields irrespective of use of systemic therapy [29]. Critics however note that given the data sets used in these studies, that the systemic therapy at that time is well known to not provide as optimal disease-free and overall survival as compared to more modern regimens. With this in mind, they caution the application of the historic meta-analysis to modern clinical practice [35].

Omission of Radiation Therapy

As our understanding of the risk and benefits to radiation therapy expands, the importance of thoughtful patient selection becomes more paramount. No better example of this exists then for those patients for whom radiation therapy might be avoided. Hughes et al. identified a group of women at low risk for local failure (age >70, T1, ER+ on tamoxifen) for whom there was little clinical benefit to adjuvant radiation therapy [36]. Despite this report in 2004, per review of Medicare data little progress has been made in the appropriate omission of radiation therapy in this well selected patient group [37]. In response to this information, the original cooperative group published updated trial data that demonstrated that the results of CALGB 9343 were durable and remained efficacious even at 12 years of follow up [38].

Other groups have studied the omission of radiation therapy in the setting of favorable cases of DCIS (low and intermediate grade, <2.5 cm mammographic extent) and have concluded that with margins >10 mm, the annual risk of recurrence is 1.9 %, or a 10-year local recurrence rate of 15 % [39]. These authors suggest that this option be candidly discussed as part of the treatment algorithm.

Conclusions

Nearly every aspect of breast cancer diagnosis and treatment has dramatically changed over the past two decades. This has led to improved survival and decreased patient morbidity. In fact much of this progress is attributable to randomized, prospective trials which provide us with Level 1 evidence. Ironically, this very success creates a very high standard for research and thus presents a significant challenge going forward given the current context of personalized care. As we better delineate the details of any one patient's breast cancer characteristics, their eligibility for any one trial will likely be narrowed. Future progress will be found in smaller, targeted trials with the focus on neoadjuvant period so as to make clinical observations and to draw conclusions in a time period appropriate for contemporary practice.

References

1. American Cancer Society. 2014. http://www.cancer.org. Accessed 20 Jul 2014.
2. US Preventative Services Task Force. Screening for breast cancer: U.S. Preventive Services Task Force recommendation statement. Ann Intern Med. 2009;151(10):716–26. W-236, doi: 10.7326/0003-4819-151-10-200911170-00008.
3. Bleyer A, Welch HG. Effect of three decades of screening mammography on breast-cancer incidence. N Engl J Med. 2012;367(21):1998–2005. doi:10.1056/NEJMoa1206809.
4. Miller AB, et al. Twenty five year follow-up for breast cancer incidence and mortality of the Canadian National Breast Screening Study: randomized screening trial. BMJ. 2014;348:g366. doi:10.1136/bmj.g366.
5. NCCN guidelines Genetic/Familial High Risk Assessment: breast and ovary. 2014. http://www.nccn.org. Accessed 20 Jul 2014.
6. McLaughlin S, et al. Ann Surg Oncol. 2014;21(1):28–36. doi:10.1245/s10434-013-3307-9. Epub 2013 Oct 22.
7. Turnball L, et al. Comparative effectiveness of MRI in breast cancer (COMICE) trial: a randomized controlled trial. Lancet. 2010;375(9714):563–71. doi:10.1016/S0140-6736(09)62070-5.
8. Silverstein MJ, et al. Special report: consensus conference III. Image-detected breast cancer: state-of-the-art diagnosis and treatment. J Am Coll Surg. 2009;209(4):504–20. doi:10.1016/j.jamcollsurg.2009.07.006. Epub 2009 Aug 20.

9. Friedewald SM, et al. Breast cancer screening using tomosynthesis in combination with digital mammography. JAMA. 2014;311(24):2499–507. doi:10.1001/jama.2014.6095.
10. Alakhras M, et al. Digital tomosynthesis: a new future for breast imaging? Clin Radiol. 2013;68(5):e225–36.
11. Hooley RJ, et al. Screening US in patients with mammographically dense breasts: initial experience with Connecticut Public Act 09-41. Radiology. 2012;265(1):59–69. Epub 2012 Jun 21.
12. Soot L, et al. Rates and indications for surgical. Am J Surg. 2014;207(4):499–503. doi:10.1016/j.amjsurg.2013.07.046. Epub 2013 Nov 10.
13. von Minckwitz G, Fontanella C. Selecting the neoadjuvant treatment by molecular subtype: how to maximize the benefit? Breast. 2013;22 Suppl 2:S149–51. doi:10.1016/j.breast.2013.07.028.
14. Early Breast Cancer Trialists Collaborative Group. Effects of radiotherapy and of differences in the extent of surgery for early breast cancer on local recurrence and 15-year survival: an overview of the randomised trials. Lancet. 2006;366(9503):2087–106.
15. Veronesi U, et al. Twenty-year follow-up of a randomized study comparing breast-conserving surgery with radical mastectomy for early breast cancer. N Engl J Med. 2002;347(16): 1227–32.
16. Poggi MM, et al. Eighteen-year results in the treatment of early breast carcinoma with mastectomy versus breast conservation therapy: the National Cancer Institute Randomized Trial. Cancer. 2003;98(4):697–702.
17. van Dongen JA, et al. Long-term results of a randomized trial comparing breast-conserving therapy with mastectomy: European Organization for Research and Treatment of Cancer 10801 trial. J Natl Cancer Inst. 2000;92(14):1143–50.
18. Arrigada R, et al. Conservative treatment versus mastectomy in early breast cancer: patterns of failure with 15 years of follow-up data. Institut Gustave-Roussy Breast Cancer Group. J Clin Oncol. 1996;14(5):1558–64.
19. Moran MS, et al. Society of Surgical Oncology – American Society for Radiation Oncology consensus guidelines on margins for breast-conserving surgery with whole-breast irradiation in stages I and II invasive breast cancer. J Clin Oncol. 2014;32(14):1507–15. doi:10.1200/JCO.2013.53.3935. Epub 2014 Feb 10.
20. Rowell NP. Are mastectomy resection margins of clinical relevance? A systematic review. Breast. 2010;19(1):14–22. doi:10.1016/j.breast.2009.10.007. Epub 2009 Nov 20.
21. Crowe JP, et al. Nipple-sparing mastectomy: technique and results of 54 procedures. Arch Surg. 2004;139(2):148–50.
22. Stolier AJ, et al. Technical considerations in nipple-sparing mastectomy: 82 consecutive cases without necrosis. Ann Surg Oncol. 2008;15(5):1341–7. doi:10.1245/s10434-007-9753-5. Epub 2008 Feb 7.
23. Eisenberg RE, et al. Pathological evaluation of nipple-sparing mastectomies with emphasis on occult nipple involvement: the Weill-Cornell experience with 325 cases. Breast J. 2014;20(1): 15–21. doi:10.1111/tbj.12199.
24. Wang F, et al. Total skin-sparing mastectomy and immediate breast reconstruction: an evolution of technique and assessment of outcomes. Ann Surg Oncol. 2014;21(10):3223–30. doi:10.1245/s10434-014-3915-z. Epub 2014 Jul 23.
25. de Alcantara FP, et al. Nipple-sparing mastectomy for breast cancer and risk-reducing surgery: the Memorial Sloan-Kettering Cancer Center experience. Ann Surg Oncol. 2011;18(11):3117–22. doi:10.1245/s10434-011-1974-y. Epub 2011 Aug 17.
26. Giuliano AE, et al. Axillary dissection vs no axillary dissection in women with invasive breast cancer and sentinel node metastasis: a randomized clinical trial. JAMA. 2011;305(6):569–75. doi:10.1001/jama.2011.90.
27. Rutgers EJ, et al. Radiotherapy or surgery of the axilla after a positive sentinel node in breast cancer patients: final analysis of the EORTC AMAROS trial. 2013 ASCO Annual Meeting. J Clin Oncol. 2013;(suppl: abstr LBA1001).

28. Boughey JC, et al. Sentinel lymph node surgery after neoadjuvant chemotherapy in patients with node-positive breast cancer: the ACOSOG Z1071 (Alliance) clinical trial. JAMA. 2013;310(14):1455–61. doi:10.1001/jama.2013.278932.

29. Clarke M, et al. Effects of radiotherapy and of differences in the extent of surgery for early breast cancer on local recurrence and 15-year survival: an overview of the randomized trials. Lancet. 2005;366(9503):2087–106.

30. Shah C, et al. The American Brachytherapy Society consensus statement for accelerated partial breast irradiation. Brachytherapy. 2013;12(4):267–77. doi:10.1016/j.brachy.2013.02.001. Epub 2013 Apr 23.

31. Ferraro DJ, et al. Comparison of accelerated partial breast irradiation via multicatheter interstitial brachytherapy versus whole breast irradiation. Radiat Oncol. 2012;7:53. doi:10.1186/1748-717X-7-53.

32. Smith BD, et al. Accelerated partial breast irradiation consensus statement from the American Society for Radiation Oncology (ASTRO). Int J Radiat Oncol Biol Phys. 2009;74(4):987–1001. doi:10.1016/j.ijrobp.2009.02.031.

33. Wilkinson JB, et al. Evaluation of current consensus statement recommendations for accelerated partial breast irradiation: a pooled analysis of William Beaumont Hospital and American Society of Breast Surgeon MammoSite Registry Trial Data. Int J Radiat Oncol Biol Phys. 2013;85(5):1179–85. doi:10.1016/j.ijrobp.2012.10.010. Epub 2012 Nov 22.

34. Zauls AJ, et al. Outcomes in women treated with MammoSite brachytherapy or whole breast irradiation stratified by ASTRO Accelerated Partial Breast Irradiation Consensus Statement Groups. Int J Radiat Oncol Biol Phys. 2012;82(1):21–9. doi:10.1016/j.ijrobp.2010.08.034. Epub 2010 Oct 15.

35. McBride A, et al. Locoregional recurrence risk for patients with T1,2 breast cancer with 1-3 positive lymph nodes treated with mastectomy and systemic treatment. Int J Radiat Oncol Biol Phys. 2014;89(2):392–8. doi:10.1016/j.ijrobp.2014.02.013. Epub 2014 Apr 7.

36. Hughes KS, et al. Lumpectomy plus tamoxifen with or without irradiation in women 70 years of age or older with early breast cancer. N Engl J Med. 2004;351(10):971–7.

37. Soulos PR, et al. Assessing the impact of a cooperative group trial on breast cancer care in the medicare population. J Clin Oncol. 2012;30(14):1601–7. doi:10.1200/JCO.2011.39.4890. Epub 2012 Mar 5.

38. Hughes KS, et al. Lumpectomy plus tamoxifen with or without irradiation in women age 70 years or older with early breast cancer: long-term follow-up of CALGB 9343. J Clin Oncol. 2013;31(19):2382–7. doi:10.1200/JCO.2012.45.2615. Epub 2013 May 20.

39. Wong JS, et al. Eight-year update of a prospective study of wide excision alone for small low- or intermediate-grade ductal carcinoma in situ (DCIS). Breast Cancer Res Treat. 2014;143(2):343–50. doi:10.1007/s10549-013-2813-6. Epub 2013 Dec 18.

40. Houssami N, et al. An individual person data meta-analysis of preoperative magnetic resonance imaging and breast cancer recurrence. J Clin Oncol. 2014;32(5):392–401. doi:10.1200/JCO.2013.52.7515. Epub 2014 Jan 6.

Current Controversies in Thyroid Cancer

Chee-Chee H. Stucky and Nancy D. Perrier

Introduction

Thyroid cancer is the most common endocrine malignancy and the eighth most common cancer diagnosed each year [1]. According to the Surveillance, Epidemiology, and End Results (SEER) data maintained by the National Cancer Institute, more than 60,000 new cases of thyroid cancer were diagnosed in 2013, comprising 3.6 % of all cancer diagnoses. The incidence of differentiated thyroid cancer (papillary, follicular, and poorly differentiated histologies) has increased significantly over the past several decades: from 4.9 cases per 100,000 individuals in 1975 to 14.3 cases per 100,000 individuals in 2009. A particularly steep rate of increase—5.1 cases per 100,000 individual—was noted between 2006 and 2013 [2]. The increasing incidence of thyroid cancer is seen not only in the United States but also throughout most of the world [3].

While the incidence has substantially increased, the mortality rate has remained low, with an estimated 1850 individuals dying of thyroid cancer in 2013 [1]. This low death rate is in part due to the indolent behavior of differentiated thyroid cancers (DTCs). Patients diagnosed with DTC have favorable survival rates nearing 98–100 % over 5 years. The incidence of medullary thyroid cancer (MTC) is lower, and while the histologic subtype carries a less favorable prognosis, survival is still around 80 % over 5 years [1]. Although the overall survival rate for patients with DTC is high, the increasing incidence calls for advances in the management of the disease. Less encouraging is the rate of DTC recurrence, which nears 25 % over the lifetime of the patient [4]. This chapter will discuss the cutting-edge therapies and current controversies surrounding the management of differentiated thyroid cancer.

C.-C.H. Stucky, M.D. • N.D. Perrier, M.D., F.A.C.S. (✉)
Department of Surgical Oncology, The University of Texas M.D. Anderson Cancer Center,
1400 Pressler Street, Faculty Tower 17.6014 Unit 1484, Houston, TX 77030-4009, USA
e-mail: chstucky@mdanderson.org; Nperrier@mdanderson.org

© Springer International Publishing Switzerland 2016
K.A. Morgan (ed.), *Current Controversies in Cancer Care for the Surgeon*, DOI 10.1007/978-3-319-16205-8_9

Preoperative Work-Up

Risk factors associated with thyroid carcinoma include a family history of the disease, radiation exposure, and a personal history of inherited syndromes associated with thyroid cancer such as hereditary nonmedullary thyroid cancer (HNMTC), multiple endocrine neoplasia type 2 (MEN 2), Cowden syndrome, familial adenomatous polyposis (FAP), Werner Syndrome, or Carney Complex [5]. Therefore, the increased incidence of thyroid cancer may not be due entirely to changes in the tumor biology, but also to awareness of risk factors leading to early detection in people with access to healthcare. Changes in environmental exposure and genetic factors may play a role in the increased incidence as well [2, 3].

Frequently, asymptomatic thyroid nodules are detected on routine physical examination or as incidental findings when an individual undergoes imaging for an unrelated indication. Other patients may present with an enlarging mass, dysphagia, dyspnea or hoarseness, but these latter symptoms are seen less frequently and may be related to a multinodular goiter or a rapidly enlarging thyroid tumor.

Once a thyroid nodule is detected, further work-up includes ultrasound (US) of the thyroid as well as a comprehensive neck US evaluating the central and lateral neck lymph nodes. Fine-needle aspiration (FNA) is indicated for cytologic evaluation of suspicious nodules based on size, imaging characteristics, and associated patient risk factors [3, 6]. Most current guidelines recommend FNA biopsy of all nodules measuring 10 mm or more. Nodules less than 10 mm in greatest dimension may still warrant cytologic evaluation if radiographic imaging demonstrates features concerning for malignancy. Ultrasonographic features suspicious for malignancy include hypoechogenicity, complex or solid nodules, vascularity, irregular borders and calcifications. Although positron emission tomography (PET) scanning is not recommended for thyroid nodule assessment, concentrated uptake of contrast in the thyroid gland may be detected when the scan is obtained for other reasons. Incidental increase in fluoro-deoxyglucose (FDG) avidity, and an increase in nodule size (more than 50 % volume) during surveillance may also be indications for FNA biopsy of nodules [6]. Patients with radiographically worrisome sub-centimeter nodules and specific risk factors (listed above) also should be considered for biopsy. Similarly, if there is a known RET mutation and rising levels of calcitonin are detected, biopsy is considered [6]. Radioactive iodine and PET scans have little utility in the contemporary work-up of thyroid nodules.

Cytologic Evaluation and Indeterminate Thyroid Nodules

As a means of standardizing the cytologic interpretation of thyroid biopsies, the Bethesda Thyroid Cytology Classification was developed. Pathologic results are now classified into one of the following six categories: Nondiagnostic or Unsatisfactory, Benign,

Atypia of Undetermined Significance (AUS) or Follicular Lesion of Undetermined Significance (FLUS), Follicular Neoplasm or Suspicious for Follicular Neoplasm, Suspicious for Malignancy, or Malignant [7]. The majority of biopsied thyroid nodules are benign, but patients with biopsy-proven malignant nodules (or nodules suspicious for malignancy) will need surgical resection as discussed below.

Nodules classified as AUS/FLUS fall into the indeterminate category because the extent of architectural or cytologic atypia excludes a benign diagnosis, but the degree of atypia is insufficient for a definitive malignant classification [7]. These lesions should be followed with repeat FNA and surgically resected only if the clinical features of the nodule change, or if biopsies repeatedly result in AUS/FLUS classification. With definitive diagnosis by surgical resection, the rate of malignancy in AUS/FLUS nodules is reported to range between 5 and 15 % [8]. At The University of Texas M.D. Anderson Cancer Center, we classify indeterminate follicular thyroid FNA biopsy findings with the terms Follicular Lesions and Follicular Neoplasms. In this classification system, the term Follicular Lesion is similar to AUS/FLUS in that the differential diagnosis ranges from hyperplasia to follicular neoplasia, favoring follicular adenoma but not ruling out follicular carcinoma. Our data show that patients with nodules classified as Follicular Lesions on FNA biopsy will have a 7 % risk of thyroid carcinoma detected upon surgical resection [9].

Both the Bethesda Classification system and the system used at The University of Texas M.D. Anderson Cancer Center use the term Follicular Neoplasm when lesions demonstrate cytomorphologic features distinctive of benign follicular nodules but indeterminate for a definitive diagnosis of malignancy. At the Center, the use of this term implies a higher suspicion of malignancy than Follicular Lesion does. We reported a 21 % rate of malignancy on final pathology after diagnostic lobectomy of Follicular Neoplasms, which is within the range of 15–30 % reported in the literature [7, 9]. Therefore, the vast majority of these thyroid lobes will be removed for benign disease. Although only 10–30 % of biopsied nodules will have an indeterminate classification on cytopathology, this still presents a clinical dilemma, as practitioners must balance the risks of further surgical intervention for a definitive diagnosis of what may ultimately be a benign nodule.

Preoperative Molecular Testing of Thyroid Nodules

Diagnostic surgery is currently indicated for nearly 25 % of cytologically indeterminate thyroid nodules as described above. The ideal goals of preoperative evaluation are to avoid unnecessary thyroid resection and to perform the correct procedure in one initial operation. Preoperative molecular testing of thyroid nodules is one way to help achieve those goals. Currently, there are two commonly used methodologies for molecular testing: gene expression classifier (GEC) and somatic mutation testing

(MT). Both are based on advancements in our understanding of molecular biomarkers. The most common mutation in papillary thyroid cancer is a point mutation in the *BRAF* V600E gene, which leads to activation of the mitogen-activated protein kinase (MAPK) pathway. Several groups have studied the *BRAF* mutation in thyroid cancer, have determined *BRAF*'s presence to be a highly specific diagnostic marker, and have even investigated the question of its possible association with more aggressive forms of the disease [10, 11]. Similarly, a point mutation of the *RAS* gene and rearrangements of the *RET/PTC1* or *3* and *TK* genes also activate the MAPK pathway, comprising 70 % of the mutations found in papillary cancer.

In follicular cancer, the predominant mutations are located in the *RAS* gene as well as in *PAX8/PPARγ* rearrangements. Point mutations of the *RET* proto-oncogene as well as the *RAS* gene are frequently identified in both the sporadic and familial types of medullary thyroid cancer. Even dedifferentiated, poorly differentiated tumors, and anaplastic thyroid cancer have been linked to specific mutations in the phosphoinositide 3-kinase (PI3K)/AKT signaling pathway, *TP53* and *CTNNB1* genes, respectively [10]. Unfortunately, the sensitivity of even well-defined mutations such as *BRAF* is low for Bethesda category III or IV nodules (3 % as reported by Kleiman et al.), and therefore, testing for the presence of these individual markers should not alter the surgical treatment of patients with indeterminate nodules [12]. However, gene expression panels have been developed to test for an array of mutational markers most commonly seen in thyroid cancer in an effort to increase the likelihood of identifying a cancerous lesion [13]. While these panels may improve accuracy in identifying cancerous nodules, a negative result from these tests does not eliminate the risk for cancer.

Gene Expression Classification (GEC) is a diagnostic test that analyzes the expression of 147 genes and classifies the indeterminate thyroid nodules as either benign or suspicious based on a proprietary algorithm. Several studies have been conducted to explore the utility of this test. The negative predictive value (NPV) of a biopsy reported as benign has been reported at 94–95 %, and the positive predictive value (PPV) of suspicious lesions is 37–38 % [14, 15]. The high sensitivity associated with GEC may improve identification of nodules with low malignancy risk and thereby select nodules that may be clinically observed. However, the test does not reliably identify those nodules at high risk for malignancy and should therefore not be used to guide the extent of initial surgical intervention. As such, current National Cancer Cooperative Network (NCCN) guidelines for the management of thyroid cancer recommend observation or ultrasound follow-up for cytopathologically indeterminate nodules diagnosed as benign on GEC testing [16]. The testing is highly dependent on the pretest probability of malignancy, and therefore, test results must be interpreted according to the risks in specific practice populations. In addition, surgery to determine the definitive diagnosis was avoided in only 28–41 % of cases (according to several studies), bringing into question the cost-effectiveness of the GEC.

In contrast, MT evaluates for somatic DNA mutations that are known to be involved in thyroid carcinoma. Specific panels assessing point mutation in *BRAF*, *RAS*, *RET/PTC1* or *3*, *PAX8/PPAR* provide testing sensitivity and specificity of 61

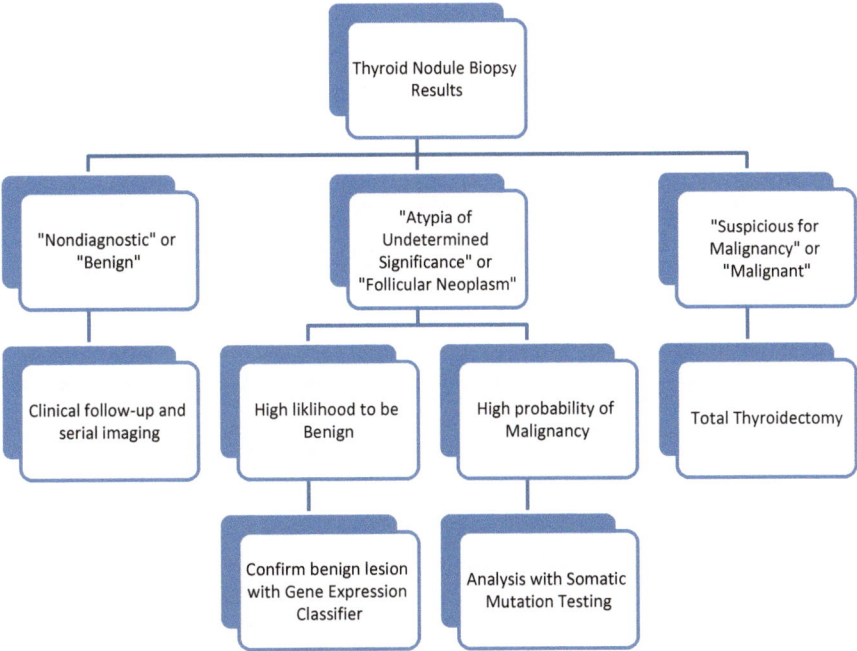

Fig. 1 Proposed algorithm for non-operative analysis with the gene expression classifier and somatic mutation testing in indeterminate thyroid nodules

and 98 %, respectively [17]. Because MT can effectively identify nodules with a high index of malignancy, it can be used to direct the extent of thyroidectomy (Fig. 1).

Surgical Treatment of Thyroid Cancer

Patients with a diagnosis of DTC should undergo total thyroidectomy as recommended by the American Thyroid Association (ATA) [18]. Patients with medullary thyroid cancer receive total thyroidectomy with central neck lymph node dissection. In instances where the tumor is within a unifocal, intrathyroidal nodule, measuring <1 cm in dimension and having low-risk features, and in the absence of a history of head or neck irradiation or lymph node involvement, thyroid lobectomy may be the appropriate treatment. Similarly, patients with clinically or radiographically positive metastatic lymph nodes should undergo total thyroidectomy and concomitant ipsilateral, compartment-oriented lymph node dissection. Comprehensive preoperative neck ultrasound not only provides the opportunity for FNA biopsy of any suspicious nodes prior to surgery but also allows the surgeon to plan the appropriate surgery and counsel the patient regarding the surgery and its associated risks [19].

Cervical Lymph Node Dissection

The risk of regional recurrence of thyroid cancer historically ranges from 20 to 59 % and most frequently presents as nodal metastases. Indeed, these recurrences may actually be residual disease left behind at the time of initial surgery. The compartment-oriented central neck dissection extends from the hyoid bone superiorly to the innominate vein inferiorly; the medial border of the carotid sheath laterally and midline trachea medially. The central neck contents include the prelaryngeal, pretracheal, and paratracheal lymph nodes (Fig. 2).

In the lateral neck, a complete compartment-oriented modified lateral neck dissection should occur if nodal disease is present. This dissection should include the superficial layer of cervical fascia wrapping of the sternocleidomastoid muscle

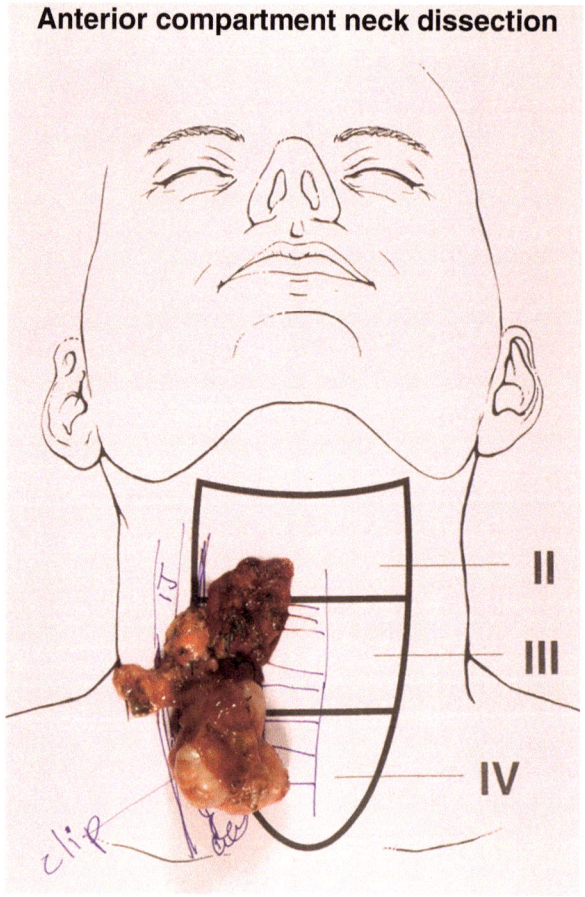

Anterior compartment neck dissection

Fig. 2 Diagram of anatomical landmarks for compartment-oriented central neck lymph node dissection

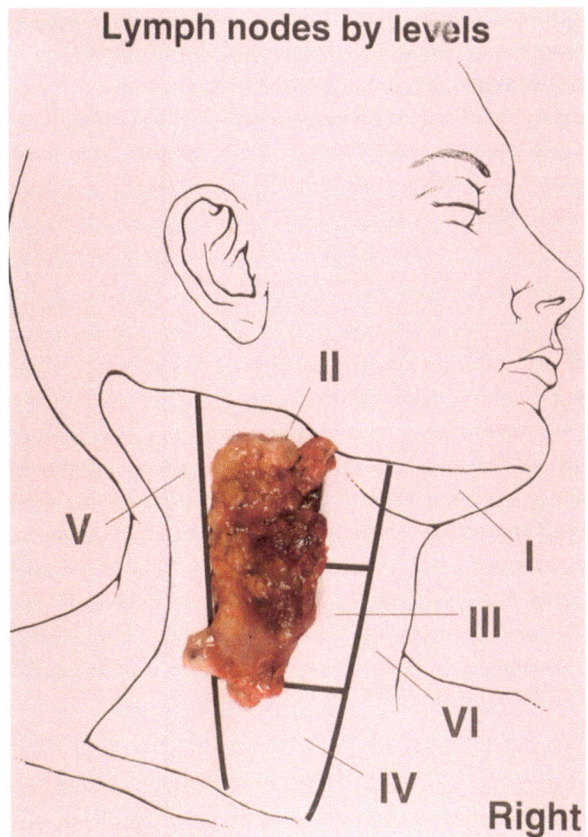

Fig. 3 Diagram of anatomical landmarks for compartment-oriented lateral neck lymph node dissection

along with identification, preservation, and dissection of the spinal accessory nerve and vascular sheath (Fig. 3). The standard nodal draining pattern of involved disease does not usually extend higher than level II, so dissection in the submental region is not necessary. Intraoperative ultrasound can be performed to identify the suspicious-appearing lymph nodes above the posterior belly of the digastric.

Prophylactic Dissection vs. Therapeutic Dissection of the Central Compartment Lymph Nodes

The majority of surgeons would agree that patients with papillary thyroid cancer and radiographically, clinically, or intraoperatively suspicious or biopsy-proven metastatic lymph nodes warrant total thyroidectomy and compartment-based removal of the lymph node basin(s). Current controversy exists, however, as to the appropriate treatment of non-enlarged lymph nodes of the central neck at the time of initial thyroidectomy. Specifically, some groups advocate routine prophylactic central node dissection (PCND) for all patients with known papillary thyroid cancer to decrease the risk of local recurrence, even recognizing that no prospective randomized data support a survival benefit [20, 21]. While two retrospective studies have reported a reduction in disease recurrence rates associated with PCND [22, 23], two recent meta-analyses have shown that PCND does not reduce recurrence rates in a clinically significant manner [24, 25]. Moo et al. endorsed PCND, arguing that those patients noted to have pathologically positive nodal metastases after PCND were upstaged and therefore received more aggressive postoperative therapy with radioactive iodine ablation. However, no studies have actually shown an improvement in long-term survival with upstaging [21].

Surgery of the neck is not without complication. Surgeons arguing against PCND are unwilling to subject patients to the risks of recurrent laryngeal nerve (RLN) injury and permanent hypocalcemia by performing a procedure that has not yet clearly been demonstrated to improve long-term outcomes. Reoperation in the neck increases the risks of hypoparathyroidism and injury to the RLN, and these risks have been used as arguments in favor of PCND. For this reason, Popadich et al. studied the rate of central neck reoperation in patients undergoing PCND with total thyroidectomy and in those undergoing total thyroidectomy alone. These investigators demonstrated a significantly lower rate of reoperation in the central neck for those patients receiving PCND, but the overall rate of reoperation between the two groups was similar. They also noted a significantly higher rate of temporary hypocalcemia and transplantation of parathyroid glands in patients receiving PCND [26]. In their meta-analysis, Shan et al. reported the rate of temporary hypocalcemia to be significantly higher in patients undergoing PCND with thyroidectomy than in patients receiving thyroidectomy alone (31 % vs. 15 %, respectively, risk difference, 0.15; 95 % confidence interval, 0.09–0.22; $P < 0.01$). However, the definition of hypocalcemia did vary among the studies analyzed, and no difference among the studies was noted in the rate of permanent hypocalcemia. Shan and colleagues found that the incidence of transient RLN injury trended to be higher in patients undergoing PCND, but that increase did not reach statistical significance [24]. There is concern that these data underreported the risks of hypocalcemia and nerve injury because the studies were conducted in high-volume tertiary care centers where PCND is more commonly performed. Surgeons performing PCND less frequently may experience higher complication rates.

The current recommendations published by the ATA state that prophylactic or bilateral Level VI lymph node dissection is recommended in patients with T3/T4 papillary tumors but may not be necessary in patients with T1, T2, N0 thyroid cancers. The ATA also states that this recommendation should be interpreted in light of available surgical expertise, acknowledging that PCND may lead to increased perioperative morbidity [18]. Ideally, a prospective randomized trial would be conducted to help determine the benefit of PCND. The ATA evaluated the design and feasibility of such a study and concluded that the required sample size would be prohibitively large and therefore this study is not readily feasible [27]. Unfortunately, high quality evidence to determine the benefit of PCND is not available at the present time. Currently, selective, rather than routine, PCND seems the most reasonable option to guide the decision process. We have noted excellent long-term regional disease control and patient survival using preoperative US and intraoperative surgeon evaluation [28].

Postoperative Therapy

Radioactive Iodine Ablation

Adjuvant therapy for patients with DTC predominantly consists of radioactive iodine ablation (RAI) and thyroid-stimulating hormone (TSH) suppression. [131]Iodine (^{131}I) is used for therapeutic ablation of any remnant or microscopic thyroid tissue that may persist after surgery. For patients with high-risk disease, the use of RAI has been associated with reduced rates of recurrence and cause-specific mortality. RAI has not been shown to be beneficial in patients at low risk for disease recurrence or cause-specific mortality [29]. The decision to treat patients with RAI in the adjuvant setting is typically reserved for papillary or follicular thyroid cancer patients who are 45 years of age or older, patients whose primary tumor is >1 cm in diameter or multifocal (at least one nodule >1 cm in greatest dimension), and for patients with extrathyroidal disease due to tissue invasion. RAI may also be used in the treatment of local recurrence or distant metastases.

Complications associated with RAI include swelling and discomfort of the salivary glands, impaired sensation of taste (frequently metallic taste), dry mouth, nausea in the acute setting, pulmonary fibrosis, bone marrow suppression, and the potential for secondary cancers [30]. Given these potential side effects, practitioners are trending toward using lower initial doses of [131]I (30–100 mCi) in patients with low-volume disease limited to the thyroid, and who have shown radioiodine uptake in only the thyroid bed on initial postoperative diagnostic whole-body scan [31]. Higher ^{131}I doses are reserved for those patients with evidence of extrathyroidal disease extension, lymph node metastases or significant radioiodine uptake in the neck on initial postoperative diagnostic thyroid scan.

After total thyroidectomy and subsequent RAI (if indicated), patients will need lifelong thyroid hormone replacement. The levothyroxine sodium starting dose is 2 µg/kg/day and is then titrated to reach an appropriate level of TSH suppression. The amount of TSH suppression is also individualized based on the patient's disease status and clinicopathological tumor features. Patients must also begin a surveillance regimen consisting of laboratory evaluation and ultrasonography. In papillary and follicular carcinoma, T4 and TSH demonstrate the level of thyroid suppression, and thyroglobulin and thyroglobulin antibody levels are important markers for possible disease recurrence or metastases. In medullary thyroid cancer, calcitonin and carcinoembryonic acid (CEA) levels should be monitored both pre- and postoperatively to identify trends suspicious for disease recurrence.

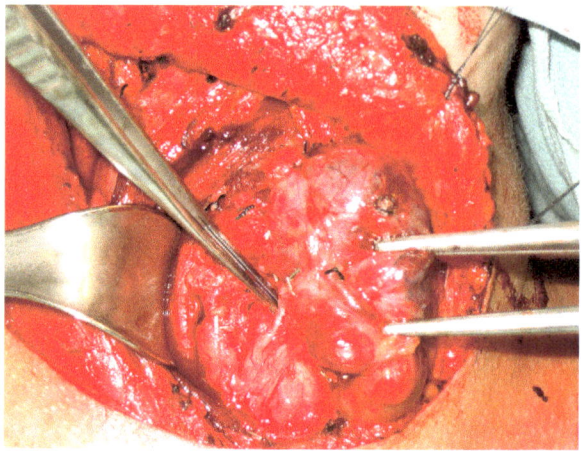

Fig. 4 Recurrent papillary thyroid cancer in the lymph nodes posterior to the right recurrent laryngeal nerve

Systemic Therapy for Metastatic and RAI-Refractory Cancers

Patients with DTC generally have a good prognosis due to the indolent nature of the disease as well as to the efficacy of standard treatment. Even those with locoregional recurrence are typically treated with further surgery (Fig. 4) or RAI and have excellent outcomes. However, a subset of patients will develop locally recurrent disease but are no longer candidates for surgical resection. Metastatic disease also is observed in 15 % of patients with DTC, of whom half have metastatic disease diagnosed at the initial presentation. Patients with metastatic disease typically do not undergo further surgery as the benefits are only palliative in nature. RAI may be used to treat metastatic disease, but unfortunately, the majority of these patients will not experience complete remission despite multiple treatments [32, 33]. Further, RAI therapy is not indicated when tumors have proven resistant to RAI by evidence of radiographic progression, if tumors are non-avid on imaging, or if patients have experienced toxicity to RAI. Overall, these tumors carry a worse prognosis but may be stable and indolent over several years. Systemic therapy is reserved for progressive or symptomatic locally advanced or metastatic disease [34].

Historically, cytotoxic chemotherapy, specifically doxorubicin, was used to treat metastatic thyroid cancers but produced a poor response. Systemic therapy is emerging in the form of antineoplastic therapies targeted at known gene mutations. Major targets involve inhibiting the kinase signaling pathways in tumor cells and vascular endothelial cells. Known mutations of the *RET/PTC*, *BRAF*, and *RAS* genes, vascular endothelial growth factor (VEGF) receptors, and epidermal growth factor (EGF) receptors and their downstream effects are of particular interest [33, 34]. Tyrosine kinase inhibitors (TKI) affect multiple signaling pathways and have shown promising results. The U.S. Food and Drug Administration (FDA) has approved the use of sorafenib for metastatic DTC and has approved vandetanib and cabozantinib for metastatic or unresectable MTC [35]. A systematic meta-analysis of eight phase II trials and retrospective studies evaluating the effects of sorafenib on disease progression, disease response and patient survival, found that sorafenib was associated with a partial response in 22 % of MTC patients, 21 % of DTC patients, and 13 % of anaplastic thyroid cancer patients. The majority of DTC and MTC patients demonstrated clinical benefit, with progression of disease noted in 6.5 % of MTC patients and 21 % of DTC patients [35].

A recent multicenter, prospective, randomized, double-blind, placebo-controlled, phase III trial entitled DECISION, was conducted to evaluate the efficacy and safety of sorafenib treatment in patients with RAI-refractory metastatic DTC. This trial included 417 patients, 207 of whom received sorafenib; however, the patients with disease progression in the placebo study arm were allowed to cross over to open-label sorafenib. The DECISION trial investigators reported a significantly longer progression-free survival in patients treated with sorafenib (10.8 months) than in patients in the placebo arm (5.8 months; hazard ratio, 0.59; 95 % confidence interval, 0.45–0.76; $P < 0.0001$). Adverse effects of sorafenib were noted in 98.6 % of treated patients and consisted mostly of the commonly reported side effects of hand–foot skin reaction, diarrhea, alopecia, and skin desquamation [36]. Of note, sorafenib has also been associated with the development of squamous cell carcinoma of the skin and therefore patients must be carefully monitored for skin cancer during and after treatment.

These promising studies have led not only to further research and development of targeted therapy in metastatic DTC, but also to expanded use of the currently approved therapies in the adjuvant setting. As more data accumulate, these therapies may be utilized in the neoadjuvant setting as well.

Special Considerations

Timing of Prophylactic Thyroidectomy for RET Mutation-Positive Patients

Unlike well-differentiated thyroid cancer, MTC is not derived from follicular cells but rather from calcitonin-producing C-cells of the thyroid. The development of MTC is sporadic in 80 % of patients; however, MTC is a distinct entity in the diagnosis of hereditary syndromes such as multiple endocrine neoplasia (MEN) type 2A and type 2B as well as familial medullary thyroid cancer (FMTC). The *RET* proto-oncogene mutation previously discussed is strongly associated with MTC and is present in 98 % of MEN 2A patients and in 95 % of FMTC individuals. Even those without an inherited etiology of MTC will frequently have a *RET* mutation identified upon genetic testing [37, 38]. Mutations in several different codons of the *RET* oncogene lead to varying degrees of transformation to MTC and to various phenotypes of the hereditary

MTCs. For this reason, relatives of patients with a *RET* mutation should undergo genetic counseling and testing to detect carriers of mutations that may not yet have manifested clinical symptoms. Given its strong association with MTC, all family members identified to carry a *RET* gene mutation are recommended to undergo thyroidectomy. The timing of thyroidectomy for prophylactic, rather than therapeutic purposes in *RET*-mutation positive individuals is debatable.

Thyroidectomy in response to rising calcitonin levels, independent of the type of *RET* mutation, is agreed upon by most. Arguments against this approach are that the ability to determine biochemical conversion is limited and that patients with micro-MTC are still at risk of having both lymph node as well as distant metastases [37]. The 2009 ATA guidelines have incorporated a classification system for RET mutations that includes consideration of mutations known to be more aggressive in determining the recommended time for prophylactic thyroidectomy [39]. Regarding prophylactic thyroidectomy based on risk stratification, invasive MTC is present in up to 22 % of patients, and the percentage of patients with invasive MTC did not differ among mutation risk levels [40]. In children, preoperative US cannot reliably distinguish MTC from other thyroid nodules. Surgical management should thus be individualized using the ATA guidelines to suggest when to operate [41].

Genetic Testing for Nonmedullary Thyroid Cancer

The vast majority of papillary or follicular thyroid cancers are sporadic in nature; however, approximately 5 % of these nonmedullary thyroid cancers (NMTCs) are hereditary in origin [42]. Familial adenomatous polyposis (FAP) and Cowden syndrome have a known association with multiple cancers in the body, including those of the breast and NMTCs. FAP is an autosomal dominant disorder due to germline mutations of the *APC* gene typically characterized by multiple colorectal polyps that develop into colorectal cancer if left untreated. Cowden syndrome is now known to be most frequently associated with PTEN tumor suppression gene mutations leading to malignant transformation of epithelial tissue-derived organs [37]. Patients diagnosed with FAP should be screened for other cancers including those of the breast and thyroid. Similarly, patients noted to have a family history of FAP or of multiple types of cancer during the initial history should be referred for genetic counseling and possibly for genetic testing to identify those at risk for germline mutations.

There have also been reports of familial nonmedullary thyroid cancers (FNMTCs) that are not associated with FAP or Cowden syndrome. Patients with FNMTC must have at least two or more first-degree relatives with well-differentiated thyroid cancer in the absence of predisposing hereditary syndromes or environmental factors. Patients with FNMTC are thought to have a more aggressive form of the disease, and early identification of at-risk family members is indicated. Some groups argue for more aggressive therapy (including prophylactic central neck dissection and radioiodine ablation despite tumor characteristics) in patients with FNMTC; however, as previously discussed, the data regarding these treatments are controversial [37].

Unfortunately, genetic markers associated with FNMTC are yet to be isolated, but studies are currently under way in hopes of better understanding the pathogenesis of this disease [37, 43]. For now, surgeons should take a detailed personal and family history when initially evaluating patients with all forms of thyroid cancer. Those with remarkable risk factors must be counseled about the risk of cancer and about appropriate screening recommendations for their relatives.

Summary

The diagnosis of DTC typically carries an excellent prognosis. Even the majority of patients with MTC will experience long-term survival rates of 80 %. Preoperative diagnosis is performed with US-guided FNA biopsy. A diagnostic dilemma occurs when the FNA biopsy results are indeterminate for cancer. Gene expression classifiers may be used to assist in the risk assessment of these indeterminate nodules to identify patients likely to have benign disease, and molecular testing can identify nodules with a high risk of malignancy.

The recommended treatment for preoperatively identified thyroid carcinoma is total thyroidectomy. In select cases involving unifocal, limited disease (<1 cm), thyroid lobectomy may be considered. A compartment-oriented lymph node dissection should be performed for radiographic or clinically evident lymph node disease. Commonly, this dissection is a central (level 6) neck dissection. Lateral neck disease is less common but if present, a compartment-oriented neck dissection should be performed. The role of PCND is less obvious but is advocated by some to reduce the risk of local recurrence. Those against PCND note that the risk-to-benefit ratio is gratuitously high, as increases in temporary hypocalcemia and nerve palsy have been noted. RAI has no long-term benefit in patients with low-risk tumors but should be considered for moderate and high-risk patients, such as those with T3-T4 or N1 disease. Adjuvant systemic chemotherapy for those patients with metastatic thyroid cancer is largely targeted to tyrosine kinase inhibitors.

References

1. Surveillance, epidemiology, and end results (SEER) stat fact sheets: thyroid cancer. National Cancer Institute. http://www.seer.cancer.gov/statfacts/html.thyro.html. Accessed 23 June 2014.
2. Davies L, Welch HG. Current thyroid cancer trends in the United States. JAMA Otolaryngol Head Neck Surg. 2014.
3. Pellegriti G, Frasca F, Regalbuto C, et al. Worldwide increasing incidence of thyroid cancer: update on epidemiology and risk factors. J Cancer Epidemiol. 2013;2013:965212.
4. Guerrero MA, Clark OH. Controversies in the management of papillary thyroid cancer revisited. ISRN Oncol. 2011;2011:303128.
5. Nose V. Familial non-medullary thyroid carcinoma: an update. Endocr Pathol. 2008;19: 226–40.
6. Kwak JY. Indications for fine needle aspiration in thyroid nodules. Endocrinol Metab (Seoul). 2013;28:81–5.

7. Cibas ES, Ali SZ. The Bethesda system for reporting thyroid cytopathology. Thyroid. 2009;19:1159–65.
8. Baloch ZW, LiVolsi VA, Asa SL, et al. Diagnostic terminology and morphologic criteria for cytologic diagnosis of thyroid lesions: a synopsis of the National Cancer Institute Thyroid Fine-Needle Aspiration State of the Science Conference. Diagn Cytopathol. 2008;36:425–37.
9. Williams MD, Suliburk JW, Staerkel GA, et al. Clinical significance of distinguishing between follicular lesion and follicular neoplasm in thyroid fine-needle aspiration biopsy. Ann Surg Oncol. 2009;16:3146–53.
10. Nikiforov YE, Nikiforova MN. Molecular genetics and diagnosis of thyroid cancer. Nat Rev Endocrinol. 2011;7:569–80.
11. Li C, Aragon Han P, Lee KC, et al. Does BRAF V600E mutation predict aggressive features in papillary thyroid cancer? Results from four endocrine surgery centers. J Clin Endocrinol Metab. 2013;98:3702–12.
12. Kleiman DA, Sporn MJ, Beninato T, et al. Preoperative BRAF(V600E) mutation screening is unlikely to alter initial surgical treatment of patients with indeterminate thyroid nodules: a prospective case series of 960 patients. Cancer. 2013;119:1495–502.
13. Nikiforov YE, Yip L, Nikiforova MN. New strategies in diagnosing cancer in thyroid nodules: impact of molecular markers. Clin Cancer Res. 2013;19:2283–8.
14. Chudova D, Wilde JI, Wang ET, et al. Molecular classification of thyroid nodules using high-dimensionality genomic data. J Clin Endocrinol Metab. 2010;95:5296–304.
15. Alexander EK, Kennedy GC, Baloch ZW, et al. Preoperative diagnosis of benign thyroid nodules with indeterminate cytology. N Engl J Med. 2012;367:705–15.
16. Network. NCC. Thyroid Carcinoma Version 2.2013. In Edition.
17. Nikiforov YE, Ohori NP, Hodak SP, et al. Impact of mutational testing on the diagnosis and management of patients with cytologically indeterminate thyroid nodules: a prospective analysis of 1056 FNA samples. J Clin Endocrinol Metab. 2011;96:3390–7.
18. Cooper DS, Doherty GM, Haugen BR, et al. Revised American Thyroid Association management guidelines for patients with thyroid nodules and differentiated thyroid cancer. Thyroid. 2009;19:1167–214.
19. Marshall CL, Lee JE, Xing Y, et al. Routine pre-operative ultrasonography for papillary thyroid cancer: effects on cervical recurrence. Surgery. 2009;146:1063–72.
20. Mazzaferri EL, Doherty GM, Steward DL. The pros and cons of prophylactic central compartment lymph node dissection for papillary thyroid carcinoma. Thyroid. 2009;19:683–9.
21. McLeod DS, Sawka AM, Cooper DS. Controversies in primary treatment of low-risk papillary thyroid cancer. Lancet. 2013;381:1046–57.
22. Moo TA, McGill J, Allendorf J, et al. Impact of prophylactic central neck lymph node dissection on early recurrence in papillary thyroid carcinoma. World J Surg. 2010;34:1187–91.
23. Perrino M, Vannucchi G, Vicentini L, et al. Outcome predictors and impact of central node dissection and radiometabolic treatments in papillary thyroid cancers < or =2 cm. Endocr Relat Cancer. 2009;16:201–10.
24. Shan CX, Zhang W, Jiang DZ, et al. Routine central neck dissection in differentiated thyroid carcinoma: a systematic review and meta-analysis. Laryngoscope. 2012;122:797–804.
25. Zetoune T, Keutgen X, Buitrago D, et al. Prophylactic central neck dissection and local recurrence in papillary thyroid cancer: a meta-analysis. Ann Surg Oncol. 2010;17:3287–93.
26. Popadich A, Levin O, Lee JC, et al. A multicenter cohort study of total thyroidectomy and routine central lymph node dissection for cN0 papillary thyroid cancer. Surgery. 2011;150:1048–57.
27. Carling T, Carty SE, Ciarleglio MM, et al. American Thyroid Association design and feasibility of a prospective randomized controlled trial of prophylactic central lymph node dissection for papillary thyroid carcinoma. Thyroid. 2012;22:237–44.
28. Moreno MA, Edeiken-Monroe BS, Siegel ER, et al. In papillary thyroid cancer, preoperative central neck ultrasound detects only macroscopic surgical disease, but negative findings predict excellent long-term regional control and survival. Thyroid. 2012;22:347–55.

29. Tala H, Tuttle RM. Contemporary post surgical management of differentiated thyroid carcinoma. Clin Oncol (R Coll Radiol). 2010;22:419–29.
30. Clarke SE. Radioiodine therapy in differentiated thyroid cancer: a nuclear medicine perspective. Clin Oncol (R Coll Radiol). 2010;22:430–7.
31. Mallick U, Harmer C, Yap B, et al. Ablation with low-dose radioiodine and thyrotropin alfa in thyroid cancer. N Engl J Med. 2012;366:1674–85.
32. Durante C, Haddy N, Baudin E, et al. Long-term outcome of 444 patients with distant metastases from papillary and follicular thyroid carcinoma: benefits and limits of radioiodine therapy. J Clin Endocrinol Metab. 2006;91:2892–9.
33. Haugen BR, Sherman SI. Evolving approaches to patients with advanced differentiated thyroid cancer. Endocr Rev. 2013;34:439–55.
34. Busaidy NL, Cabanillas ME. Differentiated thyroid cancer: management of patients with radioiodine nonresponsive disease. J Thyroid Res. 2012;2012:618985.
35. Thomas L, Lai SY, Dong W, et al. Sorafenib in metastatic thyroid cancer: a systematic review. Oncologist. 2014;19:251–8.
36. Brose MS, Nutting CM, Jarzab B, et al. Sorafenib in radioactive iodine-refractory, locally advanced or metastatic differentiated thyroid cancer: a randomised, double-blind, phase 3 trial. Lancet. 2014;384(9940):319–28.
37. Metzger R, Milas M. Inherited cancer syndromes and the thyroid: an update. Curr Opin Oncol. 2014;26:51–61.
38. Machens A, Dralle H. Multiple endocrine neoplasia type 2: achievements and current challenges. Clinics (Sao Paulo). 2012;67 Suppl 1:113–8.
39. Kloos RT, Eng C, Evans DB, et al. Medullary thyroid cancer: management guidelines of the American Thyroid Association. Thyroid. 2009;19:565–612.
40. Grubbs EG, Waguespack SG, Rich TA, et al. Do the recent American Thyroid Association (ATA) Guidelines accurately guide the timing of prophylactic thyroidectomy in MEN2A? Surgery. 2010;148:1302–9. discussion 1309–1310.
41. Morris LF, Waguespack SG, Edeiken-Monroe BS, et al. Ultrasonography should not guide the timing of thyroidectomy in pediatric patients diagnosed with multiple endocrine neoplasia syndrome 2A through genetic screening. Ann Surg Oncol. 2013;20:53–9.
42. Khan A, Smellie J, Nutting C, et al. Familial nonmedullary thyroid cancer: a review of the genetics. Thyroid. 2010;20:795–801.
43. Mazeh H, Sippel RS. Familial nonmedullary thyroid carcinoma. Thyroid. 2013;23:1049–56.

Controversies in the Surgical Management of Melanoma

Jeremiah L. Deneve, Maria C. Russell, and Keith A. Delman

Introduction

Melanoma is the third most common malignancy of the skin behind basal cell carcinoma and squamous cell carcinoma and the deadliest form of cutaneous cancer with more than 8000 deaths per year in the United States [1]. The average lifetime risk of developing melanoma in the United States increased from 1 in 1500 in 1935 to 1 in 30 in 2009 [2, 3]. The management of melanoma is based upon the Tumor-Node-Metastatsis (TNM) classification system, as described in the seventh edition of the American Joint Commission on Cancer (AJCC) published in 2009 [4].

The outcome for patients with localized (Stage I/II) melanoma without lymph node metastasis is favorable with a 92–95 % 5-year survival. Primary tumor thickness and the presence of ulceration are the primary determinants of survival for Stage I/II melanoma [5]. Emerging data from several centers has also demonstrated the mitotic rate to be an adverse prognostic determinant of outcome for localized melanoma, as evidenced by the recent inclusion of mitotic rate into the AJCC staging guidelines for thin melanomas [6–8].

J.L. Deneve, D.O.
Division of Surgical Oncology, University of Tennessee Health Science Center,
910 Madison Avenue, Suite 303, Memphis, TN 38163, USA
e-mail: jdeneve@uthsc.edu

M.C. Russell, M.D.
Division of Surgical Oncology, Emory University, 550 Peachtree Street,
NE, Suite 9000, Atlanta, GA 30308, USA
e-mail: maria.c.russell@emory.edu

K.A. Delman, M.D., F.A.C.S. (✉)
Division of Surgical Oncology, Emory University, 1365 Clifton Rd NE,
Suite C2004, Atlanta, GA 30322, USA
e-mail: kdelman@emory.edu

© Springer International Publishing Switzerland 2016
K.A. Morgan (ed.), *Current Controversies in Cancer Care for the Surgeon*, DOI 10.1007/978-3-319-16205-8_10

Patients with Stage III melanoma represent a more heterogeneous group than those with localized melanoma with regard to staging, management and prognosis. This group includes those with regional metastasis (micro- or macrometastasis) and/or in-transit metastasis. Regional lymph nodes are the most common site of metastasis for melanoma patients. The use of sentinel lymph node biopsy (SLNB) is one of the most important advances in the management of melanoma. It has significant staging and treatment implications in that it facilitates the identification of more high-risk patients (Stage IIB, IIC, or III) and identifies those with micro-metastatic disease who may benefit from earlier therapeutic lymph node dissection (LND) while sparing those node-negative patients the morbidity of an elective LND. The status of the sentinel lymph node (SLN) is the most powerful indepen-dent predictor of survival [9, 10].

Patients with Stage IV melanoma include those with metastasis to distant skin, subcutaneous tissues and/or lymph nodes (M1a), the lungs (M1b) or any non-pulmonary visceral site (M1c). The overall prognosis is generally poor with 5-year survival rates of less than 10 % [11, 12]. Historically, the treatment for this cohort has been primarily medical with surgery reserved for those with isolated resectable or symptomatic metastases. The recent discovery of targeted systemic agents for the treatment of melanoma metastasis has revolutionized the management and outcome of patients with Stage IV melanoma [13–15].

While significant advances in the management of melanoma patients have devel-oped over the past two decades, this review focuses on the current controversies in the surgical management of melanoma. For purposes of this discussion, relevant topics are segregated into lymph node-negative (Stage I/II) disease, lymph-node positive (Stage III) disease and distant metastatic melanoma (Stage IV).

Surgical Management of Node-Negative Melanoma

Is it Time to Re-address Surgical Excision Margins for Primary Cutaneous Melanoma?

Surgical excision is the primary treatment for cutaneous melanoma. Given that up to 70–85 % of patients with melanoma present with localized disease, most can be cured with surgical excision alone [4]. The margin of excision is based on the Breslow thickness of the primary melanoma and has evolved from a series of stud-ies comparing different margins. Current National Comprehensive Cancer Network (NCCN) guidelinesfor the surgical management of melanoma recommend a 0.5 cm margin for melanoma in situ (MIS) [16]. Margins >0.5 cm may be necessary for large MIS or lentigo maligna to achieve histologically negative margins. Recommended margins of excision are outlined in Table 1. It is important to note that these recommendations are based on the clinical margin mapped out at the time of surgery and not gross or histologic margins as defined by the pathologist.

Tumor thickness	Recommended margin of excision[a] (cm)
In situ[b]	0.5
≤1.0 mm	1
1.01–2.0 mm	1–2
2.01–4.0 mm	2
≥4 mm	2

Table 1 National Comprehensive Cancer Network (NCCN) guidelines for melanoma margins of excision [16]

[a]Excision recommendations are based on clinical margins taken at the time of surgery and not gross or histologic margins as measured by the pathologist
[b]For large melanoma in situ, lentigo maligna type, surgical margins >0.5 cm may be necessary to achieve histologically negative margins

The progression to the current recommendations for surgical margins of excision of invasive melanoma has continued to evolve over the last 100 years. Historically, the management of melanoma involved the removal of 2 in. (5 cm) of subcutaneous tissue down to the level of the muscle fascia with the radical removal of lymph nodes [17]. This surgical dogma perpetuated until Breslow and colleagues demonstrated a narrow excision margin was not associated with adverse events in thin melanomas (≤0.75 mm) [18]. This finding prompted the initiation of several randomized trials which have subsequently defined our current management of melanoma.

The World Health Organization (WHO) was the first to address the topic of surgical margins in a multicenter, randomized control trial (RCT) of 703 patients with melanomas no thicker than 2 mm to address the efficacy of narrow margin excision [19]. Six hundred and twelve (87 %) patients were evaluated, of which 305 underwent 1 cm excision (narrow) and 307 underwent 3 cm excision (wide). With a mean follow-up of 55 months, there was no difference in disease-free survival (DFS) or overall survival (OS) between the two groups. At 90 months follow up, only four patients had local recurrences, all within the narrow-excision group, still with no difference in OS or DFS observed [20]. The authors concluded that a narrow excision is safe and effective for patients with melanoma thinner than 1 mm with a very low rate of local recurrence.

The Swedish Melanoma Study Grouppublished their initial findings evaluating a 2 cm versus a 5 cm margin of excision for melanomas >0.8 mm and ≤2.0 mm of the trunk and extremities in 1996 [21]. A multicenter, RCT was performed of 989 patients, 476 randomized to the 2 cm group and 513 to the 5 cm group. With a median follow-up of 5.8 years, there was no difference observed between the treatment groups regarding local or regional recurrence or overall survival. At 11 years follow-up, 8 of 989 patients (<1 %) experienced a "local" recurrence in the scar or transplant [22]. There were no statistical differences in recurrence or survival between the two treatment arms. Based on these results, the authors concluded that a 2 cm margin is as safe as a 5 cm margin of resection.

Investigators of the Intergroup Melanoma Surgical Trial first reported their experience in 1993 looking at surgical excision margins for intermediate-thickness melanoma (1.0–4.0 mm) [23]. A prospective, multi-institutional surgical trial was performed in which 486 patients were randomized to 2 or 4-cm surgical margins. The local recurrence rate was 0.8 % for the 2-cm margin group and 1.7 % for the 4-cm margin group ($p=$NS). With a median follow-up of 6 years, there was no difference in local recurrence or overall survival. The authors concluded that the margin of excision for intermediate-thickness melanoma could safely be reduced to 2 cm. Subsequent long-term results reported in 1996 demonstrated a local recurrence of 3.8 % [24]. The local recurrence was not significantly affected by the margin of resection, even among thicker or ulcerated lesions. Ten-year follow up data was reported in 2001 by the Intergroup collaborators [25]. The local recurrence rate was 1.1 % for melanomas of the proximal extremities, 3.1 % for the trunk, 5.3 % for the distal extremity and 9.4 % for the head and neck. There was no difference in local recurrence or OS between a 2 or 4 cm margin of excision.

The French Group of Research on Melanoma evaluated the impact of a 2 cm versus 5 cm margin of excision for melanomas measuring less than 2.1-mm in thickness [26]. A multicenter, randomized control trial was performed in which 337 patients were randomized to a 2-cm (167 patients) or 5-cm (170 patients) margin of excision. With a median follow-up time of 192 months (16 years), there were 22 recurrences in the 2-cm arm and 33 in the 5-cm arm. The 10-year DFS was 85 % and 83 %, respectively and there was no difference in OS (87 % vs 86 %, respectively) between groups. The authors concluded that for melanoma less than 2.1-mm thick, a margin of 2 cm is sufficient and that a 5 cm margin does not appear to impact the rate or time to disease recurrence or survival.

The UK Melanoma Study Groupevaluated the impact of a 1 or 3 cm margin of excision on primary cutaneous melanoma 2 mm or greater in thickness and published their results in 2004 [27]. Nine hundred patients were randomized, 453 to the 1-cm excision group and 447 to the 3-cm excision group. A 1-cm margin of excision was associated with a significantly increased risk of local recurrence. With a median follow up of 60 months, there were 168 locoregional recurrences in the 1-cm excision group as compared with 142 in the 3-cm excision group ($p=0.05$). There was no difference in overall survival between the groups. Based on these results, the authors concluded a 1-cm margin of excision for melanoma of at least 2 mm in thickness is associated with a poor prognosis and significantly greater risk of regional recurrence than is a 3-cm margin.

In an effort to further clarify the most appropriate margin for intermediate-thickness melanoma, the Swedish Melanoma Study Group investigated whether there was a difference in survival using a 2-cm compared with a 4-cm margin of excision for melanoma thicker than 2 mm [28]. A prospective, multicenter randomized trial was performed in which 936 patients were randomized to a 2-cm margin (465 patients) or 4-cm margin (471 patients). The 5-year OS for both groups was 65 % ($p=0.69$). Based on these findings, the authors suggested that a 2-cm margin is sufficient and safe for melanoma 2 mm or thicker.

The results of the afore-mentioned studies add valuable insight into a several decade process of determining which margins are appropriate for a certain thickness melanoma. A summary of RCT outcomes for margins of excision is described in

Table 2 Randomized clinical trials for melanoma margins of excision actuarial recurrence free survival and overall survival

Clinical trial	5-year		10-Year	
	Narrow	Wide	Narrow	Wide
	Recurrence free survival			
WHO [19, 20]	NR	NR	82 %	84 %
Swedish [21, 22]	81 %	83 %	71 %	70 %
Intergroup [23–25]	75 %	70 %	NR	NR
French [26]	NR	NR	85 %	83 %
UK [27]	NR	NR	NR	NR
	Overall survival			
WHO [19, 20]	97 %	96 %	87 %	87 %
Swedish [21, 22]	86 %	89 %	79 %	76 %
Intergroup [23–25]	76 %	82 %	70 %	77 %
French [26]	93 %	90 %	87 %	86 %
UK [27]	NR	NR	NR	NR

Reproduced with permission [29]

Table 2 [29]. Several concepts are noteworthy when considering these landmark surgical clinical trials. First, in each of the five randomized control trials, no survival difference was observed based on the margin of excision. Similarly, there was no difference in local recurrence observed based on margin of excision, except for within the UK study. It is critical that we recognize that even though the UK study showed a higher local recurrence, the study did not include SLN Bx and most of the recurrences were actually in the regional nodal basin, severely limiting the applicability of this study to current practice in the United States and elsewhere. It is also important to note that many of these studies, including the most recent Swedish study, began enrollment prior to the era in which SLNB was routinely performed.

While these trials provide vital long-term follow up data and offer invaluable perspective into the current management of localized melanoma, there are currently no randomized clinical trials underway assessing the margin of resection for localized, primary melanoma. Importantly, there has never been a comparison of 1 cm vs 2 cm margins for a melanoma of any thickness, and the possibility that a 1 cm margin is acceptable for most patients is worth considering. In a review by Hudson and colleagues, a comparison of 1 cm vs 2 cm margins in T2 melanomas demonstrated that there was no difference in overall survival and that local recurrences were generally surgically salvageable without an adverse impact on survival [30]. The most recent RCT (Swedish Group) began enrollment in 1992, approximately two decades ago. Given the lack of association between an impact on survival and the margin of excision, is it time to address whether there is a difference between a 1 and 2-cm margin of resection for intermediate-thickness and/or thick melanoma? This effort would require a large patient population and a multicenter, international collaborative effort but is certainly worth addressing and would have a similar far-reaching impact as each of the above studies have so nicely demonstrated.

Should All Melanoma Patients Undergo SLNB?

The prognostic implication of the status of the sentinel lymph node cannot be over-stated. SLNB has become the standard of care for melanoma >1.0 mm in thickness and provides valuable staging and prognostic information. Similarly, it identifies those with clinically occult melanoma micro-metastasis who may benefit from early elective LND and those who may be eligible for clinical trials or adjuvant therapies [31]. The technique of SLNB is a low-risk procedure with minimal morbidity and low false negativity [32]. Several clinicopathologic factors have been investigated and associated with increased risk of SLN metastasis. Breslow thickness is not only a significant predictor of overall outcome but also of risk of development of regional lymph node metastasis [33, 34]. Other factors such as gender [35], Clark level [36], ulceration [37], age [38, 39] and other tumor-related factors also have an association with lymph node metastasis [40].

While there is general consensus on indications for SLNB, there remains some debate for patients on the extreme ends of the spectrum of disease. Similarly, there are several considerations for when to omit the SLNB. When the likelihood of SLN-positivity is low or of minimal staging benefit, the cost and potential SLNB-related side effects may be prohibitive when compared with wide local excision alone. Thin melanomas (thickness < 1.0 mm) fall within this category. Similarly, patient factors such as extremes of age or significant medical comorbidities may impact the decision to perform SLNB. Specifically, the risk associated with general anesthesia or therapeutic lymphadenectomy may be prohibitive in these instances. These patients may be followed with close observation and expectant management of clinical disease if it is to develop. Previous treatment also has an impact on the utilization of SLNB. Ideally, SLNB occurs in conjunction with excision of the primary tumor. In situations such as prior excision or flap/wound coverage, ambiguous drainage and impaired accuracy of the SLNB may result which may impact diagnostic yield and additional treatment recommendations. In situations of an unsuccessful SLNB or contraindication to SLNB, other surveillance options exist. Ultrasonography (US) has been used to follow and detect sub-clinical recurrence of melanoma. US imaging is the most sensitive and specific imaging modality for detecting nodal melanoma metastasis [41]. Furthermore, US imaging and US-guided fine needle aspiration can accurately identify SLN metastasis in up to 65 % of patients and guide treatment recommendations for those who can avoid SLNB and proceed to therapeutic lymphadenectomy [42]. The role of US surveillance is currently being addressed in Multicenter Selective Lymphadenectomy Trial-II (MSLT-II).

No randomized trial has demonstrated a survival benefit for SLNB. Indeed, less than 20 % of patients who undergo SLNB are found to have metastatic disease and therefore are considered for completion LND [43]. One could certainly suggest that a majority of patients are unaffected by SLNB and therefore undergo an unnecessary procedure, placing them at increased risk for complication. Nonetheless, for patients with regional metastasis, there is a survival advantage (72 % vs 52 % OS) in undergoing early therapeutic LND when compared to those who develop clinical regional disease and are managed expectantly [43]. Data from the Multicenter Selective Lymphadenectomy Trial-1 (MSLT-1) demonstrated that lymphadenectomy performed for a positive SLN was associated with fewer and less severe complications, and in particular less risk of long-term lymphedema [43, 44].

Thin Melanoma (<1 mm Breslow Thickness)

Patients with thin melanomas comprise a majority of those encountered in clinical practice [45]. Generally, patients with thin melanoma have a favorable prognosis and low risk of metastasis and melanoma-related death. Primary tumors less than 1 mm in thickness have less than a 5 % risk of metastasis overall [46]. It is recognized, however, that even for those with thin melanoma, a certain percentage of patients may recur.

The routine use of SLNB in thin melanoma is controversial. Determination of which patients are at highest risk for nodal recurrence and possibly subsequent melanoma-related death is important given the number of new melanoma diagnoses yearly in this category. Several potential predictors of SLN metastasis have been identified including but not limited to gender, Breslow thickness, Clark level, age, mitotic rate and tumor infiltrating lymphocytes [47–51]. The mitotic rate has been identified to be an extremely important variable in the outcome of thin melanoma, so much so that it was added to the seventh edition of the AJCC staging system. However, by itself, mitotic rate has not been shown to be a predictor of nodal metastases in the AJCC analysis [4, 52–54]. Ulceration has been associated with higher propensity for nodal metastasis and overall worse outcome. While the presence of ulcerative lesions warrants further investigation, it is an infrequent finding in thin melanoma, affecting less than 3 % of patients [55, 56]. Age is also a risk factor for thin melanoma and several predictive models identify it as prognostic for increased risk of nodal involvement [56, 57]. No appropriate age cut off has been identified of when to offer SLNB and therefore cannot be used alone to pursue the procedure. Interestingly, while prognosis is worse with advancing age, the incidence of nodal metastases is lower. Similarly, while prognosis is better with younger age, the incidence of nodal metastases is higher [39, 58]. Nomograms are clinically helpful in identifying which patients with thin melanoma may be at increased risk for lymph node metastasis and may benefit from SLNB. However, while nomograms may be useful, it should also be recognized that a surgeon selection bias exists in which patients with thin melanoma are considered for SLNB testing and therefore may have an impact on which factors are ultimately included as selection criteria.

There has been considerable debate on the management of thin melanoma (AJCC Stage IA/IB) with respect to SLNB testing. The NCCN guidelines recommend SLNB for melanoma ≥ 1.0 mm in thickness. For melanomas less than 0.76 mm without adverse features, SLNB is not recommended. For lesions 0.76–1.0 mm, discussion of SLNB is at the discretion of the treating physician and patient [16, 59]. Recently, the American Society of Clinical Oncology (ASCO) and Society of Surgical Oncology (SSO) published consensus guidelines with evidence-based recommendations for SLNB in melanoma [60]. Four key recommendations were issued. With regard to thin melanomas, specifically, they reported there to be insufficient evidence to support routine SLNB for melanoma <1 mm in Breslow thickness, but suggest that it may be considered in select high-risk individuals.

Discussion of SLNB for patients with thin melanoma is highly individualized and must take into account the available pathology report, the patient's level of anxiety and expectations and growing body of emerging published data. Long-term data on outcome for SLNB in thin melanoma requires longer follow up and randomized clinical trials to clarify this issue.

Intermediate Thickness Melanoma (1–4 mm Breslow Thickness)

There is agreement and uniformity on the role of SLNB for intermediate thickness melanoma. Our understanding of the importance of SLNB on staging and prognosis and ultimately overall outcome is due to the work of Dr. Morton and colleagues of the MSLT Cooperative Group [32, 61, 62]. A large, multicenter randomized trial was conducted in which patients with clinically localized melanoma were assigned to wide excision and sentinel-node biopsy (biopsy group) or wide excision and postoperative observation of the regional nodal basin (observation group). Patients in the biopsy group underwent immediate lymphadenectomy if micro-metastasis were detected at the time of SLNB. Patients in the observation group underwent delayed lymphadenectomy if nodal recurrences developed. Patients with melanomas 1.2–3.5 mm were selected as the primary study group based on prospective database analysis from the John Wayne Cancer Institute [63]. With a median follow-up of 59.8 months, there was no difference in melanoma-specific survival between groups (86.6 % and 87.1 %; $p = 0.58$). For patients with a positive sentinel node, the disease-free survival was 53.4 %, compared to 83.2 % if the sentinel node was free of metastases ($p < 0.001$).

The third interim analysis suggested a survival benefit for patients with intermediate-thickness melanoma who were found to be node-positive and underwent immediate lymphadenectomy (72.3 % vs 52.4 % 5-year survival) [43]. Seventy-eight patients in the observation group developed nodal relapse in the regional basin. The median time to development of nodal recurrence was 1.33 years. Furthermore, the mean number of clinically involved tumor-positive nodes in patients who underwent delayed lymphadenectomy (observation group) was 3.3 compared to 1.4 involved nodes for those who underwent immediate lymphadenectomy ($p < 0.001$), suggesting that even in the absence of clinically evident disease, micro-metastatic disease continues to grow and if left untreated will eventually develop into significant disease.

Subsequent long-term follow-up data was recently reported [64]. There was no difference in 10-year melanoma-specific survival between the biopsy or observation group. The overall rate of nodal disease was 20.8 %, suggesting that 79.2 % of patients did not derive a benefit from SLNB. On subset analysis, for patients with nodal disease and intermediate-thickness melanoma (1.2–3.5 mm), early treatment following a positive SLNB was associated with improved 10-year distant DFS and melanoma-specific survival.

Others have demonstrated similar findings with the use of SLNB testing for intermediate thickness melanoma. Post hoc analysis of study data from patients enrolled in the Sunbelt Melanoma Trial was performed looking at the use of SLNB in melanoma intermediate thickness (1–2 mm) melanoma [65]. Over 1100 patients were evaluated and divided into two groups: Group A (1.0–1.59 mm) and Group B (1.60–2.0 mm). The SLN was positive in 133 (12 %), including 8.7 % in Group A (66/672) and 19.3 % of Group B (67/348). Patient age, Breslow thickness and lymphovascular invasion were independently predictive of a positive SLN on multivariate analysis. The DFS and OS were significantly better for Group A than Group B. Based on review of the data, the authors were not able to identify or reasonably predict which patients with melanoma between 1 and 2 mm in thickness would be at minimal risk for SLN metastasis and therefore unlikely to benefit from SLNB. The authors recommend SLNB for all patients with intermediate thickness melanoma.

Thick Melanoma (>4 mm Breslow Thickness)

Just as with the role of SLNB in thin lesions, there is lack of unanimity with the use of SLNB in thick (>4 mm) melanoma. The risk of SLN metastasis increases as primary tumor thickness increases, with tumors greater than 4 mm in depth having a risk of metastasis of greater than 30 % [33, 66]. Some clinicians, however, contend that SLNB may not provide the same benefit in patients with thick melanoma as these patients have a high rate of occult systemic disease at the time of presentation [67]. The SLN would not provide useful prognostic information and completion lymph node dissection would not have a significant impact on outcome in the presence of distant disease.

Several series have demonstrated conflicting results with the use of SLNB in thick melanomas. For instance, Jacobs et al. identified no statistical difference in overall survival (OS) in 43 patients with thick melanomas (median thickness 6.4 mm) [68]. Essner and colleagues, similarly, identified no difference in OS but there was a disease free survival (DFS) observed for node-negative patients with thick melanomas who underwent SLNB ($N=135$ patients, median thickness 5.9 mm) [69]. Cherpelis also identified no difference in OS between node-negative and node-positive patients as identified by SLNB in thick melanomas ($N=201$ patients, median thickness 5.2 mm) [70]. These results have led some clinicians to suggest that the routine use of SLNB in thick melanomas may not have the same clinical significance as in intermediate thickness melanoma.

Other series have demonstrated a benefit to the routine use of SLNB in thick melanoma. Gershenwald and colleagues at MD Anderson Cancer Center identified the status of the SLN (along with ulceration) to be the most significant predictor of DFS and OS in 131 patients with T4N0 melanoma and recommended routine use of SLNB in this patient population [66]. Similarly, Carlson and colleagues from Emory University, identified that 37 of 114 patients (32.5 %) with thick melanomas had a positive SLNB, 18 patients (48.6 %) of which had a single tumor-positive lymph node after lymphadenectomy [71]. The status of the SLN was the strongest independent predictor of OS. The authors recommended routine SLN mapping for those with thick ($\geq$ 4 mm) melanoma. The authors of a study from the University of Michigan reported on one of the largest experiences with the use of SLNB for patients with thick melanoma [72]. Of 227 patients with thick melanomas, 107 (47 %) were found to be SLN-positive. Angiolymphatic invasion, satellitosis and ulceration of the primary tumor were the strongest predictors of a positive-SLN. The SLN status was the most significant predictor of distant DFS (DDFS) and OS in that population. Patients with T4 melanoma who were node-negative had a significantly better DDFS (85 % vs 48 %, $p < 0.0001$) and OS (80 % vs 47 %, $p < 0.0001$) compared to those who were found to have metastasis on SLNB. The authors recommended strongly considering SLNB, regardless of Breslow depth, for patients with clinically node-negative T4 melanoma.

The use of SLNB for patients with thick melanoma is generally less controversial than for thin melanoma. While there is some conflicting data regarding the impact and outcome for patients who undergo SLNB with thick melanoma, the standard practice for most high-volume melanoma centers is offer SLNB and treat based on results of the biopsy. No randomized clinical trials are currently underway addressing this issue specifically.

Adjuvant Therapy for Node Negative Melanoma

At present, adjuvant therapy is reserved for patients with metastatic disease (stage III/in transit disease) or those with thick primary tumors (T4N0) who bear a high likelihood of harboring occult metastatic disease [16]. Interferon-alpha (IFN-alpha) is the only FDA approved agent for adjuvant use in melanoma. The use of INF-alpha is associated with severe toxicity which is limits its routine use for high-risk patients. Unfortunately, as many as 50 % of patients are unable to complete the recommended course of therapy due to its side effects.

Further complicating the issue, Interferon has only a marginal benefit in patients. Numerous randomized clinical trials have been performed, many with conflicting results. While an extensive body of interferon-related literature exists, in short, a DFS advantage exists (mainly over observation) but no definitive evidence suggest a OS benefit for the adjuvant use of INF-alpha for melanoma [73, 74]. As a result its use remains controversial, particularly in patients without active disease and especially those without metastatic disease. At present, this agent remains the only off-protocol, approved agent for adjuvant therapy and most clinicians recommend it with considerable trepidation. It is important to note though, that in the past 5 years, several agents have been newly approved for the treatment of melanoma and while none are yet accepted for use in the adjuvant therapy, their utility is currently under investigation [13, 15, 75–77].

Surgical Management of Node-Positive Melanoma

Observation of Sentinel Lymph Node-Positive Melanoma

Lymphadenectomy is the standard of care for patients with clinically node-positive or SLN-positive melanoma [4, 16]. For patients who have a positive SLNB, up to 15 % of patients will have occult disease identified in non-SLNs at the time of completion of lymphadenectomy [78, 79]. Perhaps more accurately, data from MSLT-1 has demonstrated that 88 % of patients who have a single tumor-containing sentinel node will have no additional metastasis identified at the time of CLND by hematoxylin and eosin staining [43]. This suggests that the majority of patients derive no benefit in undergoing CLND and, therefore, undergo a potentially unnecessary procedure with concomitant increased risk for complications. While the NCCN recommendation is for patients with a positive SLN to undergo CLND, at least one study demonstrated that up to 50 % of patients forego CLND [80]. Currently, the natural history of patients with a positive-SLN who do not undergo CLND is unknown.

Because a majority of patients have no additional disease identified in non-sentinel lymph nodes (NSLNs),several centers have begun to assess predictive factors that may provide information on who may avoid CLND after a positive SLNB. Sabel and authors from University of Michigan queried their prospective melanoma database and identified 980 patients who underwent SLNB for cutaneous melanoma [81]. A positive SLN was identified in 24 % of patients (232). At CLND, 34 patients (15 %) had one or more positive NSLN. Three or more positive SLNs, male gender, Breslow thickness and extranodal extension were all associated with likelihood of finding additional positive nodes on CLND. The authors at Emory University reviewed their experience of 70 patients with a positive SLN and drainage to a single nodal basin [82]. Nineteen patients (24 %) were found to have NSLNs after CLND. Breslow thickness, ulceration, SLN tumor burden, number of positive SLNs and number of SLNs removed were examined and a predictive model developed to identify positive NSLNs was developed. Neither comparison of the tumor factors examined, nor the predictive model could accurately predict NSLN involvement. Others have been likewise unsuccessful in identification of a group of patients at zero-risk for NSLN metastasis when using algorithms or predictive models [83].

Frankel and colleagues examined whether size and location of metastases within the SLN may help better stratify the likelihood of finding additional positive NSLNs [84]. The presence of a head/neck or lower extremity primary, angiolymphatic invasion, mitosis, Breslow thickness >4 mm, extranodal extension, ≥3 positive SLNs and tumor burden involving >1 % of SLN surface area were significantly associated with finding additional disease on CLND. Location of metastases within the SLN (capsular, subcapsular, or parenchymal) did not correlate with a positive NSLN. The Swiss performed a retrospective analysis of 392 patients and investigated whether SLN tumor load had an effect on NSLN positivity or DFS, possibly sparing some patients from CLND [85]. A total of 114 positive SLNs were identified and at the time of CLND, 22 % were found to have additional positive NSLNs. Of those with SLN micrometastasis, 16.4 % had a positive NSLN identified at CLND ($p=0.09$). SLN tumor burden, however, did not correlate with NSLN-positivity. Similarly, the authors were not able to reliably or reproducibly predict NSLN-positivity at the time of CLND.

The lack of uniform results has led some authors to question the utility of CLND for positive SLN patients. Kingham and authors reviewed the Memorial Sloan-Kettering Cancer Center experience for patients who hade a positive SLN and did not undergo CLND [86]. Of 2269 patients who underwent SLNB, 313 (13.7 %) had a positive SLN of which 271 (87 %) underwent CLND and 42 (13 %) did not (no-CLND). Patients in the no-CLND group were older, had a higher percentage of lower extremity melanomas, and a trend toward thicker melanomas. The most common reason (45 %) for not performing CLND was refusal by the patient. The patterns and rates of recurrences were similar between groups, suggesting that possibly CLND may not need to be performed in all melanoma patients with a positive SLN. Bamboat and colleagues recently reported updated information on 4310 patients undergoing SLNB over a 20-year period [87]. A positive SLN was observed in 495 (11 %) of which 328 (66 %) underwent immediate CLND and 167 (34 %) underwent nodal observation. There were no differences in Breslow thickness, Clark level, ulceration or SLN tumor burden between groups. Nodal disease was the site of first recurrence in 15 % of patients in the no-CLND group and 6 % of the CLND group ($p=0.002$). There was no difference in local and in-transit recurrence between groups. Systemic recurrences occurred in 8 % of the no-CLND patients compared with 27 % of the CLND patients ($p<0.001$). Immediate CLND after a positive-SLNB was associated with fewer initial nodal basin recurrences but no difference in melanoma-specific survival when compared with those who were observed and did not undergo CLND. The authors concluded that these results further validate the ongoing, pending results of the Multicenter Selective Lymphadenectomy Trial II (MSLT-II).

MSLT-II is a phase III multicenter, randomized trial of SLNB followed by CLND or SLNB followed by observation for node-positive melanoma (Clinicaltrials.gov, NCT000297895). Because most patients with SLN positive disease have no additional nodal involvement, this suggest that nodal metastasis may be limited to only 1 or 2 sentinel nodes and that SLNB may be therapeutic as well as diagnostic. The underlying hypothesis of MSLT-II is that CLND can be avoided in most patients with SLN metastasis. Enrollment of a planned 1925 subjects began in 2005. SLN positive patients are randomized to CLND or ultrasound observation (+ delayed CLND if recurrence is detected) and are followed for 10 years with a primary outcome measure of melanoma-specific survival. The results from this large clinical trial will hopefully provide valuable insight and demonstrate the true impact of CLND for node-positive melanoma.

When to Consider Ilioinguinal (Deep) versus Inguinal (Superficial) LND

For metastasis to the inguinal lymph nodes, disagreement exists about the extent of surgical dissection required. Specifically, whether a superficial (inguinal) groin dissection is sufficient or whether a combined superficial and deep (ilioinguinal) LND is necessary. Arguments against performing a deep groin dissection are valid as complication rates after combined superficial and deep groin dissection have been reported to be as high as 50 % [88]. Furthermore, several studies support the argument that ilioinguinal metastatic involvement represents more systemic disease and an aggressive surgical approach or the extent of surgery may not have an impact on outcome [89, 90]. Conversely, others support the routine surgical practice of performing deep pelvic LND as there is no difference in OS for involved versus negative deep pelvic nodes. These supporters maintain that metastatic pelvic nodal disease behaves as stage III disease rather than stage IV disease [91]. A recent survey demonstrated that only 30 % of melanoma surgeons routinely perform ilioinguinal lymph node dissection [92]. These issues demonstrate some of the uncertainty and lack of uniformity of when to perform a deep lymphadenectomy for ilioinguinal disease.

Several issues are central to the discussion of when to perform a deep pelvic lymphadenectomy for metastatic disease to the groin. Preoperative lymphoscintigraphy of the lower extremity for SLNB will at times identify selective drainage to the pelvis. This may represent drainage via separate lymphatic channels or second-echelon lymph node drainage from superficial groin nodes. Kaoutzanis and colleagues reviewed their experience of 82 patients over a 3-year period that underwent SLNB of the groin, pelvis or both [93]. Of the 82 patients, 19 (24 %) had positive SLNs. Eleven patients underwent pelvic SLNB, none of which had a positive node. Pre-operative lymphoscintigraphy identified that for primary tumors located below the knee, pelvic nodes appeared to be second level nodes. For primary tumors located on the thigh/trunk, lymphoscintigraphy identified individual tracks draining directly to the pelvis. The complication rate was higher following SLNB in the pelvis but was not statistically significant when compared with SLNB of the groin alone. Soteldo and authors of the European Institute of Oncology (Milan, Italy) reviewed their experience for patients who underwent pelvic SLNB or developed recurrent pelvic disease after a negative inguinal SLNB [94]. One hundred four patients with stage I/II melanoma with primary tumors of the lower extremity or trunk underwent SLNB and were found to have hot spots both in the superficial (groin) and deep (iliac-obturator) areas during dynamic lymphoscintigraphy. Of the 104 patients, 21 patients (20 %) had a positive SLNB and all underwent superficial and deep inguinal dissection. Three patients who underwent ilioinguinal dissection were found to have positive pelvic lymph nodes. Two patients (2.4 %) who were initially SLN negative developed pelvic recurrence. With a 60-month follow up, the DFS was 69 % for SLN-negative patients and 53 % for SLN-positive patients, which was not significant ($p = 0.15$). Chu and colleagues from Emory University reviewed a single-surgeon experience of 40 patients with positive inguinal SLNB who underwent 42 complete inguinopelvic lymphadenectomies [95]. The median Breslow thickness was 2.3 mm and 79 % had lower extremity primaries. Five patients (11.9 %) had synchronous pelvic disease. All five cases with pelvic metastases had extremity primaries (4 distal, 1 proximal). Three of the five patients (60 %) had ≥3 total involved inguinal lymph nodes. The inguinal node ratio (ratio of positive to total number inguinal lymph nodes retrieved) was >0.2 in 80 % of cases with pelvic disease compared to 8.6 % of cases without pelvic disease ($p = 0.002$).

The authors noted that more involved inguinal LNs and inguinal ratio >0.2 appear more likely to harbor pelvic disease. The impact of lymph node ratio provides prognostic information, with a lower ratio as a marker for better outcome [96, 97]. Karakousis evaluated the prognostic significance of drainage to pelvic nodes at SLN mapping in 325 patients with melanomas of the lower extremity or buttocks [98]. Drainage to pelvic nodes (DPN) was identified in 23 % of cases and associated with increased Breslow thickness ($p=0.007$) and age ($p=0.01$) on multivariate analysis. Patients with DPN were not more likely to have a positive SLN. The pelvic recurrence rates were similar in patients with recurrence with DPN compared to those without DPN (39 % in both groups, $p=NS$). SLN negative patients with DPN showed a shorter time to melanoma recurrence in a multivariable analysis model when considering tumor thickness and ulceration ($p=0.002$) but marginally when age was included ($p=0.08$).

Management of clinical (palpable) lymph node metastasis to the groin consists of a superficial and deep inguinal lymphadenectomy. In practice, however, some perform only a superficial or inguinal groin dissection and forego performing an ilioinguinal (deep) dissection. Proponents of this approach only perform a combined superficial and deep inguinal lymphadenectomy when multiple positive nodes are involved in the groin or the evidence of pelvic nodal involvement as identified on computed tomography (CT) imaging [99]. The Dutch reported their experience on 169 melanoma patients with palpable groin metastases [100]. Of the 169 patients, 121 underwent combined (superficial and deep) groin dissection and 48 underwent superficial groin dissection (SGD). Patients were clinically diagnosed by CT, fine-needle aspiration and/or ultrasound (US). In general, patients with palpable nodes underwent CGD. The indication for SGD was surgeon preference. Thirty patients (24.8 %) who underwent CGD for palpable groin metastasis had involved deep pelvic nodes. CGD patients had significantly more patients with large superficial nodes (≥ 3 cm) than SGD patients (70.8 % vs 50 %, $p=0.002$), more harvested superficial lymph nodes (15 nodes vs 8 nodes, $p<0.001$) and lower superficial lymph node ratio (11 % vs 20 %, $p=0.0004$). There was no difference in morbidity rates between groups, although patients undergoing CGD did have a trend toward more chronic lymphedema. There was no difference in local control rates, DFS or OS between SGD or CGD patients. CGD patients with involved deep lymph nodes (24.8 %) had an estimated 5-year OS of 12 % compared with 40 % without involved deep lymph nodes ($p=0.001$). The authors noted that survival and recurrence do not differ between patients with palpable groin metastases who are treated by CGD or SGD. They suggest that patients without iliac nodes on CT may undergo SGD and CGD reserved for patients with multiple positive nodes on SGD or deep nodes evident on CT imaging. Authors from the National Institute of Cancer in Naples, Italy also came to similar conclusions [101]. One hundred thirty-three patients underwent superficial and deep groin dissection for melanoma groin metastasis (84 had clinically positive inguinal nodes at diagnosis, 49 patients had tumor-positive SLN). None of the 133 patients had clinical evidence of involvement of deep lymph nodes at initial staging with CT or US. Of the 49 patients with a positive SLNB, 3 (6.1 %) had evidence of disease in deep nodes and 27/84 (20.3 %) with clinically positive inguinal nodes had positive deep nodes identified. The 5-year DFS and melanoma-specific survival was significantly better for patients with superficial lymph node metastasis than both superficial and deep lymph nodes, respectively (34.9 % vs 19 %, $p=0.001$ and 55.6 % vs 33.3 %, $p=0.001$). Metastasis to the deep nodes was found to be the strongest predictor of DFS and melanoma-specific survival. The authors commented that a deep groin dissection should be considered for all patients with clinical nodal involvement but may be spared in patients with only a positive sentinel lymph node.

NCCN recommendations for performing an ilioinguinal dissection are category 2B, noting that the risk of pelvic LN involvement is increased when there are more than three superficial LNs involved, when the superficial nodes are clinically positive, or when Cloquet's node is positive [90, 102]. The decision to perform a superficial inguinal or a deep pelvic lymph node dissection is patient-specific and requires a discussion of risks and benefits between counseling physicians and their patients. A multicenter, randomized clinical trial would be required to more adequately address which patients with groin nodal metastasis (either clinical or identified on SLNB) may safely undergo superficial inguinal dissection and forego deep pelvic lymphadenectomy.

Minimally Invasive Management of Regional Nodal Metastasis

One of the more recent technical advances in the field of melanoma has been the minimally invasive approach to inguinal lymphadenectomy for nodal metastasis. The rationale to pursue other alternatives to open lymphadenectomy originates from the desire to minimize associated wound-healing complications. Open inguinal lymphadenectomy, while offering excellent regional control, is associated with chronic lymphedema and in the short-term with wound healing complications, skin flap loss and seroma rates as high as 50 % [103–105]. Bishoff et al. were the first to investigate the use of endoscopic technology for metastatic groin disease for squamous cell carcinoma of the penis [106]. Sotelo subsequently reported no wound-related complications observed in a series of 14 minimally invasive lymphadenectomies for penile carcinoma [107]. Delman and colleagues were the first to address the feasibility of minimally invasive groin dissection for melanoma [108]. Five patients underwent minimally invasive lymphadenectomy with a median operative time of 180 min (median Breslow thickness 3 mm, three patients had ulceration). An average of ten lymph nodes were harvested (4–13) and the median duration of drain usage was 8 days. One patient with clinical nodal metastasis underwent minimally invasive superficial groin dissection and open deep pelvic dissection (surgeon preference). Two patients developed cellulitis and no wound dehiscence was observed. Two recurrences were observed: one distant (patient with clinical lymphadenopathy who underwent deep pelvic LND) and one in-transit. The authors concluded that minimally invasive lymphadenectomy is feasible in melanoma as demonstrated by nodal yield and may reduce complication rates/wound dehiscence and obviate the need for sartorius muscle transposition.

The same authors subsequently published their initial experience with video-scopic inguinal lymphadenectomy (VIL) in 32 patients who underwent 45 VIL procedures [109]. A variety of disease processes including extramammary Paget's disease, neuroendocrine, genitourinary and melanoma diseases were treated. Median nodes collected was 11 (range 4–24), the largest of which was 5.6 cm in size. Wound complications were observed in eight cases (18 %) and included: cellulitis (6), seroma (1) and diabetic-associated skin flap necrosis (1) which was managed conservatively.

Other centers have since validated the utility of minimally invasive inguinal lymph node dissection (MILND) for metastatic melanoma [110]. Abbott and colleagues from two separate academic centers performed 13 MILND cases and retrospectively compared them with 28 patients who underwent open inguinal LND (OILND). They were able to demonstrate a decreased wound dehiscence rate, hospital readmission rate and hospital length of stay in patients who underwent MILND compared to traditional OILND. Lymph node harvest was also greater for those who underwent MILND compared with OILND (11 vs 8, $p=0.03$). The authors commented that MILND offers an equivalent lymphadenectomy while minimizing the severity of postoperative complications, but suggested that further research is needed to determine if oncologic outcomes are similar. Martin et al. recently reported updated oncologic outcomes for patients undergoing VIL for metastatic melanoma [111]. Forty VIL patients were compared to a retrospective cohort of open superficial inguinal lymphadenectomy patients and outcomes reviewed. The median follow up was 19.1 months versus 33.9 months, respectively. There were no differences in demographic or histologic features between groups. The lymph node yield was similar (12.6 nodes vs 14.2 nodes, $p=0.131$) as was overall recurrence rates (27.5 % vs 30 %, $p=0.81$) between groups. Analysis of wound complications including infection, skin necrosis and seroma, patients undergoing VIL had markedly less morbidity (47.5 % vs 80 %, $p=0.002$). While median survival was not reached in the VIL group, on Kaplan-Meier estimates, there was no difference in DFS or OS between groups. The authors concluded that, when compared with open inguinal lymphadenectomy, VIL is associated with similar oncologic outcomes with reduced wound complications and may be the preferred method of inguinal lymphadenectomy for metastatic melanoma.

Others have begun to explore the use of minimally invasive techniques to address deep pelvic node involvement [112]. While this methodology has been well described for gynecologic and urologic malignancies, it has previously not been addressed for melanoma. Sohn and colleagues reported on the robot-assisted use of pelvic lymphadenectomy for metastatic melanoma [113]. The authors report two case reports of isolated metastatic melanoma who successfully underwent robot-assisted pelvic lymphadenectomy for isolated, pelvic metastases. The authors noted that patients were safely managed without complication and robot-assistance provides excellent visibility and minimum morbidity.

As refinements in the technique and surgeon experience increases with the technology, additional results will emerge. The long-term impact and oncologic outcome for patients undergoing minimally invasive metastatectomy for melanoma remains to be determined and will require a randomized clinical trial to clarify this issue.

Surgical Management of Distant Metastatic Melanoma

The prognosis for patients with distant melanoma metastasis is poor. The median OS is in the range of 7–8 months with a 5 year survival of less than 5 % [114, 115]. Surgery is rarely considered as primary treatment, except in situations of palliation or symptomatic metastases, and rarely for curative intent. Primary treatment of stage IV metastases has been reserved to systemic chemotherapy, immunotherapy, biochemotherapy, intralesional therapy, radiation or any combination of these. Unfortunately, complete cures are rarely observed and these therapies have been unable to successfully prolong survival. Dacarbazine (DTIC) was approved by the Food and Drug Administration (FDA) over 30 years ago for the treatment of stage IV melanoma. DTIC demonstrates a response rate of approximately 20 % with a median duration of response of 5–6 months and complete responses observed in less than 5 % of patients [116]. Combining DTIC with other agents such as BOLD (bleomycin, vincrisitine, lomustine and DTIC), CVD (cisplatin, vinblastine and DTIC) and the "Dartmouth Regimen" (cisplatin, carmustine, DTIC and tamoxifin) demonstrated initially higher response rates but with no improvement in overall survival [117–119]. Interleukin-2 (IL-2),a biologic agent FDA approved for metastatic melanoma, offers a response in up to 16 %, but with a median response of less than 6 months for responders and a median survival of 11.4 months [120]. The addition of interferon-alpha to IL-2 and/or biochemotherapy (multi-agent chemotherapy + biologic modifiers), while demonstrating favorable initial response rates, does so at the expense of increased toxicity with a failure to demonstrate an improvement in overall survival [121–123].

Mestatectomy for Stage IV Disease

The role of the surgeon has historically been limited to occasional complete resection of solitary visceral metastasis or for palliative resection of symptomatic metastases. While the role of surgical resection for stage IV melanoma has been greatly debated, it should still be considered a viable potential treatment modality in the multidisciplinary management of metastatic melanoma. Although most patients succumb from disease involving multiple organ sites, the majority of patients initially present with distant disease limited to only a single-organ site [11, 124]. Early surgical intervention offers the potential for eradication of distant disease and patients with fewer sites of disease are more likely to benefit from surgical resection. Median survival for involvement of a single-organ site is approximately 29 months; this drops to 14 months if ≥4 sites are involved [125, 126]. Numerous reports of long-term survivors have been reported following resection for stage IV disease with survivors observed beyond 10 years [127–129]. Patients in good overall health who have limited disease and respond favorably to medical (non-surgical) approaches are more likely to benefit from aggressive resection [125, 126]. Furthermore, several studies have demonstrated a survival benefit to repeat resection of recurrent stage IV metastases [128].

The most common sites of melanoma metastasis are the lung, skin, lymph nodes, brain, liver and gastrointestinal tract. Survival decreases as metastasis progress from skin/subcutaneous to visceral-sites. Surgical resection of distant metastases can extend survival. Resection of skin or subcutaneous metastases, for instance, can be associated with excellent results with median survivals of 24 months [128]. It is important to resect metastases early, before they become bulky or symptomatic. A margin of 1 cm is generally adequate to minimize local recurrences. Distant lymph node metastases should be managed with complete dissection of the affected basin. Additional treatment alternatives to surgical resection include: hyperthermic isolated limb perfusion, isolated limb infusion, topical therapy or intralesional therapy for dermal metastases.

Patients with pulmonary metastases tend to survive longer than those with other visceral metastases. Complete resection may extend median survival to 28 months [126]. Unfortunately, most patients present with multiple, bilateral metastases. This underscores the importance of proper patient selection for potential candidates for pulmonary metastectomy [130]. In patients undergoing resection of isolated pulmonary metastases, complete resection, prolonged disease-free interval, ≤2 pulmonary nodules, prior chemotherapy and lack of lymph node involvement are associated with improved survival [131].

Gastrointestinal (GI) metastases often originate from a cutaneous primary and present with widespread metastases. Without surgery, the median survival is only 5–11 months [132]. Sanki and colleagues reported on 117 patients who underwent surgical resection of GI melanoma metastases, 63 % for therapeutic intent, 37 % for palliative indications [133]. The most common symptoms were anemia and bowel obstruction. The overall 5-year survival was 27 % and, on multivariate analysis, the presence of residual intra-abdominal disease and presence of non-GI metastases at the time of surgery were the most significant prognostic indicators of survival. The authors of the John Wayne Cancer Institute reported on 124 patients with GI metastases [134]. Sixty-nine patients (55 %) underwent exploration: 66 % curative resection, 34 % for palliative indications. They reported that 97 % of patients experienced postoperative relief of their presenting GI symptoms. The median disease-free interval prior to development of GI tract metastasis was 23 months. The median survival for patients undergoing curative resection was 49 months versus only 5 months for those undergoing palliative procedures or no surgery at all. Complete resection of the GI tract metastases and the GI tract as the initial site of distant metastasis were the two most important prognostic factors for long-term survival. These studies demonstrate that, in appropriately selected patients, curative resection is possible and can be associated with long-term survival. Metastectomy has also been described for other organ-specific sites including: liver [135], central nervous system [136], genitourinary [137], skeletal system [138] and others [139–141].

The treatment of metastatic melanoma changed dramatically in 2010 with the discovery of ipilimumab and vemurafenib. Ipilimumab, a human monoclonal antibody which inhibits cytotoxic T lymphocyte-associated antigen 4 (CTLA-4), was evaluated in phase III clinical trial for unresectable stage III or stage IV melanoma (MDX010-20) [13]. When administered at 3 mg/kg with glycoprotein 100 vaccine (gp100), the median overall survival was 10.0 months compared to 6.4 months for patients receiving gp100 alone ($p < 0.001$). Vemurafenib (PLX4032), a potent inhibitor of mutated BRAF, demonstrated response rates of more than 50 % in patients with metastatic melanoma with the BRAF V600E mutation in phase I and II clinical trials [14, 142]. A phase III randomized clinical trial was performed comparing vemurafenib with dacarbazine in 675 patients with previously untreated, metastatic melanoma with the BRAF V600E [15]. The OS was 84 % at 6 months in the vemurafenib group and 64 % in the dacarbazine group. Based on these results, these two agents, as well the subsequent agents dabrafenib (BRAF inhibitor) and trametinib (MEK inhibitor), were approved for the treatment of unresectable, metastatic melanoma. Several new agents, including anti-programmed death 1 (anti-PD1) antibodies, are currently undergoing investigation in phase III clinical trial [75–77].

Dramatic recent advances have changed the treatment paradigm for the management of patients with metastatic melanoma and the eagerly awaited results of ongoing phase III trials of combinations of targeted or immunologic agents will certainly have an impact on future treatment. For the first time ever, advances in the medical management of stage IV melanoma have begun to approach or even exceed the best results observed with surgical resection. While surgical resection will continue to have a role for symptomatic disease and/or resectable metastases, it is possible that with ongoing research and advances, the role of surgery may diminish in the future for patients with asymptomatic stage IV melanoma.

Conclusion

The surgical management of melanoma has continued to evolve over the last several decades. The results of randomized clinical trials that have progressively shaped our understanding of the appropriate margins of excision, the role of sentinel lymph node biopsy and therapeutic lymphadenectomy for metastatic disease. The role of the surgeon-scientist has been instrumental in the design and implementation of several of these clinical trials and has been integral to our understanding and current management of melanoma. Ongoing results of these studies will continue to provide valuable insight and have a future impact on the surgical management of this complex disease. Moving forward, randomized clinical trials will be necessary to definitively address unanswered questions such as the impact of a 1 cm vs 2 cm margin for melanoma excision and the use of SLNB for thin/thick melanoma.

Newer targeted therapies will continue to be investigated and have an increasing role in the multimodality management of metastatic melanoma. As molecular profiling and the identification of higher-risk individuals improves, the role of adjuvant, targeted therapy for early stage node-negative disease will also certainly be addressed. Our hope is that this review adequately addresses several issues involving the surgical management of melanoma and will lead to further clinical trial development and, ultimately, treatment recommendations for melanoma.

References

1. Jemal A, Siegel R, Xu J, Ward E. Cancer statistics, 2010. CA Cancer J Clin. 2010;60: 277–300.
2. Rigel DS. Trends in dermatology: melanoma incidence. Arch Dermatol. 2010;146:318.
3. Mulliken JS, Russak JE, Rigel DS. The effect of sunscreen on melanoma risk. Dermatol Clin. 2012;30:369–76.
4. Balch CM, Gershenwald JE, Soong SJ, et al. Final version of 2009 AJCC melanoma staging and classification. J Clin Oncol. 2009;27:6199–206.
5. Balch CM, Buzaid AC, Soong SJ, et al. Final version of the American Joint Committee on Cancer staging system for cutaneous melanoma. J Clin Oncol. 2001;19:3635–48.
6. Azzola MF, Shaw HM, Thompson JF, et al. Tumor mitotic rate is a more powerful prognostic indicator than ulceration in patients with primary cutaneous melanoma: an analysis of 3661 patients from a single center. Cancer. 2003;97:1488–98.
7. Gimotty PA, Elder DE, Fraker DL, et al. Identification of high-risk patients among those diagnosed with thin cutaneous melanomas. J Clin Oncol. 2007;25:1129–34.
8. Busam KJ. The prognostic importance of tumor mitotic rate for patients with primary cutaneous melanoma. Ann Surg Oncol. 2004;11:360–1.
9. Gershenwald JE, Colome MI, Lee JE, et al. Patterns of recurrence following a negative sentinel lymph node biopsy in 243 patients with stage I or II melanoma. J Clin Oncol. 1998;16: 2253–60.
10. Thompson JF, Uren RF. Lymphatic mapping and sentinel node biopsy for melanoma. Expert Rev Anticancer Ther. 2001;1:446–52.
11. Barth A, Wanek LA, Morton DL. Prognostic factors in 1,521 melanoma patients with distant metastases. J Am Coll Surg. 1995;181:193–201.
12. Manola J, Atkins M, Ibrahim J, Kirkwood J. Prognostic factors in metastatic melanoma: a pooled analysis of Eastern Cooperative Oncology Group trials. J Clin Oncol. 2000;18: 3782–93.
13. Hodi FS, O'Day SJ, McDermott DF, et al. Improved survival with ipilimumab in patients with metastatic melanoma. N Engl J Med. 2010;363:711–23.
14. Flaherty KT, Puzanov I, Kim KB, et al. Inhibition of mutated, activated BRAF in metastatic melanoma. N Engl J Med. 2010;363:809–19.
15. Chapman PB, Hauschild A, Robert C, et al. Improved survival with vemurafenib in melanoma with BRAF V600E mutation. N Engl J Med. 2011;364:2507–16.
16. Coit DG, Thompson JA, Andtbacka R, et al. Melanoma, version 4.2014. J Natl Compr Canc Netw. 2014;12:621–9.
17. Handley WS. The pathology of melanotic growths in relation to their operative treatment. Lancet. 1907;1:927–33.
18. Breslow A, Macht SD. Optimal size of resection margin for thin cutaneous melanoma. Surg Gynecol Obstet. 1977;145:691–2.
19. Veronesi U, Cascinelli N, Adamus J, et al. Thin stage I primary cutaneous malignant melanoma. Comparison of excision with margins of 1 or 3 cm. N Engl J Med. 1988;318:1159–62.

20. Veronesi U, Cascinelli N. Narrow excision (1-cm margin). A safe procedure for thin cutaneous melanoma. Arch Surg. 1991;126:438–41.
21. Ringborg U, Andersson R, Eldh J, et al. Resection margins of 2 versus 5 cm for cutaneous malignant melanoma with a tumor thickness of 0.8 to 2.0 mm: randomized study by the Swedish Melanoma Study Group. Cancer. 1996;77:1809–14.
22. Cohn-Cedermark G, Rutqvist LE, Andersson R, et al. Long term results of a randomized study by the Swedish Melanoma Study Group on 2-cm versus 5-cm resection margins for patients with cutaneous melanoma with a tumor thickness of 0.8-2.0 mm. Cancer. 2000;89:1495–501.
23. Balch CM, Urist MM, Karakousis CP, et al. Efficacy of 2-cm surgical margins for intermediate-thickness melanomas (1 to 4 mm). Results of a multi-institutional randomized surgical trial. Ann Surg. 1993;218:262–7. discussion 267–269.
24. Karakousis CP, Balch CM, Urist MM, et al. Local recurrence in malignant melanoma: long-term results of the multiinstitutional randomized surgical trial. Ann Surg Oncol. 1996;3:446–52.
25. Balch CM, Soong SJ, Smith T, et al. Long-term results of a prospective surgical trial comparing 2 cm vs. 4 cm excision margins for 740 patients with 1-4 mm melanomas. Ann Surg Oncol. 2001;8:101–8.
26. Khayat D, Rixe O, Martin G, et al. Surgical margins in cutaneous melanoma (2 cm versus 5 cm for lesions measuring less than 2.1-mm thick). Cancer. 2003;97:1941–6.
27. Thomas JM, Newton-Bishop J, A'Hern R, et al. Excision margins in high-risk malignant melanoma. N Engl J Med. 2004;350:757–66.
28. Gillgren P, Drzewiecki KT, Niin M, et al. 2-cm versus 4-cm surgical excision margins for primary cutaneous melanoma thicker than 2 mm: a randomised, multicentre trial. Lancet. 2011;378:1635–42.
29. Sladden MJ, Balch C, Barzilai DA et al. Surgical excision margins for primary cutaneous melanoma. Cochrane Database Syst Rev 2009; (4):CD004835.
30. Hudson LE, Maithel SK, Carlson GW, et al. 1 or 2 cm margins of excision for T2 melanomas: do they impact recurrence or survival? Ann Surg Oncol. 2013;20:346–51.
31. McMasters KM, Reintgen DS, Ross MI, et al. Sentinel lymph node biopsy for melanoma: controversy despite widespread agreement. J Clin Oncol. 2001;19:2851–5.
32. Morton DL, Cochran AJ, Thompson JF, et al. Sentinel node biopsy for early-stage melanoma: accuracy and morbidity in MSLT-I, an international multicenter trial. Ann Surg. 2005;242:302–11. discussion 311–303.
33. Balch CM, Soong SJ, Gershenwald JE, et al. Prognostic factors analysis of 17,600 melanoma patients: validation of the American Joint Committee on Cancer melanoma staging system. J Clin Oncol. 2001;19:3622–34.
34. Wagner JD, Gordon MS, Chuang TY, et al. Predicting sentinel and residual lymph node basin disease after sentinel lymph node biopsy for melanoma. Cancer. 2000;89:453–62.
35. Scoggins CR, Ross MI, Reintgen DS, et al. Gender-related differences in outcome for melanoma patients. Ann Surg. 2006;243:693–8. discussion 698–700.
36. Balch CM, Murad TM, Soong SJ, et al. A multifactorial analysis of melanoma: prognostic histopathological features comparing Clark's and Breslow's staging methods. Ann Surg. 1978;188:732–42.
37. Balch CM, Wilkerson JA, Murad TM, et al. The prognostic significance of ulceration of cutaneous melanoma. Cancer. 1980;45:3012–7.
38. McMasters KM, Wong SL, Edwards MJ, et al. Factors that predict the presence of sentinel lymph node metastasis in patients with melanoma. Surgery. 2001;130:151–6.
39. Chao C, Martin 2nd RC, Ross MI, et al. Correlation between prognostic factors and increasing age in melanoma. Ann Surg Oncol. 2004;11:259–64.
40. McMasters KM, Noyes RD, Reintgen DS, et al. Lessons learned from the Sunbelt Melanoma Trial. J Surg Oncol. 2004;86:212–23.
41. Xing Y, Cromwell KD, Cormier JN. Review of diagnostic imaging modalities for the surveillance of melanoma patients. Dermatol Res Pract. 2012;2012:941921.
42. Voit C, Van Akkooi AC, Schafer-Hesterberg G, et al. Ultrasound morphology criteria predict metastatic disease of the sentinel nodes in patients with melanoma. J Clin Oncol. 2010;28:847–52.

43. Morton DL, Thompson JF, Cochran AJ, et al. Sentinel-node biopsy or nodal observation in melanoma. N Engl J Med. 2006;355:1307–17.

44. Faries MB, Thompson JF, Cochran A, et al. The impact on morbidity and length of stay of early versus delayed complete lymphadenectomy in melanoma: results of the Multicenter Selective Lymphadenectomy Trial (I). Ann Surg Oncol. 2010;17:3324–9.

45. Andtbacka RH, Gershenwald JE. Role of sentinel lymph node biopsy in patients with thin melanoma. J Natl Compr Canc Netw. 2009;7:308–17.

46. Gershenwald JE, Thompson W, Mansfield PF, et al. Multi-institutional melanoma lymphatic mapping experience: the prognostic value of sentinel lymph node status in 612 stage I or II melanoma patients. J Clin Oncol. 1999;17:976–83.

47. Cecchi R, Buralli L, Innocenti S, De Gaudio C. Sentinel lymph node biopsy in patients with thin melanomas. J Dermatol. 2007;34:512–5.

48. Bedrosian I, Faries MB, Guerry D, et al. Incidence of sentinel node metastasis in patients with thin primary melanoma (< or = 1 mm) with vertical growth phase. Ann Surg Oncol. 2000;7:262–7.

49. Puleo CA, Messina JL, Riker AI, et al. Sentinel node biopsy for thin melanomas: which patients should be considered? Cancer Control. 2005;12:230–5.

50. Kesmodel SB, Karakousis GC, Botbyl JD, et al. Mitotic rate as a predictor of sentinel lymph node positivity in patients with thin melanomas. Ann Surg Oncol. 2005;12:449–58.

51. Bleicher RJ, Essner R, Foshag LJ, et al. Role of sentinel lymphadenectomy in thin invasive cutaneous melanomas. J Clin Oncol. 2003;21:1326–31.

52. Sondak VK, Taylor JM, Sabel MS, et al. Mitotic rate and younger age are predictors of sentinel lymph node positivity: lessons learned from the generation of a probabilistic model. Ann Surg Oncol. 2004;11:247–58.

53. Gimotty PA, Van Belle P, Elder DE, et al. Biologic and prognostic significance of dermal Ki67 expression, mitoses, and tumorigenicity in thin invasive cutaneous melanoma. J Clin Oncol. 2005;23:8048–56.

54. Paek SC, Griffith KA, Johnson TM, et al. The impact of factors beyond Breslow depth on predicting sentinel lymph node positivity in melanoma. Cancer. 2007;109:100–8.

55. Gimotty PA, Guerry D, Ming ME, et al. Thin primary cutaneous malignant melanoma: a prognostic tree for 10-year metastasis is more accurate than American Joint Committee on Cancer staging. J Clin Oncol. 2004;22:3668–76.

56. Faries MB, Wanek LA, Elashoff D, et al. Predictors of occult nodal metastasis in patients with thin melanoma. Arch Surg. 2010;145:137–42.

57. Gershenwald JE, Coit DG, Sondak VK, Thompson JF. The challenge of defining guidelines for sentinel lymph node biopsy in patients with thin primary cutaneous melanomas. Ann Surg Oncol. 2012;19:3301–3.

58. Page AJ, Li A, Hestley A, et al. Increasing age is associated with worse prognostic factors and increased distant recurrences despite fewer sentinel lymph node positives in melanoma. Int J Surg Oncol. 2012;2012:456987.

59. Coit DG, Andtbacka R, Anker CJ, et al. Melanoma. J Natl Compr Canc Netw. 2012;10: 366–400.

60. Wong SL, Balch CM, Hurley P, et al. Sentinel lymph node biopsy for melanoma: American Society of Clinical Oncology and Society of Surgical Oncology joint clinical practice guideline. J Clin Oncol. 2012;30:2912–8.

61. Morton DL, Thompson JF, Essner R, et al. Validation of the accuracy of intraoperative lymphatic mapping and sentinel lymphadenectomy for early-stage melanoma: a multicenter trial. Multicenter Selective Lymphadenectomy Trial Group. Ann Surg. 1999;230:453–63. discussion 463–455.

62. Morton DL, Hoon DS, Cochran AJ, et al. Lymphatic mapping and sentinel lymphadenectomy for early-stage melanoma: therapeutic utility and implications of nodal microanatomy and molecular staging for improving the accuracy of detection of nodal micrometastases. Ann Surg. 2003;238:538–49. discussion 549–550.

63. Morton DL, Wanek L, Nizze JA, et al. Improved long-term survival after lymphadenectomy of melanoma metastatic to regional nodes. Analysis of prognostic factors in 1134 patients from the John Wayne Cancer Clinic. Ann Surg. 1991;214:491–9. discussion 499–501.
64. Durham AB, Wong SL. Sentinel lymph node biopsy in melanoma: final results of MSLT-I. Future Oncol. 2014;10:1121–3.
65. Mays MP, Martin RC, Burton A, et al. Should all patients with melanoma between 1 and 2 mm Breslow thickness undergo sentinel lymph node biopsy? Cancer. 2010;116:1535–44.
66. Gershenwald JE, Mansfield PF, Lee JE, Ross MI. Role for lymphatic mapping and sentinel lymph node biopsy in patients with thick (> or =4 mm) primary melanoma. Ann Surg Oncol. 2000;7:160–5.
67. Perrott RE, Glass LF, Reintgen DS, Fenske NA. Reassessing the role of lymphatic mapping and sentinel lymphadenectomy in the management of cutaneous malignant melanoma. J Am Acad Dermatol. 2003;49:567–88. quiz 589–592.
68. Jacobs IA, Chang CK, Salti GI. Role of sentinel lymph node biopsy in patients with thick (>4 mm) primary melanoma. Am Surg. 2004;70:59–62.
69. Essner R, Chung MH, Bleicher R, et al. Prognostic implications of thick (>or =4-mm) melanoma in the era of intraoperative lymphatic mapping and sentinel lymphadenectomy. Ann Surg Oncol. 2002;9:754–61.
70. Cherpelis BS, Haddad F, Messina J, et al. Sentinel lymph node micrometastasis and other histologic factors that predict outcome in patients with thicker melanomas. J Am Acad Dermatol. 2001;44:762–6.
71. Carlson GW, Murray DR, Hestley A, et al. Sentinel lymph node mapping for thick (>or =4-mm) melanoma: should we be doing it? Ann Surg Oncol. 2003;10:408–15.
72. Gajdos C, Griffith KA, Wong SL, et al. Is there a benefit to sentinel lymph node biopsy in patients with T4 melanoma? Cancer. 2009;115:5752–60.
73. Pirard D, Heenen M, Melot C, Vereecken P. Interferon alpha as adjuvant postsurgical treatment of melanoma: a meta-analysis. Dermatology. 2004;208:43–8.
74. Wheatley K, Ives N, Hancock B, et al. Does adjuvant interferon-alpha for high-risk melanoma provide a worthwhile benefit? A meta-analysis of the randomised trials. Cancer Treat Rev. 2003;29:241–52.
75. Hamid O, Robert C, Daud A, et al. Safety and tumor responses with lambrolizumab (anti-PD-1) in melanoma. N Engl J Med. 2013;369:134–44.
76. Hauschild A, Grob JJ, Demidov LV, et al. Dabrafenib in BRAF-mutated metastatic melanoma: a multicentre, open-label, phase 3 randomised controlled trial. Lancet. 2012;380:358–65.
77. Patel JD, Krilov L, Adams S, et al. Clinical cancer advances 2013: annual report on progress against cancer from the American Society of Clinical Oncology. J Clin Oncol. 2014;32:129–60.
78. Cascinelli N, Bombardieri E, Bufalino R, et al. Sentinel and nonsentinel node status in stage IB and II melanoma patients: two-step prognostic indicators of survival. J Clin Oncol. 2006;24:4464–71.
79. Lee JH, Essner R, Torisu-Itakura H, et al. Factors predictive of tumor-positive nonsentinel lymph nodes after tumor-positive sentinel lymph node dissection for melanoma. J Clin Oncol. 2004;22:3677–84.
80. Bilimoria KY, Balch CM, Bentrem DJ, et al. Complete lymph node dissection for sentinel node-positive melanoma: assessment of practice patterns in the United States. Ann Surg Oncol. 2008;15:1566–76.
81. Sabel MS, Griffith K, Sondak VK, et al. Predictors of nonsentinel lymph node positivity in patients with a positive sentinel node for melanoma. J Am Coll Surg. 2005;201:37–47.
82. Page AJ, Carlson GW, Delman KA, et al. Prediction of nonsentinel lymph node involvement in patients with a positive sentinel lymph node in malignant melanoma. Am Surg. 2007;73:674–8. discussion 678–679.
83. Roka F, Mastan P, Binder M, et al. Prediction of non-sentinel node status and outcome in sentinel node-positive melanoma patients. Eur J Surg Oncol. 2008;34:82–8.

84. Frankel TL, Griffith KA, Lowe L, et al. Do micromorphometric features of metastatic deposits within sentinel nodes predict nonsentinel lymph node involvement in melanoma? Ann Surg Oncol. 2008;15:2403–11.

85. Guggenheim M, Dummer R, Jung FJ, et al. The influence of sentinel lymph node tumour burden on additional lymph node involvement and disease-free survival in cutaneous melanoma--a retrospective analysis of 392 cases. Br J Cancer. 2008;98:1922–8.

86. Kingham TP, Panageas KS, Ariyan CE, et al. Outcome of patients with a positive sentinel lymph node who do not undergo completion lymphadenectomy. Ann Surg Oncol. 2010;17:514–20.

87. Bamboat ZM, Konstantinidis IT, Kuk D, et al. Observation after a positive sentinel lymph node biopsy in patients with melanoma. Ann Surg Oncol. 2014;21:3117.

88. Poos HP, Kruijff S, Bastiaannet E, et al. Therapeutic groin dissection for melanoma: risk factors for short term morbidity. Eur J Surg Oncol. 2009;35:877–83.

89. Singletary SE, Shallenberger R, Guinee VF. Surgical management of groin nodal metastases from primary melanoma of the lower extremity. Surg Gynecol Obstet. 1992;174:195–200.

90. Coit DG, Brennan MF. Extent of lymph node dissection in melanoma of the trunk or lower extremity. Arch Surg. 1989;124:162–6.

91. Badgwell B, Xing Y, Gershenwald JE, et al. Pelvic lymph node dissection is beneficial in subsets of patients with node-positive melanoma. Ann Surg Oncol. 2007;14:2867–75.

92. Pasquali S, Spillane AJ, de Wilt JH, et al. Surgeons' opinions on lymphadenectomy in melanoma patients with positive sentinel nodes: a worldwide web-based survey. Ann Surg Oncol. 2012;19:4322–9.

93. Kaoutzanis C, Barabas A, Allan R, et al. When should pelvic sentinel lymph nodes be harvested in patients with malignant melanoma? J Plast Reconstr Aesthet Surg. 2012;65:85–90.

94. Soteldo J, Ratto EL, Gandini S, et al. Pelvic sentinel lymph node biopsy in melanoma patients: is it worthwhile? Melanoma Res. 2010;20:133–7.

95. Chu CK, Delman KA, Carlson GW, et al. Inguinopelvic lymphadenectomy following positive inguinal sentinel lymph node biopsy in melanoma: true frequency of synchronous pelvic metastases. Ann Surg Oncol. 2011;18:3309–15.

96. Xing Y, Badgwell BD, Ross MI, et al. Lymph node ratio predicts disease-specific survival in melanoma patients. Cancer. 2009;115:2505–13.

97. Spillane AJ, Cheung BL, Winstanley J, Thompson JF. Lymph node ratio provides prognostic information in addition to american joint committee on cancer N stage in patients with melanoma, even if quality of surgery is standardized. Ann Surg. 2011;253:109–15.

98. Karakousis GC, Pandit-Taskar N, Hsu M, et al. Prognostic significance of drainage to pelvic nodes at sentinel lymph node mapping in patients with extremity melanoma. Melanoma Res. 2013;23:40–6.

99. Mann GB, Coit DG. Does the extent of operation influence the prognosis in patients with melanoma metastatic to inguinal nodes? Ann Surg Oncol. 1999;6:263–71.

100. van der Ploeg AP, van Akkooi AC, Schmitz PI, et al. Therapeutic surgical management of palpable melanoma groin metastases: superficial or combined superficial and deep groin lymph node dissection. Ann Surg Oncol. 2011;18:3300–8.

101. Mozzillo N, Caraco C, Marone U, et al. Superficial and deep lymph node dissection for stage III cutaneous melanoma: clinical outcome and prognostic factors. World J Surg Oncol. 2013;11:36.

102. Shen P, Conforti AM, Essner R, et al. Is the node of Cloquet the sentinel node for the iliac/obturator node group? Cancer J. 2000;6:93–7.

103. Coit DG, Peters M, Brennan MF. A prospective randomized trial of perioperative cefazolin treatment in axillary and groin dissection. Arch Surg. 1991;126:1366–71. discussion 1371–1362.

104. Karakousis CP, Driscoll DL. Groin dissection in malignant melanoma. Br J Surg. 1994;81:1771–4.

105. Guggenheim MM, Hug U, Jung FJ, et al. Morbidity and recurrence after completion lymph node dissection following sentinel lymph node biopsy in cutaneous malignant melanoma. Ann Surg. 2008;247:687–93.

106. Bishoff JT, Basler JW, Teichman JM, Thompson IM. Endoscopic subcutaneous modified inguinal lymph node dissection (ESMIL) for squamous cell carcinoma of the penis. J Urol. 2003;169:78.

107. Sotelo R, Sanchez-Salas R, Carmona O, et al. Endoscopic lymphadenectomy for penile carcinoma. J Endourol. 2007;21:364–7. discussion 367.

108. Delman KA, Kooby DA, Ogan K, et al. Feasibility of a novel approach to inguinal lymphadenectomy: minimally invasive groin dissection for melanoma. Ann Surg Oncol. 2010;17:731–7.

109. Delman KA, Kooby DA, Rizzo M, et al. Initial experience with videoscopic inguinal lymphadenectomy. Ann Surg Oncol. 2011;18:977–82.

110. Abbott AM, Grotz TE, Rueth NM, et al. Minimally invasive inguinal lymph node dissection (MILND) for melanoma: experience from two academic centers. Ann Surg Oncol. 2013;20:340–5.

111. Martin BM, Etra JW, Russell MC, et al. Oncologic outcomes of patients undergoing videoscopic inguinal lymphadenectomy for metastatic melanoma. J Am Coll Surg. 2014;218:620–6.

112. Pellegrino A, Damiani GR, Terruzzi M, et al. Robot-assisted laparoscopic transperitoneal deep pelvic lymphadenectomy for metastatic melanoma of the lower limb: initial report of four cases and outcomes at 1-year follow-up. Updates Surg. 2013;65:339–40.

113. Sohn W, Finley DS, Jakowatz J, Ornstein DK. Robot-assisted laparoscopic transperitoneal pelvic lymphadenectomy and metastasectomy for melanoma: initial report of two cases. J Robot Surg. 2010;4:129–32.

114. Tsao H, Atkins MB, Sober AJ. Management of cutaneous melanoma. N Engl J Med. 2004;351:998–1012.

115. Feun LG, Gutterman J, Burgess MA, et al. The natural history of resectable metastatic melanoma (Stage IVA melanoma). Cancer. 1982;50:1656–63.

116. Serrone L, Zeuli M, Sega FM, Cognetti F. Dacarbazine-based chemotherapy for metastatic melanoma: thirty-year experience overview. J Exp Clin Cancer Res. 2000;19:21–34.

117. Chapman PB, Einhorn LH, Meyers ML, et al. Phase III multicenter randomized trial of the Dartmouth regimen versus dacarbazine in patients with metastatic melanoma. J Clin Oncol. 1999;17:2745–51.

118. Legha SS, Ring S, Papadopoulos N, et al. A prospective evaluation of a triple-drug regimen containing cisplatin, vinblastine, and dacarbazine (CVD) for metastatic melanoma. Cancer. 1989;64:2024–9.

119. Verschraegen CF, Legha SS, Hersh EM, et al. Phase II study of vindesine and dacarbazine with or without non-specific stimulation of the immune system in patients with metastatic melanoma. Eur J Cancer. 1993;29A:708–11.

120. Atkins MB, Lotze MT, Dutcher JP, et al. High-dose recombinant interleukin 2 therapy for patients with metastatic melanoma: analysis of 270 patients treated between 1985 and 1993. J Clin Oncol. 1999;17:2105–16.

121. Keilholz U, Martus P, Punt CJ, et al. Prognostic factors for survival and factors associated with long-term remission in patients with advanced melanoma receiving cytokine-based treatments: second analysis of a randomised EORTC Melanoma Group trial comparing interferon-alpha2a (IFNalpha) and interleukin 2 (IL-2) with or without cisplatin. Eur J Cancer. 2002;38:1501–11.

122. Eton O, Legha SS, Bedikian AY, et al. Sequential biochemotherapy versus chemotherapy for metastatic melanoma: results from a phase III randomized trial. J Clin Oncol. 2002;20:2045–52.

123. Bajetta E, Del Vecchio M, Nova P, et al. Multicenter phase III randomized trial of polychemotherapy (CVD regimen) versus the same chemotherapy (CT) plus subcutaneous interleukin-2 and interferon-alpha2b in metastatic melanoma. Ann Oncol. 2006;17:571–7.

124. Lee ML, Tomsu K, Von Eschen KB. Duration of survival for disseminated malignant melanoma: results of a meta-analysis. Melanoma Res. 2000;10:81–92.

125. Allen PJ, Coit DG. The role of surgery for patients with metastatic melanoma. Curr Opin Oncol. 2002;14:221–6.

126. Essner R, Lee JH, Wanek LA, et al. Contemporary surgical treatment of advanced-stage melanoma. Arch Surg. 2004;139:961–6. discussion 966–967.
127. Balch CM, Soong SJ, Murad TM, et al. A multifactorial analysis of melanoma. IV. Prognostic factors in 200 melanoma patients with distant metastases (stage III). J Clin Oncol. 1983;1: 126–34.
128. Ollila DW, Hsueh EC, Stern SL, Morton DL. Metastasectomy for recurrent stage IV melanoma. J Surg Oncol. 1999;71:209–13.
129. Wornom 3rd IL, Smith JW, Soong SJ, et al. Surgery as palliative treatment for distant metastases of melanoma. Ann Surg. 1986;204:181–5.
130. Leo F, Cagini L, Rocmans P, et al. Lung metastases from melanoma: when is surgical treatment warranted? Br J Cancer. 2000;83:569–72.
131. Harpole Jr DH, Johnson CM, Wolfe WG, et al. Analysis of 945 cases of pulmonary metastatic melanoma. J Thorac Cardiovasc Surg. 1992;103:743–8. discussion 748–750.
132. Schuchter LM, Green R, Fraker D. Primary and metastatic diseases in malignant melanoma of the gastrointestinal tract. Curr Opin Oncol. 2000;12:181–5.
133. Sanki A, Scolyer RA, Thompson JF. Surgery for melanoma metastases of the gastrointestinal tract: indications and results. Eur J Surg Oncol. 2009;35:313–9.
134. Ollila DW, Essner R, Wanek LA, Morton DL. Surgical resection for melanoma metastatic to the gastrointestinal tract. Arch Surg. 1996;131:975–9. 979–980.
135. Wood TF, DiFronzo LA, Rose DM, et al. Does complete resection of melanoma metastatic to solid intra-abdominal organs improve survival? Ann Surg Oncol. 2001;8:658–62.
136. Tarhini AA, Agarwala SS. Management of brain metastases in patients with melanoma. Curr Opin Oncol. 2004;16:161–6.
137. Demirkesen O, Yaycioglu O, Uygun N, et al. A case of metastatic malignant melanoma presenting with hematuria. Urol Int. 2000;64:118–20.
138. DeBoer DK, Schwartz HS, Thelman S, Reynolds VH. Heterogeneous survival rates for isolated skeletal metastases from melanoma. Clin Orthop Relat Res 1996; (323): 277–283.
139. Haigh PI, Essner R, Wardlaw JC, et al. Long-term survival after complete resection of melanoma metastatic to the adrenal gland. Ann Surg Oncol. 1999;6:633–9.
140. Plesnicar A, Kovac V. Breast metastases from cutaneous melanoma: a report of three cases. Tumori. 2000;86:170–3.
141. Zografos L, Ducrey N, Beati D, et al. Metastatic melanoma in the eye and orbit. Ophthalmology. 2003;110:2245–56.
142. Ribas A, Flaherty KT. BRAF targeted therapy changes the treatment paradigm in melanoma. Nat Rev Clin Oncol. 2011;8:426–33.

Peritoneal Carcinomatosis

Michelle L. Bryan, Shuja Ahmed, Konstantinos I. Votanopoulos, Perry Shen, Edward A. Levine, and John H. Stewart

Introduction to Peritoneal Carcinomatosis

The intraabdominal dissemination of neoplasm to the peritoneal surface is referred to as peritoneal carcinomatosis or peritoneal surface disease (PSD). PSD represents localized metastasis that may occur as the initial presentation or as recurrent disease in a number of intraabdominal neoplasms including appendiceal, colon, ovarian, and gastric carcinomas, as well as peritoneal mesothelioma and sarcomas (Table 1). This seeding and subsequent spread may occur secondary to spontaneous tumor rupture or tumor disruption during the initial resection. Intraperitoneal free tumor cells then preferentially deposit on peritoneal surfaces, the diaphragm, and the small bowel mesentery (Fig. 1). As dictated by the aggressiveness of the origin tumor, the number, size, and distribution of the individual tumor deposits on peritoneal surfaces vary greatly. For many causes of PSD, the disease may remain contained in the abdomen, with modest risk of extra-abdominal metastasis. This regional pattern

M.L. Bryan, M.D., Ph.D. • K.I. Votanopoulos, M.D., Ph.D. • P. Shen, M.D.
E.A. Levine, M.D.
Department of Surgery, Wake Forest School of Medicine,
Medical Center Boulevard, Winston-Salem, NC 27157, USA
e-mail: mbryan@wakehealth.edu; kvotanop@wakehealth.edu;
pshen@wakehealth.edu; elevine@wakehealth.edu

S. Ahmed, M.D.
Department of Surgery, Louisiana State University Health Sciences Center,
1501 Kings Highway, New Orleans, LA 71103, USA
e-mail: shuja_ahmed2003@yahoo.com

J.H. Stewart IV, M.D., M.B.A (✉)
Department of Surgery, Duke University School of Medicine,
P.O. Box 3118, Durham, LC 27710, USA
e-mail: john.stewart@duke.edu

© Springer International Publishing Switzerland 2016
K.A. Morgan (ed.), *Current Controversies in Cancer Care
for the Surgeon*, DOI 10.1007/978-3-319-16205-8_11

185

Table 1 Sources of peritoneal surface disease

Malignancies causing peritoneal surface disease (PSD)
Primary Peritoneal
Mesothelioma
Locoregional metastasis
Appendiceal
Colon
Ovarian
Gastric
Small bowel
Sarcoma
Distant metastasis
Breast
Other

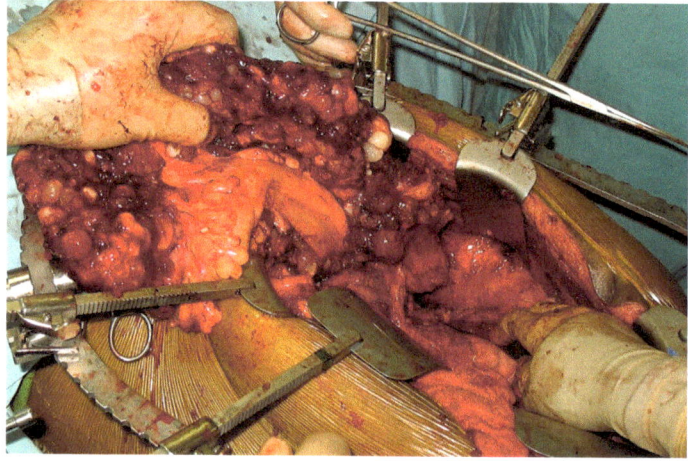

Fig. 1 Intraoperative image of peritoneal surface disease. Patient's head is at left. Note the large tumor nodules throughout the omentum, which is held in the surgeon's hand

of recurrence makes aggressive therapy in the abdomen with cytoreduction an attractive therapy for many patients with PSD.

In most cases, peritoneal carcinomatosis is diagnosed incidentally during surgical exploration, evaluation of abdominal pain, or on radiographic imaging for other indications. Unfortunately, these patients have a dismal prognosis without treatment, with median survival reported between 3 and 7 months [1]. This chapter describes the staging, treatment, and current patient outcomes in peritoneal carcinomatosis as well as controversies in the management of this disease.

Staging of Peritoneal Surface Malignancies

Imaging

The most commonly used imaging modality for both diagnosis and preoperative evaluation is contrast enhanced computed tomography (CT) scan of the chest, abdomen, and pelvis. The first objective evaluation of this modality in 1993 by Sugarbaker and colleagues demonstrated an overall sensitivity of 79 % in detecting peritoneal lesions [2]. In that study, sensitivity was lowest in the pelvis and decreased with decreasing tumor volume, with a sensitivity of only 28 % obtained for tumor nodules less than 5 mm in size. Although CT technology has progressed since 1993, the sensitivity for gross detection of peritoneal lesions remains similar, with more recently described overall sensitivity of detection rates of 60–76 % [3]. Again, the sensitivity of CT scans is highly dependent on implant size, with sensitivities of upwards of 94 % for nodules >5 cm in size [4]. Despite its shortcomings, CT is appropriate for the detection of solid organ involvement, retroperitoneal spread, overall operability, and prognosis, making it the continued imaging modality of choice [5, 6] (Fig. 2).

Magnetic resonance imaging (MRI) with both oral and intravenous contrast has been reported to have an overall sensitivity of detection of peritoneal implants of between 84 and 100 % [7, 8]. In many patients with peritoneal surface malignancies,

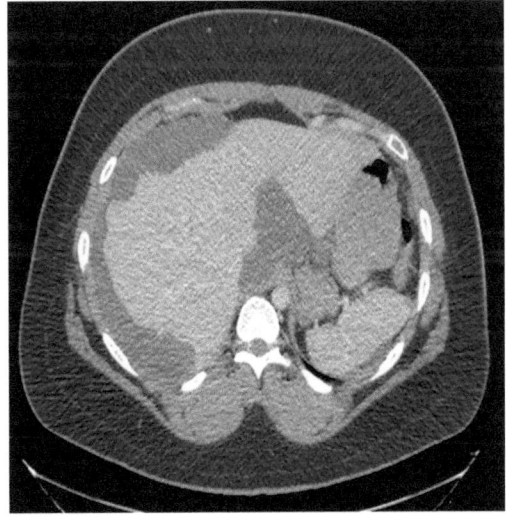

Fig. 2 Contrast enhanced computed tomography of a patient with large volume pseudomyxoma peritonei. Tumor encases the lateral liver and porta hepatis. A smaller amount of disease is deposited on the spleen. With kind permission from Springer Science + Business Media: Surgical Oncology, Cytoreductive Surgery and Hyperthermic Intraperitoneal Chemotherapy, 2015, Randle RW et al., Figure 27.2

prior operative management makes MRI a poor imaging modality as it cannot discern between postoperative scar and peritoneal implants, resulting in a high false positive rate in this group of patients [9]. Overall, the increased cost, time, and lack of prognostic significance of MRI have not made it a preferred imaging choice for PSD.

The role of positron emission tomography (PET) in patients with peritoneal surface dissemination is mainly to detect extra-abdominal disease in planning treatment. Sensitivity is reported at approximately 10 % in low volume disease. Unlike contrast CT, which has a specificity of >90 %, PET specificity remains approximately 42 % in patients with low volume disease [10, 11]. In addition, not all histological subtypes of carcinomas that present as diffuse PSD have sufficient glucose uptake of 18F-FDG. Despite these shortcomings, PET may be warranted to rule out extra-abdominal disease in patients being considered for aggressive surgical therapy. PET imaging is of limited utility for patients with low grade appendiceal disease [12].

Staging

Given the aforementioned findings, the two primary staging algorithms are based on CT scan and operative findings. The Peritoneal Carcinomatosis Index (PCI) is the most widely used staging system for peritoneal carcinomatosis. This system divides the abdomen into nine regions and the small bowel into four regions. A score is assigned to each region based on the amount of tumor present. A score of 0 (no tumor), 1 (tumor up to 0.5 cm), 2 (tumor up to 5 cm), or 3 (tumor >5 cm) is applied to each region and the scores for the 12 regions are then tabulated to give a final score [13] (Fig. 3). The PCI has become the most widely cited scoring system as it can be used both pre and postoperatively, and correlates with likelihood of complete resection and prognosis [14–16]. The Gilly Carcinomatosis Staging Scale is an alternative staging system with scoring ranging between Stage 0 to Stage 4 [17]. Stage 0 is applied for patients with no macroscopic disease, Stage 1 designates localized tumor implants less than 0.5 cm in diameter, Stage 2 disease represents non-localized tumor implants less than 0.5 cm, Stage 3 identifies implants 0.5–2 cm, and Stage 4 represents any implants greater than 2 cm in diameter. As with the the PCI, higher stage correlates with worse prognosis [18–20].

Surgical Staging

Laparoscopic staging has been suggested as a more sensitive form of staging than the imaging modalities above over the last 10 years. Denzer et al. conducted a comparison of CT scan versus "minilaparoscopy" in the detection of peritoneal surface malignancies. They reported that diagnostic laparoscopy detected PSD in 100 % of the treated

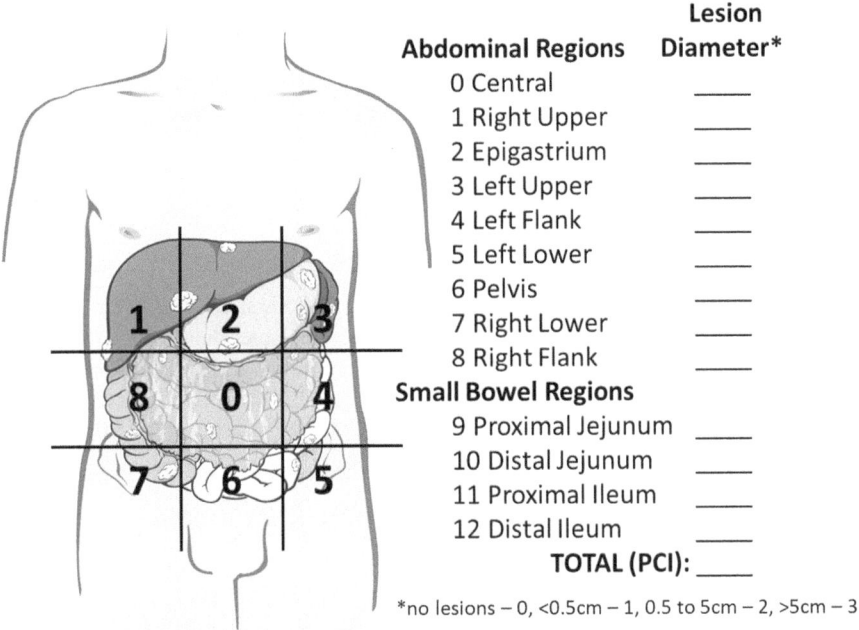

	Abdominal Regions	Lesion Diameter*
	0 Central	____
	1 Right Upper	____
	2 Epigastrium	____
	3 Left Upper	____
	4 Left Flank	____
	5 Left Lower	____
	6 Pelvis	____
	7 Right Lower	____
	8 Right Flank	____
Small Bowel Regions		
	9 Proximal Jejunum	____
	10 Distal Jejunum	____
	11 Proximal Ileum	____
	12 Distal Ileum	____
	TOTAL (PCI):	____

*no lesions – 0, <0.5cm – 1, 0.5 to 5cm – 2, >5cm – 3

Fig. 3 Schematic for calculating the peritoneal carcinomatosis index (PCI) staging system. Scores based on lesion size for each of nine abdominal regions plus four small bowel regions are added together to reach the PCI. With kind permission from Springer Science + Business Media: Surgical Oncology, Cytoreductive Surgery and Hyperthermic Intraperitoneal Chemotherapy, 2015, Randle RW et al., Figure 27.3

cases, whereas only 47.8 % had been revealed by a CT scan previously performed on the same patients [21]. Taking this further, Valle and colleagues described the use of 2–3 port video laparoscopy in assessing PCI and resectability in 97 patients [22]. They reported that 16/97 (16 %) patients presented with disease that was deemed unresectable based upon laparoscopic staging, while two patients were under-staged by laparoscopy. They also noted that while there was no tumor seeding of the trocar sites, there was a 2 % superficial soft tissue infection of the trocar sites. This study, however, did not include evaluation of preoperative CT scans to assess whether all of the enrolled patients would have been eligible for laparotomy by radiographic criteria. This question was more directly addressed by Pomel and colleagues in an assessment of 11 patients of uncertain resectability [23]. Laparotomy was avoided in three patients (27 %); one patient was deemed to have completely resectable disease at laparoscopy could not be completely debulked (9 %); and seven patients underwent successful resections (63.6 %). On the other hand, 20 % of patients who went directly to laparotomy in their comparative study could not undergo a complete resection. Based on these limited studies, it remains to be determined whether laparoscopy has a role in determining staging and potential resectability in patients for whom imaging is inconclusive. At present, the use of laparoscopy remains an area of controversy.

Current Treatment Modalities

Currently, the best management of patients with peritoneal surface disease remains an area of debate. Options for treatment include systemic chemotherapy, surgical debulking alone, or surgical debulking with adjuvant intraperitoneal chemotherapy. These approaches are described below.

Cytoreductive Surgery with Hyperthermic Intraperitoneal Chemotherapy (CRS/HIPEC)

Surgical resection is recommended for removal of the primary lesion, and peritoneal debulking is undertaken for disseminated peritoneal surface disease. The cytoreduction procedure removes macroscopic tumor deposits but if microscopic disease is not addressed, traditionally 90 % of patients developed disease progression and death, typically from bowel obstruction. In 1980 a method of combining debulking surgery with heated intraperitoneal chemotherapy was first described [24]. The administration of cytotoxic chemotherapy directly into the peritoneal cavity has been shown to achieve higher local concentrations at the site of disease than could be achieved systemically [25]. The addition of heat was found to be synergistic with the chemotherapy [9]. As a complete technique, CRS/HIPEC targets both macroscopic and microscopic disease.

The surgical technique involves both the cytoreduction and the perfusion step. Cytoreduction is the key intervention, and is undertaken in a manner similar to exploratory laparotomy. If still in place, the primary lesion is removed as well as any involved organs. Tumor deposits are then stripped from peritoneal surfaces, including the abdominal wall and diaphragm. Bowel and organ resection may be undertaken if the peritoneum is unable to be stripped. Anastomoses can be performed prior to or following HIPEC, while stomas are created following the chemoperfusion. Following cytoreduction, perfusion is performed by either a closed abdomen or open or "coliseum" technique. Inflow and outflow catheters are placed through the abdominal wall and connected to the heat exchanger and pump of the perfusion circuit. In the closed technique, the abdomen is temporarily closed with a running watertight suture. In the open or coliseum approaches, a temporary plastic sheet is sewn onto the abdomen. Perfusion is generally maintained for 30–120 min dependent on the individual cen-

Table 2 Comparison of cytoreductive surgery scoring systems

Residual disease (cm)	Residual disease (R) status	Completeness of cytoreduction (CC) score
0	R0-Negative margins on final pathology	CC-0: No visible disease following cytoreduction
	R1-Positive margins on final pathology	
0.25	R2a	CC-1
0.5		CC-2
>0.5–2	R2b	
>2–2.5	R2c	
>2.5		CC-3

ter's protocol for the tumor type. Following perfusion, the cannulas and/or plastic sheet are removed, stomas created if required, and the abdomen is closed.

The goal of CRS/HIPEC is complete surgical removal of macroscopic disease and chemical destruction of microscopic disease by the chemotherapeutic agent. Disease-free progression and survival have been correlated with the completeness of resection, as judged by the surgeon. Two classification systems are utilized in the reporting of the completeness of resection in both clinical documentation and research. The R status of resection (from the AJCC staging manual) or the CC score for completeness of cytoreduction can be used as shown in Table 2. Complete cytoreduction of all macroscopic disease is designated as R0 or R1 on the R scale and CC-0 on the CC scale. R0 versus R1 allows the distinction of negative versus positive margins on pathology. R2 resection or >CC-0 indicate residual macroscopic disease. Regardless of the origin of the tumor, the resection status is the main independent predictor of survival across multiple studies [26–31].

In addition to resection status, patient factors prior to surgery have a significant impact on overall survival. Preoperative performance status is a significant prognostic factor. Patients with ECOG scores of 0 or 1 have been shown to have better outcomes after CRS/HIPEC then those with scores of 2 or 3. For example, in one study of patients with PSD from a variety of primaries, median survival was 21.7 months with an ECOG of 0–1 and 9.5 months with ECOG 2–3 [32].

Many chemotherapeutic agents have been utilized for intraperitoneal chemotherapy. At present, the most widely utilized agents are oxaliplatin and mitomycin C. A prospective randomized controlled trial of these two agents is ongoing for appendiceal cancer at Wake Forest University and should complete accrual in 2015. Randomized trials for intraperitoneal chemotherapeutic agents are otherwise lacking in this setting, and agents have historically been chosen based on large molecular weight conveying an ability to achieve higher intraperitoneal concentrations with low systemic absorption and associated toxicities.

Systemic Chemotherapy

Peritoneal surface disease represents a unique challenge for systemic chemotherapy. It has long been understood that the permeability of the peritoneal cavity to many systemic chemotherapy drugs is less than the plasma clearance, therefore allowing little of the systemically delivered drug to reach the PSD tumor nodules [33–35]. The capacity of the peritoneal cavity to serve as a barrier to drug transport is thought to lie mainly in the transport properties of the blood capillary wall and interstitial matrix [36]. This is supported by the fact that surgical peritonectomy of the peritoneal membrane itself does not alter intraperitoneal concentrations of chemotherapeutic agents [37]. Given this information, it is not surprising that the clinical response of patients with PSD to systemic chemotherapy is modest at best. As will be discussed below, the most widely studied patients with PSD undergoing systemic chemotherapy are those with PSD from colorectal carcinoma (CRC). In this select group, median survival is approximately 19–22 months with modern systemic chemotherapy combined with biologics, with 5 year survival rates <5 % [38, 39]. The role of systemic chemotherapy, if applicable, will be discussed within each disease specific section below.

Overview of Peritoneal Carcinomatosis of Select Cancers

Appendiceal Neoplasms

Epithelial neoplasms of the appendix represent a rare disease and are estimated to be diagnosed in approximately 1 % of all appendectomy specimens [40]. Those not diagnosed in appendectomy specimens often present late with peritoneal surface disease due to the nonspecific nature of appendiceal neoplasm symptoms. In peritoneal surface disease, the lumen becomes obstructed by tumor, which is often mucin producing, and subsequent rupture leads to peritoneal dissemination.

Pseudomyxoma peritonei, or malignant mucinous ascites, develops in approximately 10 % of patients with an epithelial appendiceal neoplasm. In those who develop PSD, patient prognosis correlates with pathologic classification. At present, two potential pathologic classification schemes exist, indicating an area of controversy. The system proposed by Ronnett et al. in 1995 is a staging system consisting of three categories; Diffuse peritoneal adenomucinosis (DPAM) consisting of low-grade tumors with low numbers of mitotic figures and cytologic atypia; peritoneal mucinous carcinomatosis (PMCA) consisting of high-grade tumors and characterized by atypia and more prominent mitotic figures; and, PMCA-I/D marked by intermediate or discordant features [20]. A subsequent study showed that indeed, these categories correlated with both 5 and 10-year survival. Survival for patients with DPAM (75 %, 68 %) was significantly better than that for PMCA-I/D (50 %, 21 %) or PMCA (14 %, 3 %) [41]. More recently, the group at Wake Forest has proposed a two-tiered classification system based upon a pathologic review of 101 patients with mucinous ascites related to primary appendiceal tumors. The 5-year survival for DPAM and PMCA-I/D was found to be similar, at 68 % and 61 %, respectively. PMCA, however, was associated with a statistically significant 5-year survival of 37 % ($p=0.004$) [42]. Based upon this information, the two categories proposed were low grade mucinous carcinoma peritonei (MCP-L) and high-grade mucinous carcinoma peritonei (MCP-H). Low grade mucinous carcinoma encompasses DPAM, PMCA I/D, and well differentiated variants of mucinous adenocarcinoma. High grade mucinous carcinoma includes PMCA, histologically moderate or poorly differentiated adenocarcinoma, and cases with signet ring cell components. Categorizing PSD from appendiceal tumors into two categories has remained more consistent with response to CRS-HIPEC as well [43]. Approximately 16 % of low grade lesions are thought to dedifferentiate into higher-grade lesions during the course of the disease [44].

Despite their rarity, outcomes from appendiceal neoplasms have been extensively studied due to their role as the classic indication for CRS/HIPEC. A 2008 consensus statement from the Fifth International Workshop on Peritoneal Surface Malignancy supported CRS/HIPEC as the standard of care for perforated appendiceal tumor with PSD, based on a review of the evidence [45]. Due to the rarity of this entity, randomized studies have not been undertaken directly comparing cytoreduction versus CRS/HIPEC. Cytoreduction alone is known to confer a significant survival benefit. Gough et al. reported 5 years and 10 years survival rates of 53 % and 32 % respectively with serial debulking alone [46]. While no direct comparisons exist, studies investigating survival post CRS/HIPEC have shown 5 year survival rates ranging from 60 to 97 %, with a recent study reporting a 15-year survival rate of 59 % [42, 47–50].

The importance of cytoreduction is emphasized by the fact that the extent of the resection is a large factor in the wide range of survival rates. In a series of 481 appendiceal carcinoma patients, the extent of cytoreduction was independently associated with survival ($p<0.001$) with median survival times of 175 months, 73 months, 29 months, and 17 months for R0/1, R2a, R2b, or R2c resections, respectively [51]. This significant correlation of R0/1 resection with increased survival correlates with findings from other studies [50, 52]. The wide range of survival percentages also indicates that survival is likely not dependent on surgery alone, but with multiple patient factors. The largest retrospective study to date on CRS/HIPEC for appendiceal cancer was a recent large multi-institutional study involving 2298 patients from 16 institutions. Multivariate analysis from this study indicated that preoperative PCI score, prior chemotherapy, PMCA histopathologic subtype, incomplete debulking, major (Grade 3, 4) post operative complications, and not including HIPEC were predictors of shorter progression-free survival [29].

The role of perioperative systemic chemotherapy in appendiceal carcinoma remains an area of controversy. An initial study by Sugarbaker and colleagues evaluated 34 patients with PMCA and found a 29 % histopathologic response after 3–6 months of FOLFOX with or without bevacizumab [52]. However, they found that there was no overall survival advantage to neoadjuvant chemotherapy ($p=0.56$) in this same population of patients in a follow-up study [53]. Not surprisingly, however, patients who had a histopathological response to neoadjuvant therapy had a significant survival advantage (median survival NR) versus those who did not (median survival 29.5 months, $p=0.034$). In addition, perioperative chemotherapy was associated with a lower preoperative PCI ($p=0.003$) and decreased number of visceral resections ($p<0.001$), but not with completeness of resection ($p=0.78$) or complications ($p=0.16$). This study excluded patients with low grade disease (MCP-L), classified as DPAM or PMCA I/D. In contrast Chua et al. performed a registry review which implicated prior chemotherapy in the setting of CRS/HIPEC was associated with poorer progression free and overall survival [31]. Our group studied both MCP-L and MCP-H patients and found no improvement in median progression free survival (PFS) in patients with MCP-L treated with perioperative chemotherapy versus those not (29.5 months vs 37 months, $p=0.18$). In those patients with MCP-H, postoperative chemotherapy was associated with longer PFS (13.6 months, $p<0.01$) than preoperative chemotherapy (6.8 months) or CRS/HIPEC alone (7 months, $p=0.03$) [54].

Modern chemotherapy may offer modest benefit in patients with unresectable disease. Similar to the histopathologic response reported in surgical patients, Farquharson et al. reported that 38 % of patients with unresectable PSD from appendiceal carcinoma experienced a reduction in ascites or stabilization of disease with systemic chemotherapy consisting of mitomycin c and capecitabine [55]. Shapiro et al. additionally reported a 55.6 % total disease control rate in patients deemed unresectable and receiving at least two cycles of systemic chemotherapy. Disease control included complete response, partial response, and stabilization of disease in this study [56]. While CRS/HIPEC remains the standard of care in appropriate surgical patients, in patients deemed suboptimal candidates for surgical resection, systemic chemotherapy offers an option for potential disease and symptom control. Further, it clearly has a role in high grade appendiceal cancer with PSD.

Colorectal Cancer (CRC)

Colorectal cancer is the third most common cancer in the United States. Despite the significant improvements in systemic chemotherapy, CRC continues to have high rates of recurrence. While the liver and lung remain the most common sites of recurrence, peritoneal surface disease (PSD)*is the only site of recurrence in up to 25 %* of patients [56]. In a retrospective study of 3019 patients with CRC, Jayne et al. reported peritoneal surface disease in 349 (13 %) patients. The majority of the patients (214 out of 349) had synchronous metastasis and 58 % of that subset having PSD as the only site of metastasis [57].

PSD from CRC, like those from other primary tumors, was traditionally considered a terminal disease, all too frequently approached with therapeutic nihilism. PSD from CRC has been shown to be somewhat responsive to chemotherapy. Franko et al., compared outcomes of patients with PSD from CRC enrolled in two prospective randomized trials of chemotherapy with those of non-peritoneal metastatic CRC [58]. Both the median overall survival (12.7 months versus 17.6 months) and progression-free survival (5.8 months vs 7.2 months) were inferior for PSD compared to non-peritoneal metastasis for CRC. However, this survival was a marked improvement from the median 6-month survival for PSD noted in the EVOCAPE-1 trial, and it is noteworthy that approximately 3 % of patients were alive 5 years after diagnosis [1]. Furthermore, it substantiated the role of CRS/HIPEC in improving outcomes for PSD from CRC.

The only randomized trial comparing outcomes of CRS/HIPEC with systemic chemotherapy for PSD from CRC was reported in 2003 [59]. The trial involved 105 patients with PSD from CRC randomly assigned to either systemic chemotherapy (5-fluorouracil and leucovorin) or CRS/HIPEC with the same chemotherapy. After a median follow-up of 21.6 months, the median survival was 12.6 months in the systemic chemotherapy arm versus 22.3 months in the CRS/HIPEC arm ($p=0.032$). A more recent update of the study, after a median follow-up of 8 years, reported superior progression-free survival ($p=0.020$) as well as disease-specific survival ($p=0.028$) in the CRS/HIPEC group [60]. Although this study was criticized for the use of 5-fluorouracil and leucovorin as the systemic chemotherapy regimen instead of the now more standard FOLFOX regimen and for including some appendiceal cancers in the cohort, the significant difference in (the more than doubled) survival related to CRS/HIPEC could not be denied. A subsequent retrospective study by Franko et al. showed that, for best outcomes, CRS/HIPEC should be used in conjunction with systemic chemotherapy and not in lieu of it [61]. Encouraged by the solid evidence, a multi-institutional consensus statement was issued by an international peritoneal surface group, delineating the treatment algorithm for PSD from CRC with particular emphasis on CRS/HIPEC in 2007 [62].

Since that landmark trial, several studies/centers have reported their outcomes with CRS/HIPEC for CRC-related PSD [63]. Glehen et al. reported a median survival of 19 months after median follow-up of 53 months with 5 year survival of 31 % in a multi-institutional study involving 506 patients from 28 international centers [64]. Several other studies have corroborated these improved outcomes associated with CRS/HIPEC [65, 66]. Based on these encouraging results, a multi-institutional consensus statement was issued proposing guidelines regarding the indication and technique of CRS/HIPEC for PSD from CRC [67].

Similar to outcomes of CRS/HIPEC for other primary malignancies, several prognostic factors have been identified for PSD from CRC. These include completeness of cytoreduction/residual disease (R) score, performance status of the patient and PCI score. The impact of PCI score on outcome of PSD for CRC is particularly well documented. Sugarbaker showed a 50 % 5-year survival for PCI < 10 which dropped to 20 % for PCI between 11 and 20. There were no survivors after 5 years amongst patients with PCI >20 [68]. The PCI is also related to the completeness of cytoreduction scores (R or CC); with the PCI and cytoreductions scores being inversely related.

Progressively improving outcomes associated with CRS/HIPEC for PSD for CRC has encouraged more aggressive surgical approaches in quest of even better outcomes. Although synchronous resection of liver metastasis at the time of CRS/HIPEC for PSD from CRC was initially noted to have negative prognostic value, subsequent studies have shown similar outcomes for CRS/HIPEC with and without liver metastatectomy. Chua et al. reported a 2-year survival rate of 68 % in the nonliver metastatic group versus 65 % for the liver metastatic group after complete cyto-reduction/metastatectomy [69]. Their results are consistent with studies from Elias et al. and Kianmanesh et al. both of which showed no difference in survival between the two groups [70, 71]. At the 5th International Workshop on Peritoneal Surface Malignancy, it was recommended that in carefully selected patients it was feasible and potentially beneficial to perform CRS/HIPEC with simultaneous metastatec-tomy provided there were three or fewer liver metastases [69, 72]. This presumed that all hepatic lesions were resected or ablated at the time of surgery and that the hepatic resections/ablations could be performed without lobar hepatectomy.

Ovarian Neoplasms

Epithelial ovarian cancer (EOC) affects approximately 22,000 women annually in the United States, resulting in approximately 15,000 deaths per year [73]. Despite advances in treatment, 5 year survival rates for women with advanced cancer remain less than 50 %. The presenting symptoms of EOC may remain vague and thus diag-nosis is often at a late stage. Advanced disease is often confined to the peritoneal cavity, with PSD being a substantial clinical problem in these women [74].

Munnell's early description of the benefit of "maximum surgical effort" in EOC patients belays the early history of cytoreduction [75]. In his 1968 report, he showed survival benefit for cytoreduction in EOC patients with intraperitoneal disease, which we would now refer to as PSD. Since that time, the definition of "maximum surgical effort" in EOC has evolved. While standards of CRS for EOC at one time called for removal of all disease to <2 cm dimension of the largest lesion, this has now evolved to a standard of <1 cm [76, 77]. A large meta-analysis of 6885 patients found maximal cytoreduction to be an independent predictor of survival among patients with stage III or IV ovarian carcinoma [78].

While CRS is accepted as standard of care, the role of CRS/HIPEC in EOC remains debated. Randomized clinical trials have shown the benefit of the addi-tion of intraperitoneal chemotherapy to CRS. Armstrong et al. randomized 415 patients with Stage III ovarian cancer who had undergone maximal CRS to <1 cm to receive either IV paclitaxel and cisplatin or IV paclitaxel with intraperitoneal cisplatin. The addition of intraperitoneal cisplatin was associated with longer pro-gression free survival (23.8 months vs 18.3 months, $p = 0.05$) and overall survival (65.6 months vs 49.7 months, $p = 0.03$) [79]. While this study referred to catheter based early post-operative intraperitoneal chemotherapy (EPIC), studies have also reviewed the role of CRS/HIPEC in EOC. A systemic review of CRS/HIPEC outcomes for PSD from ovarian cancer included 19 studies and was published in 2009 by Chua et al. [80]. They found a wide range of reported outcomes, with 5 year survival ranging from 12 to 66 %. Despite prior descriptions of increased Grade 3/4 complications with intraperitoneal cisplatin, peri-operative morbidity (0–40 %) and mortality (0–10 %) were similar to that reported for CRS/HIPEC in other cancers.

Unlike other PSD of gastrointestinal origin, systemic chemotherapy plays a more important role in EOC. Initial response of EOC to platinum based chemotherapy is often high (>60 %), but development of platinum resistance is all too common [81]. The benefit of CRS has been shown in multiple studies, therefore the current approach is CRS followed by adjuvant therapy with a combination platinum and taxane regimen [82]. However, whether to approach chemotherapy from a neoadjuvant or adjuvant standpoint with CRS has been debated. Several studies have attempted to address this question. A randomized study of 632 patients with Stage IIIC and IV ovarian cancer showed no difference in overall survival between those who were assigned to initial CRS followed by chemotherapy, versus those undergoing neoadjuvant chemotherapy and interval CRS (hazard ratio for death 0.98, CI 0.84–1.13) [83]. Proponents of neoadjuvant chemotherapy site benefits such as pre-operative improvement in performance status and reduced CRS leading to lower morbidity [84, 85]. At present, this remains a topic of ongoing trials.

Diffuse Malignant Peritoneal Mesothelioma (DMPM)

DMPM is a rare but locally aggressive malignancy that arises from the serosal lining of the peritoneum. It is rapidly fatal, if left untreated, with median survival of less than 1 year [86]. The aggressive tumor biology and late presentation both contribute to the dismal prognosis. Its presenting symptoms are also vague such as abdominal pain and weight loss leading to delayed diagnosis. Fortunately, however, DMPM has an annual incidence of only 300–400 cases in the US [87]. Unlike pleural mesothelioma, DMPM is not as strongly linked to asbestos exposure and is broadly divided into three main subtypes. Epithelioid subtype is the most prevalent and has the best prognosis, while biphasic and sarcomatoid variants are less common but have worse outcomes [88, 89]. It is noteworthy that we are unaware of a single long term survivor in the literature from a sarcomatoid subtype and we do not offer cytoreduction and HIPEC to these patients.

Like other peritoneal malignancies, DMPM has a poor response to systemic chemotherapy as well as radiation therapy. If left untreated, it has OS of 4–12 months [90]. However, systemic chemotherapy with the combination regimen of cisplatin and pemetrexed has shown to marginally improve median OS to 10–26.8 months, and is the only FDA approved regimen for the disease [91, 92]. In the context of the poor response of DMPM to most modalities of treatment, CRS/HIPEC has emerged as an important modality to significantly extend survival in patients with DMPM. It is important to mention, however, that, unlike CRC, there are no randomized trials comparing systemic chemotherapy with CRS/HIPEC for DMPM. In a multi-institutional registry study involving leading HIPEC centers of the world, CRS/HIPEC for DMPM was associated with median survival of 53 months with 3- and 5-year survivals of 60 % and 47 %, respectively [93]. Similar to HIPEC for other tumor types, 31 % of patients developed significant peri-operative morbidity while the peri-operative mortality was 2 %. Similarly, a recently published meta-analysis involving 1047 patients showed 1-, 3- and 5-year survivals of 84 %, 59 % and 42 %, respectively [92]. Sugarbaker, et al. took this a step further and reported 3- and 5-year survival of 60 % and 52 %, respectively for iterative CRS/HIPEC in patients with DMPM [94].

Prognostic factors associated with improved outcomes in DMPM include epithelioid subtype, negative lymph nodes, completeness of cytoreduction and HIPEC [91]. The results of an Italian study epitomized the significance of complete cytoreduction in DMPM. Forty-four percent of the 108 patients in the study were alive 7 years after undergoing complete cytoreduction and HIPEC [93]. In the presence of complete cytoreduction, the study identified other prognostic clinicopathological variables including epithelioid subtype, negative lymph nodes and ≤10 % Ki-67 positive cells.

With respect to intraperitoneal chemotherapy, mitomycin and cisplatin, used alone or in various combinations, have been the two most common chemotherapy agents used for DMPM [95, 96]. Recent data point to a survival benefit with cisplatin-based therapy. Wake Forest University compared outcomes of cisplatin with mitomycin and showed a trend toward improved disease-free and progression-free survival with cisplatin [97]. Alexander et al. subsequently showed statistically significant improvement in survival with cisplatin-based intraperitoneal chemotherapy [28]. Results of a meta-analysis by Johnston et al. also confirmed better 5-year survival with cisplatin-based chemotherapy [92]. Importantly, however, whether cisplatin is used alone or in combination regimen, remains a matter of institutional preference.

The role of perioperative chemotherapy for DMPM, like appendiceal cancer, remains controversial. Based on evidence of a 26 % partial response rate of DMPM to combination regimen systemic chemotherapy of cisplatin and pemetrexed, a consensus statement recommended induction systemic chemotherapy for patients not deemed suitable for immediate cytoreduction and adjuvant systemic chemotherapy for patients considered high-risk for post-operative failure [98]. A recent study from an Italian group, however, showed no survival benefit for chemotherapy at the induction or adjuvant stage [99]. Most centers currently reserve systemic chemotherapy for patients unable to undergo cytoreduction and/or patients who recur after it.

Quality of Life

In conditions such as PSD in which the median survival is measured in months, the consideration of quality of life in the choice of therapeutic regimen becomes paramount. Peritoneal surface disease itself is associated with a significant decrease in functional status. CRS/HIPEC may improve some quality of life factors, but bring with it new issues such as: wound healing, ostomy, bowel changes due to resections, exacerbation of comorbid conditions, and complications with a morbidity rate of approximately 40 % in most studies. Over the years since CRS/HIPEC introduction, multiple studies have been designed to determine the effect of CRS/HIPEC on patient quality of life. A recent study of 216 patients post CRS/HIPEC found that quality of life was decreased at 3–6 months postoperatively, but returned to (or surpassed) baseline at 1 year [100]. Statistically significant determinants of quality of life were found to be; origin of PSD (3 months), presence of stoma (6 and 12 months), length of surgery >270 min (12 months), and recurrence (12 months). Increased length of surgery may be associated with increased PCI and attendant morbidity and likelihood of a bowel resection requiring stoma. This is in agreement with prior studies which indicate that despite an initial impairment in quality of life, there is improvement over starting baseline QOL in long term survivors [101, 102]. One report shows similar findings to those cited above, with decreased well-being scores at 3–12 months, but goes further in investigating depression symptoms, which were found to persist at 12 months [103]. Another indicates that in those surviving greater than 12 months, scores of physical impairment remain lower than the general population, but those indicating mental components were higher than the general population. Though, at greater than 12 months the majority of patients (56 %) reported continued sleep disturbances [104].

Together these studies indicate the need for multifaceted cancer care including psychosocial support in following patients with PSD. Given the early impairment of quality of life following CRS/HIPEC, the choice to pursue this surgery must be weighed against the potential for cure. The studies above and others indicate that in long term survivors, there is a statistical increase in QOL. This would indicate that in PSD from carcinomas in which CRS/HIPEC carries a high chance for cure such as low grade appendiceal lesions, there may be benefit. In those with lower probability of cure, the benefits and risks must be explicitly discussed with the patients, allowing them to factor in the information above on QOL. Follow up of patients who are long term survivors should include screening for sleep disturbances and depression.

Conclusions

- Peritoneal surface disease represents a form of regional metastasis that may occur as the initial presentation or as recurrent disease for a number of intraabdominal neoplasms.
- The peritoneal cavity presents barriers to effective systemic chemotherapy, requiring unique treatment strategies win patients with peritoneal surface disease, such as CRS/HIPEC.
- Outcomes differ for treatment depending on the origin of the cancer, but all require a multidisciplinary approach combining surgery and medical therapy.
- Patients with good performance status and resectable peritoneal disease should be considered for cytoreductive surgery and HIPEC.
- Cytoreductive surgery and HIPEC should be administered with systemic chemotherapy (except for low grade appendiceal carcinoma and mesothelioma) and not in lieu of it.

References

1. Sadeghi B, Arvieux C, Glehen O, Beaujard AC, Rivoire M, Baulieux J, et al. Peritoneal carcinomatosis from non-gynecologic malignancies: results of the EVOCAPE 1 multicentric prospective study. Cancer. 2000;88:358–63.
2. Jacquet P, Jelinek JS, Steves MA, Sugarbaker PH. Evaluation of computed tomography in patients with peritoneal carcinomatosis. Cancer. 1993;72(5):1631–6.
3. de Bree E, Koops W, Kröger R, van Ruth S, Witkamp AJ, Zoetmulder FA. Peritoneal carcinomatosis from colorectal or appendiceal origin: correlation of preoperative CT with intraoperative findings and evaluation of interobserver agreement. J Surg Oncol. 2004;86(2):64–73.
4. Koh JL, Yan TD, Glenn D, Morris DL. Evaluation of preoperative computed tomography in estimating peritoneal cancer index in colorectal peritoneal carcinomatosis. Ann Surg Oncol. 2009;16(2):327–33.
5. Stewart 4th JH, Shen P, Levine EA. Intraperitoneal hyperthermic chemotherapy for peritoneal surface malignancy current status and future directions. Ann Surg Oncol. 2005;12(10):765–77.
6. Esquivel J, Chua TC, Stojadinovic A, Melero JT, Levine EA, Gutman M, et al. Accuracy and clinical relevance of computed tomography scan interpretation of peritoneal cancer index in colorectal cancer peritoneal carcinomatosis: a multi-institutional study. J Surg Oncol. 2010;102(6):565–70.
7. Kubik-Huch RA, Dorffler W, von Schulthess GK, Marincek B, Kochli OR, Seifert B, et al. Value of (18F)-FDG positron emission tomography, computed tomography, and magnetic resonance imaging in diagnosing primary and recurrent ovarian carcinoma. Eur Radiol. 2000;10(5):761–7.
8. Low RN, Barone RM, Lacey C, Sigeti JS, Alzate GD, Sebrechts CP. Peritoneal tumor: MR imaging with dilute oral barium and intravenous gadolinium-containing contrast agents compared with unenhanced MR imaging and CT. Radiology. 1997;204(2):513–20.
9. Sugarbaker PH. Intraperitoneal chemotherapy and cytoreductive surgery for the prevention and treatment of peritoneal carcinomatosis and sarcomatosis. Semin Surg Oncol. 1998;14(3):254–61.
10. Rose PG, Faulhaber P, Miraldi F, Abdul-Karim FW. Positive emission tomography for evaluating a complete clinical response in patients with ovarian or peritoneal carcinoma: correlation with second-look laparotomy. Gynecol Oncol. 2001;82(1):17–21.
11. Esquivel J, Elias D, Baratti D, Kusamura S, Deraco M. Consensus statement on the loco regional treatment of colorectal cancer with peritoneal dissemination. J Surg Oncol. 2008;98(4):263–7.
12. Rohani P, Scotti SD, Shen P, Stewart JH, Russell GB, Cromer M, et al. Use of FDG-PET imaging for patients with disseminated cancer of the appendix. Am Surg. 2010;76(12):1338–44.
13. Sebbag G, Sugarbaker PH. Peritoneal mesothelioma proposal for a staging system. Eur J Surg Oncol. 2001;27(3):223–4.
14. Berthet B, Sugarbaker TA, Chang D, Sugarbaker PH. Quantitative methodologies for selection of patients with recurrent abdominopelvic sarcoma for treatment. Eur J Cancer. 1999;35(3):413–9.
15. Tentes AA, Tripsiannis G, Markakidis SK, Karanikiotis CN, Tzegas G, Georgiadis G, et al. Peritoneal cancer index: a prognostic indicator of survival in advanced ovarian cancer. Eur J Surg Oncol. 2003;29(1):69–73.
16. Harmon RL, Sugarbaker PH. Prognostic indicators in peritoneal carcinomatosisfrom gastrointestinal cancer. Int Semin Surg Oncol. 2005;2(1):3.
17. Gilly FN, Carry PY, Sayag AC, Brachet A, Panteix G, Salle B, et al. Regional chemotherapy (with mitomycin C) and intra-operative hyperthermia for digestive cancers with peritoneal carcinomatosis. Hepatogastroenterology. 1994;41(2):124–9.
18. Beaujard AC, Glehen O, Caillot JL, Francois Y, Bienvenu J, Panteix G, et al. Intraperitoneal chemohyperthermia with mitomycin C for digestive tract cancer patients with peritoneal carcinomatosis. Cancer. 2000;88(11):2512–9.

19. Rey Y, Porcheron J, Talabard JN, Szafnicki K, Balique JG. Peritoneal carcinomatosis treated by cytoreductive surgery and intraperitoneal chemohyperthermia. Ann Chir. 2000;125(7): 631–42.

20. Ronnett BM, Zahn CM, Kurman RJ, Kass ME, Sugarbaker PH, Shmookler BM. Disseminated peritoneal adenomucinosis and peritoneal mucinous carcinomatosis. A clinicopathologic analysis of 109 cases with emphasis on distinguishing pathologic features, site of origin, prognosis, and relationship to "pseudomyxoma peritonei". Am J Surg Pathol. 1995;19(12):1390–408.

21. Denzer U, Hoffmann S, Helmreich-Becker I, Kauczor HU, Thelen M, Kanzler S, et al. Minilaparoscopy In the diagnosis of peritoneal tumor spread: prospective controlled comparison with computed tomography. Surg Endosc. 2004;18:1067–70.

22. Valle M, Garofalo A. Laparoscopic staging of peritoneal surface malignancies. Eur J Surg Oncol. 2006;32(6):625–7.

23. Pomel C, Appleyard TL, Gouy S, Rouzier R, Elias D. The role of laparoscopy to evaluate candidates for complete cytoreduction of peritoneal carcinomatosis and hyperthermic intraperitoneal chemotherapy. Eur J Surg Oncol. 2005;31(5):540–3.

24. Spratt JS, Adcock RA, Muskovin M, Sherrill W, McKeown J. Clinical delivery system for intraperitoneal hyperthermic chemotherapy. Cancer Res. 1980;40(2):256–60.

25. Glockzin G, Schlitt HJ, Piso P. Peritoneal carcinomatosis: patients selection, perioperative complications and quality of life related to cytoreductive surgery and hyperthermic intraperitoneal chemotherapy. World J Surg Oncol. 2009;7:5–12.

26. Levine EA, Stewart JH, Russell GB, Geisinger KR, Loggie BL, Shen P. Cytoreductive surgery and intraperitoneal hyperthermic chemotherapy for peritoneal surface malignancy: experience with 501 procedures. J Am Coll Surg. 2007;204(5):943–53.

27. Levine EA, Stewart JH, Shen P, Russell GB, Loggie BL, Votanopoulos KI. Cytoreductive surgery and intraperitoneal hyperthermic chemotherapy for peritoneal surface malignancy: experience with 1,000 patients. J Am Coll Surg. 2014;518:573–87.

28. Alexander Jr HR, Bartlett DL, Pingpank JF, Libutti SK, Royal R, Hughes MS, et al. Treatment factors associated with long-term survival after cytoreductive surgery and regional chemotherapy for patients with malignant peritoneal mesothelioma. Surgery. 2013;153(6):779–86.

29. Van Sweringen HL, Hanseman DJ, Ahmad SA, Edwards MJ, Sussman JJ. Predictors of survival in patients with high-grade peritoneal metastases undergoing cytoreductive surgery and hyperthermic intraperitoneal chemotherapy. Surgery. 2012;152(4):617–24.

30. Spiliotis J, Vaxevanidou A, Sergouniotis F, Lambropoulou E, Datsis A, Christopoulou A. The role of cytoreductive surgery and hyperthermic intraperitoneal chemotherapy in the management of recurrent advanced ovarian cancer: a prospective study. J BUON. 2011;16(1):74–9.

31. Chua TC, Moran BJ, Sugarbaker PH, Levine EA, Glehen O, Gilly FN, et al. Early- and long-term outcome data of patients with pseudomyxoma peritonei from appendiceal origin treated by a strategy of cytoreductive surgery and hyperthermic intraperitoneal chemotherapy. J Clin Oncol. 2012;30(20):2449–56.

32. Shen P, Levine EA, Hall J, Case D, Russell G, Fleming R, et al. Factors predicting survival after intraperitoneal hyperthermic chemotherapy with mitomycin C after cytoreductive surgery for patients with peritoneal carcinomatosis. Arch Surg. 2003;138(1):26–33.

33. Dedrick RL, Myers CE, Bungay PM, et al. Pharmacokinetic rationale for peritoneal drug administration in the treatment of ovarian cancer. Cancer Treat Rep. 1978;62(1):1–11.

34. Dedrick RL. Theoretical and experimental bases of intraperitoneal chemotherapy. Semin Oncol. 1985;12(3 Suppl 4):1–6.

35. Flessner MF, Fenstermacher JD, Dedrick RL, Blasberg RG. A distributed model of peritoneal-plasma transport: tissue concentration gradients. Am J Physiol. 1985;248(3):F425–35.

36. Sugarbaker PH, Van der Speeten K, Anthony Stuart O, Chang D. Impact of surgical and clinical factors on the pharmacology of intraperitoneal doxorubicin in 145 patients with peritoneal carcinomatosis. Eur J Surg Oncol. 2011;37(8):719–26.

37. de Lima Vazquez V, Stuart OA, Mohamed F, Sugarbaker PH. Extent of parietal peritonectomy does not change intraperitoneal chemotherapy pharmacokinetics. Cancer Chemother Pharmacol. 2003;52(2):108–12.

38. Saltz LB, Clarke S, Díaz-Rubio E, Scheithauer W, Figer A, Wong R, et al. Bevacizumab in combination with oxaliplatin-based chemotherapy as first-line therapy in metastatic colorectal cancer: a randomized phase III study. J Clin Oncol. 2008;26:1013–9.
39. Klaver YL, Lemmens VE, Creemers GJ, Rutten HJ, Nienhuijs SW, de Hingh IH. Population-based survival of patients with peritoneal carcinomatosis from colorectal origin in the era of increasing use of palliative chemotherapy. Ann Oncol. 2011;22:2250–6.
40. Collins DC. 71,000 human appendix specimens. A final report, summarizing forty years' study. Am J Proctol. 1963;14:265–81.
41. Ronnett BM, Yan H, Kurman RJ, Shmookler BM, Wu L, Sugarbaker PH. Patients with pseudomyxoma peritonei associated with disseminated peritoneal adenomucinosis have a significantly more favorable prognosis than patients with peritoneal mucinous carcinomatosis. Cancer. 2001;92(1):85–91.
42. Bradley RF, Stewart 4th JH, Ruseell GB, Levine EA, Geisinger KR. Pseudomyxoma peritonei of appendiceal origin: a clinicopathologic analysis of 101 patients uniformly treated at single institution, with literature review. Am J Surg Pathol. 2006;30(5):551–9.
43. Votanopoulos KI, Russell G, Randle RW, Shen P, Stewart JH, Levine EA. Peritoneal surface disease (PSD) from appendiceal cancer treated with cytoreductive surgery (CRS) and hyperthermic intraperitoneal chemotherapy (HIPEC): overview of 481 cases. Ann Surg Oncol. 2015;22(4):1274–9.
44. Chua TC, Al-Zahrani A, Saxena A, Liauw W, Zhao J, Morris DL. Secondary cytoreduction and perioperative intraperitoneal chemotherapy after initial debulking of pseudomyxoma peritonei: a study of timing and the impact of malignant dedifferentiation. J Am Coll Surg. 2010;211(4):526–35.
45. Moran B, Baratti D, Yan TD, Kusamura S, Deraco M. Consensus statement on the loco-regional treatment of appendiceal mucinous neoplasms with peritoneal dissemination (pseudomyxoma peritonei). J Surg Oncol. 2008;98(4):277–82.
46. Gough DB, Donohue JH, Schutt AJ, Gonchoroff N, Goellner JR, Wilson TO, et al. Pseudomyxoma peritonei. Long-term patient survival with an aggressive regional approach. Ann Surg. 1994;219(2):112–9.
47. Sugarbaker PH, Chang D. Results of treatment of 385 patients with peritoneal surface spread of appendiceal malignancy. Ann Surg Oncol. 1999;6(8):727–31.
48. Deraco M, Baratti D, Inglese MG, Allaria B, Andreola S, Gavazzi C, et al. Peritonectomy and intraperitoneal hyperthermic perfusion (IPHP): a strategy that has confirmed its efficacy in patients with pseudomyxoma peritonei. Ann Surg Oncol. 2004;11(4):393–8.
49. Yan TD, Links M, Xu ZY, Kam PC, Glenn D, Morris DL. Cytoreductive surgery and perioperative intraperitoneal chemotherapy for pseudomyxoma peritonei from appendiceal mucinous neoplasms. Br J Surg. 2006;93(10):1270–6.
50. Smeenk RM, Verwaal VJ, Antonini N, Zoetmulder FA. Survival analysis of pseudomyxoma peritonei patients treated by cytoreductive surgery and hyperthermic intraperitoneal chemotherapy. Ann Surg. 2007;245(1):104–9.
51. Chua TC, Yan TD, Smigielski ME, Zhu KJ, Ng KM, Zhao J, Morris DL. Long-term survival in patients with pseudomyxoma peritonei treated with cytoreductive surgery and perioperative intraperitoneal chemotherapy: 10 years of experience from a single institution. Ann Surg Oncol. 2009;16(7):1903–11.
52. Sugarbaker PH, Bijelic L, Chang D, Yoo D. Neoadjuvant FOLFOX chemotherapy in 34 consecutive patients with mucinous peritoneal carcinomatosis of appendiceal origin. J Surg Oncol. 2010;102:576–81.
53. Bijelic L, Kumar AS, Stuart OA, Sugarbaker PH. Systemic chemotherapy prior to cytoreductive surgery and HIPEC for carcinomatosis from appendix cancer: impact on perioperative outcomes and short-term survival. Gastroenterol Res Pract. 2012;2012:163284.
54. Blackham AU, Swett K, Eng C, Sirintrapun J, Bergman S, Geisinger KR, et al. Perioperative systemic chemotherapy for appendiceal mucinous carcinoma peritonei treated with cytoreductive surgery and hyperthermic intraperitoneal chemotherapy. J Surg Oncol. 2014;109(7):740–5.

55. Farquharson AL, Pranesh N, Witham G, Swindell R, Taylor MB, Renehan A, et al. A phase II study evaluating the use of concurrent mitomycin C and capecitabine in patients with advanced unresectable pseudomyxoma peritonei. Br J Cancer. 2008;99:591–6.
56. Shapiro JF, Chase JL, Wolff RA, Lambert LA, Mansfield PF, Overman MJ, et al. Modern systemic chemotherapy in surgically unresectable neoplasms of appendiceal origin: a single-institution experience. Cancer. 2010;116:316–22.
57. Confuorto G, Giuliano ME, Grimaldi A, Viviano C. Peritoneal carcinomatosis from colorectal cancer: HIPEC? Surg Oncol. 2007;16 Suppl 1:S149–52.
58. Franko J, Shi Q, Goldman CD, Pockaj BA, Nelson GD, Goldberg RM, et al. Treatment of colorectal peritoneal carcinomatosis with systemic chemotherapy: a pooled analysis of north central cancer treatment group phase III trials N9741 and N9841. J Clin Oncol. 2012;30(3):263–7.
59. Verwaal VJ, van Ruth S, de Bree E, van Sloothen GW, van Tinteren H, Boot H, et al. Randomized trial of cytoreduction and hyperthermic intraperitoneal chemotherapy versus systemic chemotherapy and palliative surgery in patients with peritoneal carcinomatosis of colorectal cancer. J Clin Oncol. 2003;21(20):3737–43.
60. Verwaal VJ, Bruin S, Boot H, van Slooten G, van Tinteren H. 8-year follow-up of randomized trial: cytoreduction and hyperthermic intraperitoneal chemotherapy versus systemic chemotherapy in patients with peritoneal carcinomatosis of colorectal cancer. Ann Surg Oncol. 2008;15(9):2426–32.
61. Franko J, Ibrahim Z, Gusani NJ, Holtzman MP, Bartlett DL, Zeh 3rd HJ. Cytoreductive surgery and hyperthermic intraperitoneal chemoperfusion versus systemic chemotherapy alone for colorectal peritoneal carcinomatosis. Cancer. 2010;116(16):3756–62.
62. Esquivel J, Sticca R, Sugarbaker P, Levine E, Yan TD, Alexander R, et al. Society of Surgical Oncology Annual Meeting. Cytoreductive surgery and hyperthermic intraperitoneal chemotherapy in the management of peritoneal surface malignancies of colonic origin: a consensus statement. Society of Surgical Oncology. Ann Surg Oncol. 2007;14(1):128–33.
63. Shen P, Hawksworth J, Lovato J, Loggie BW, Geisinger KR, Fleming RA, et al. Cytoreductive surgery and intraperitoneal hyperthermic chemotherapy with mitomycin C for peritoneal carcinomatosis from nonappendiceal colorectal carcinoma. Ann Surg Oncol. 2004;11(2):178–86.
64. Glehen O, Kwiatkowski F, Sugarbaker PH, Elias D, Levine EA, De Simone M, et al. Cytoreductive surgery combined with perioperative intraperitoneal chemotherapy for the management of peritoneal carcinomatosis from colorectal cancer: a multi-institutional study. J Clin Oncol. 2004;22(16):3284–92.
65. Elias D, Gilly F, Boutitie F, Quenet F, Bereder JM, Mansvelt B, et al. Peritoneal colorectal carcinomatosis treated with surgery and perioperative intraperitoneal chemotherapy: retrospective analysis of 523 patients from a multicentric French study. J Clin Oncol. 2010;28(1):63–8.
66. Elias D, Lefevre JH, Chevalier J, Brouquet A, Marchal F, Classe JM, et al. Complete cytoreductive surgery plus intraperitoneal chemohyperthermia with oxaliplatin for peritoneal carcinomatosis of colorectal origin. J Clin Oncol. 2009;27(5):681–5.
67. Turaga K, Levine E, Barone R, Sticca R, Petrelli N, Lambert L, et al. Consensus guidelines from The American Society of Peritoneal Surface Malignancies on standardizing the delivery of hyperthermic intraperitoneal chemotherapy (HIPEC) in colorectal cancer patients in the United States. Ann Surg Oncol. 2014;21(5):1501–5.
68. Sugarbaker PH. Successful management of microscopic residual disease in large bowel cancer. Cancer Chemother Pharmacol. 1999;43:S15–25.
69. Chua TC, Yan TD, Zhao J, Morris DL. Peritoneal carcinomatosis and liver metastases from colorectal cancer treated with cytoreductive surgery perioperative intraperitoneal chemotherapy and liver resection. Eur J Surg Oncol. 2009;35(12):1299–305.
70. Elias D, Benizri E, Pocard M, Ducreux M, Boige V, Lasser P. Treatment of synchronous peritoneal carcinomatosis and liver metastases from colorectal cancer. Eur J Surg Oncol. 2006;32(6):632–6.

71. Kianmanesh R, Scaringi S, Sabate JM, Castel B, Pons-Kerjean N, Coffin B, et al. Iterative cytoreductive surgery associated with hyperthermic intraperitoneal chemotherapy for treatment of peritoneal carcinomatosis of colorectal origin with or without liver metastases. Ann Surg. 2007;245(4):597–603.

72. Verwaal VJ, Kusamura S, Baratti D, Deraco M. The eligibility for local-regional treatment of peritoneal surface malignancy. J Surg Oncol. 2008;98(4):220–3.

73. Howlader N, Noone AM, Krapcho M, Garshell J, Miller D, Altekruse SF, et al. SEER cancer statistics review, 1975–2012. Bethesda, MD: National Cancer Institute; 2015. http://seer.cancer.gov/csr/1975_2012/.

74. Cannistra SA. Cancer of the ovary. N Engl J Med. 2004;351(24):2519–29.

75. Munnell EW. The changing prognosis and treatment in cancer of the ovary. A report of 235 patients with primary ovarian carcinoma 1952-1961. Am J Obstet Gynecol. 1968;100:790–805.

76. Hoskins WJ, Bundy BN, Thigpen JT, Omura GA. The influence of cytoreductive surgery on recurrence-free interval and survival in small-volume stage III epithelial ovariancancer: a Gynecologic Oncology Group study. Gynecol Oncol. 1992;47:159–66.

77. Eisenkop SM, Spirtos NM. What are the current surgical objectives, strategies, and technical capabilities of gynecologic oncologists treating advanced epithelial ovarian cancer? Gynecol Oncol. 2001;82:489–97.

78. Bristow RE, Tomacruz RS, Armstrong DK, Trimble EL, Montz FJ. Survival effect of maximal cytoreductive surgery for advanced ovarian carcinoma during the platinum era: a meta-analysis. J Clin Oncol. 2002;20:1248–59.

79. Armstrong DK, Bundy B, Wenzel L, Huang HQ, Baergen R, Lele S, et al. Gynecologic Oncology Group. Intraperitoneal cisplatin and paclitaxel in ovarian cancer. N Engl J Med. 2006;354(1):34–43.

80. Chua TC, Robertson G, Liauw W, Farrell R, Yan TD, Morris DL. Intraoperative hyperthermic intraperitoneal chemotherapy after cytoreductive surgery in ovarian cancer peritoneal carcinomatosis: systematic review of current results. J Cancer Res Clin Oncol. 2009;135(12):1637–45.

81. McGuire WP, Hoskins WJ, Brady MF, Kucera PR, Partridge EE, Look KY, et al. Cyclophosphamide and cisplatin compared with paclitaxel and cisplatin in patients with stage III and stage IV ovarian cancer. N Engl J Med. 1996;334(1):1–6.

82. du Bois A, Quinn M, Thigpen T, Vermorken J, Avall-Lundqvist E, Bookman M, et al. 2004 consensus statements on the management of ovarian cancer: final document of the 3rd International Gynecologic Cancer Intergroup Ovarian Cancer Consensus Conference (GCIG OCCC 2004). Ann Oncol. 2005;16 Suppl 8:viii7–12.

83. Vergote I, Tropé CG, Amant F, Kristensen GB, Ehlen T, Johnson N, et al. Neoadjuvant chemotherapy or primary surgery in stage IIIC or IV ovarian cancer. N Engl J Med. 2010;363:943–53.

84. Kang S, Nam BH. Does neoadjuvant chemotherapy increase optimal cytoreduction rate in advanced ovarian cancer? Meta-analysis of 21 studies. Ann Surg Oncol. 2009;16:2315–20.

85. Huober J, Meyer A, Wagner U, Wallwiener D. The role of neoadjuvant chemotherapy and interval laparotomy in advanced ovarian cancer. J Cancer Res Clin Oncol. 2002;128:153–60.

86. Baratti D, Kusamura S, Deraco M. Diffuse malignant peritoneal mesothelioma: systemic review of clinical management and biologic research. J Surg Oncol. 2011;103(8):822–31.

87. Yan TD, Welch L, Black D, Sugarbaker PH. A systematic review on the efficacy of cytoreductive surgery combined with perioperative intraperitoneal chemotherapy for diffuse malignant peritoneal mesothelioma. Ann Oncol. 2007;18:827–34.

88. Blackham AU, Levine EA. Cytoreductive surgery with hyperthermic intraperitoneal chemotherapy for malignant peritoneal mesothelioma. Eur J Clin Med Oncol. 2012;4(2):25–32.

89. Faig J, Howard S, Levine EA, Casselman G, Hesdorffer M, Ohar JA. Changing pattern in malignant mesothelioma survival. Transl Oncol. 2015;8(1):35–9.

90. Chua TC, Yan TD, Morris DL. Outcomes of cytoreductive surgery and hyperthermic intraperitoneal chemotherapy for peritoneal mesothelioma: the Australian experience. J Surg Oncol. 2009;99:109–13.

91. Jänne PA, Wozniak AJ, Belani CP, Keohan ML, Ross HJ, Polikoff JA, et al. Open-label study of pemetrexed alone or in combination with cisplatin for the treatment of patients with peritoneal mesothelioma: outcomes of an expanded access program. Clin Lung Cancer. 2005;7(1):40–6.

92. Helm JH, Miura JT, Glenn JA, Marcus RK, Larrieux G, Jayakrishnan TT, et al. Cytoreductive surgery and hyperthermic intraperitoneal chemotherapy for malignant peritoneal mesothelioma: a systematic review and meta-analysis. Ann Surg Oncol. 2015;22(5):1686–93.

93. Yan TD, Deraco M, Baratti D, Kusamura S, Elias D, Glehen O, et al. Cytoreductive surgery and hyperthermic intraperitoneal chemotherapy for malignant peritoneal mesothelioma: multi-institutional experience. J Clin Oncol. 2009;27(36):6237–42.

94. Ihemelandu C, Bijelic L, Sugarbaker PH. Iterative cytoreductive surgery and hyperthermic intraperitoneal chemotherapy for recurrent or progressive diffuse malignant peritoneal mesothelioma: clinicopathologic characteristics and survival outcome. Ann Surg Oncol. 2015; 22(5):1680–5.

95. Deraco M, Nonaka D, Baratti D, Casali P, Rosai J, Younan R, et al. Prognostic analysis of clinicopathologic factors in 49 patients with diffuse malignant peritoneal mesothelioma treated with cytoreductive surgery and intraperitoneal hyperthermic perfusion. Ann Surg Oncol. 2006;13(2):229–37.

96. Brigand C, Monneuse O, Mohamed F, Sayag-Beaujard AC, Isaac S, Gilly FN, et al. Peritoneal mesothelioma treated by cytoreductive surgery and intraperitoneal hyperthermic chemotherapy: results of a prospective study. Ann Surg Oncol. 2006;13(3):405–12.

97. Blackham AU, Shen P, Stewart JH, Russell GB, Levine EA. Cytoreductive surgery with intraperitoneal hyperthermic chemotherapy for malignant peritoneal mesothelioma: mitomycin versus cisplatin. Ann Surg Oncol. 2010;17(10):2720–7.

98. Deraco M, Bartlett D, Kusamura S, Baratti D. Consensus statement on peritoneal mesothelioma. J Surg Oncol. 2008;98(4):268–72.

99. Deraco M, Baratti D, Hutanu I, Bertuli R, Kusamura S. The role of perioperative systemic chemotherapy in diffuse malignant peritoneal mesothelioma patients treated with cytoreductive surgery and hyperthermic intraperitoneal chemotherapy. Ann Surg Oncol. 2013;20(4):1093–100.

100. Passot G, Bakrin N, Roux AS, Vaudoyer D, Gilly FN, Glehen O, et al. Quality of life after cytoreductive surgery plus hyperthermic intraperitoneal chemotherapy: a prospective study of 216 patients. Eur J Surg Oncol. 2014;40(5):529–35.

101. Schmidt U, Dahlke MH, Klempnauer J, Schlitt HJ, Piso P. Perioperative morbidity and quality of life in long-term survivors following cytoreductive surgery and hyperthermic intraperitoneal chemotherapy. Eur J Surg Oncol. 2005;31(1):53–8.

102. McQuellon RP, Loggie BW, Lehman AB, Russell GB, Fleming RA, Shen P, et al. Long-term survivorship and quality of life after cytoreductive surgery plus intraperitoneal hyperthermic chemotherapy for peritoneal carcinomatosis. Ann Surg Oncol. 2003;10(2):155–62.

103. Duckworth KE, McQuellon RP, Russell GB, Cashwell CS, Shen P, Stewart JH, et al. Patient reported outcomes and survivorship following cytoreductive surgery plus hyperthermic intraperitoneal chemotherapy (CS + HIPEC). J Surg Oncol. 2012;106(4):376–80.

104. Hill AR, McQuellon RP, Russell GB, Shen P, Stewart JH, Levine EA. Survival and quality of life following cytoreductive surgery plus hyperthermic intraperitoneal chemotherapy for peritoneal carcinomatosis of colonic origin. Ann Surg Oncol. 2011;18(13):3673–9.

Index

© Springer International Publishing Switzerland 2016
K.A. Morgan (ed.), *Current Controversies in Cancer Care*
for the Surgeon, DOI 10.1007/978-3-319-16205-8